D0809199

HANDBOOK OF MATERNAL-NEWBORN NURSING

HANDBOOK OF MATERNAL-NEWBORN NURSING

Edited by

Kathleen A. Buckley, M.S.N., C.N.M.

and

Nancy W. Kulb, M.S., C.N.M.

Associates in Nursing
Columbia University
School of Nursing
New York, New York

A WILEY MEDICAL PUBLICATION
JOHN WILEY & SONS
New York • Chichester • Brisbane • Toronto • Singapore

FLESCHNER PUBLISHING CO.
Bethany, Connecticut

Library of Congress Cataloging in Publication Data:

Main entry under title:

Handbook of maternal-newborn nursing.

(A Wiley medical publication)   (Wiley red book series)

Includes index.
1. Obstetrical nursing. I. Buckley, Kathleen A. II. Kulb, Nancy W.
III. Series. IV. Series: Wiley red book series. [DNLM: 1. Obstetrical
nursing—Handbooks. 2. Pediatric nursing—Handbooks. WY 157 H236]
RG951.H36   1983   610.73'678   82-20048
ISBN 0-471-86984-8

Printed in the United States of America

10 9 8 7 6 5 4 3 2 1

This book is dedicated to David and Tia.

CONTRIBUTORS

Dorothy J. Allbritten, RN, C, MSN, PNP
Associate in Nursing
School of Nursing
Columbia University
New York, New York

Kathleen A. Buckley, MSN, CNM
Associate in Nursing
School of Nursing
Columbia University
New York, New York

Nancy J. Burton, CNM, MSN
Nurse-Midwife
Mount Sinai Hospital
Hartford, Connecticut
Clinical Faculty
School of Nursing
Yale University
New Haven, Connecticut

Barbara Decker, CNM, MA
Assistant Professor
School of Nursing
Columbia University
New York, New York

Margherita M. Hawkins, RN, MS
Director of Education
Regional Center for Tertiary Perinatal Care
Columbia-Presbyterian Medical Center
New York, New York
Senior Staff Associate
Department of Obstetrics
College of Physicians & Surgeons
Columbia University
New York, New York

Nancy W. Kulb, MS, CNM
Associate in Nursing
School of Nursing
Columbia University
New York, New York

Elizabeth R. Luginbuhl, RN, BSN, MS
Clinical Coordinator
Department of Pediatrics
Hartford Hospital
Hartford, Connecticut
Assistant Clinical Professor
School of Nursing
University of Connecticut
Storrs, Connecticut

Judith S. Melson, CNM, MS
Assistant Professor
School of Nursing
Georgetown University
Washington, D. C.

Smriti Panwar, RN, EdD
Assistant Professor
School of Nursing
Columbia University
New York, New York

Susan Papera, RN, MS, CNM
Associate in Nursing
School of Nursing
Columbia University
New York, New York
Staff Nurse-Midwife
North Central Bronx Hospital
Bronx, New York

Angela Portale, RN, MS
Clinical Specialist
Department of Maternal-Fetal Medicine
Harlem Hospital Center
New York, New York

Sister M. Rose Carmel Scalone, RSM, CNM, MPH
Associate in Nursing
School of Nursing
Columbia University
New York, New York

Suzanne M. Smith, CNM, MS, MPH
Private Midwifery Practice
St. Vincent's Hospital and Medical Center
New York, New York
Clinical Faculty
New York Medical College
New York, New York

CONTENTS

PREFACE

Health care professionals in obstetric practice today have a changing and ever-expanding volume of knowledge on which to base their clinical practice. As the knowledge base has grown, the clinical expertise and skills required of the practitioner have become more complex. This book has evolved out of the need for an easily available reference for clinical information. It is intended for obstetric nurses, nurse practitioners, and other health professionals who are actively involved in delivering health care to the childbearing family.

The substantive content assumes a basic knowledge of anatomy and physiology as well as nursing principles and skills. The focus is on theoretical content and technical skills that the practicing nurse is called on to use but may not learn in school.

Because pregnancy itself is a normal physiological process, and because most pregnancies are normal, the text focuses on the nurse's role in the normal childbearing process. Information that is necessary in screening for and managing complications is included because we believe the nurse is in a unique position to identify complications early and to coordinate the efforts of the health care team in promoting the best possible outcome for both the mother and her baby.

The editors envision the obstetric nurse's role as being an essential partner in the provision of health care — a partner with other health care professionals who are committed to promoting the health and well-being of the mother, infant, and family, and who work with the client in meeting her health care goals. The fact that nurses work with clients from different cultures in a variety of settings and in various nursing roles is also recognized.

It is hoped that the small size of this book will make it convenient for clinicians to carry with them, and that the many tables and charts will help make readily available the specific information that the user needs. Most of all, it is hoped that this book will contribute to the health and well-being of mothers, babies, and families by enhancing the knowledge base of the health care professionals who serve them.

KAB and NWK

CHAPTER 1

MATERNAL ANATOMY, THE FETAL HEAD, AND CATEGORIES OF PRESENTATION AND POSITION

Sister Rose Scalone

Examination of the pregnant woman is based on a thorough knowledge of how pregnancy affects each of the body's systems and of how each of these systems adapts to the growing fetus. This chapter is concerned primarily with maternal anatomy and includes discussions of the antepartal/intrapartal abdominal examination, two methods used in measuring fundal height, the procedures for abdominal palpation and Leopold's maneuvers, and the probable location of the fetal heart tones. A discussion of the anatomy of female external and internal organs of reproduction and the bony pelvis is also included.

THE ABDOMEN

The amount and degree of nursing assessment of the maternal abdomen, genitalia, and pelvis depends on the protocols used by the institution or agency where the nurse practices. An understanding of maternal anatomy will help the nurse to teach and explain procedures to the pregnant woman.

The **Schuchardt charts** published by the Maternity Center Association in New York City (Fig. 1-1) illustrate the nonpregnant abdomi-

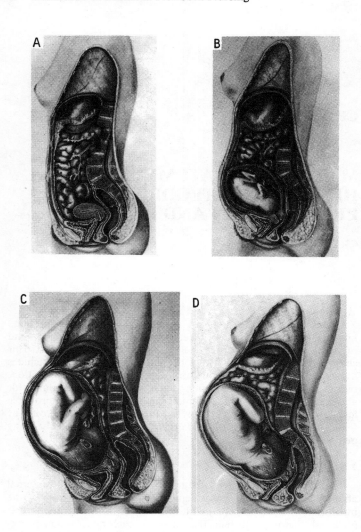

Figure 1-1. The Schuchardt charts for the maternal abdomen. (A) Nonpregnant, (B) fifth lunar month, (C) ninth lunar month, and (D) just before labor. *Reprinted with permission from* the Maternity Center Association, New York.

nal organs and the changing position of these organs as the abdominal space is filled with the enlarging uterus. Many of the normal discomforts of pregnancy can be understood when these pictures are reviewed. The purpose, nursing actions, and materials for an obstetric abdominal examination are listed in Table 1-1.

General factors to remember

The woman's abdomen is completely exposed from just below the breast to the symphysis pubis. The woman should be supine on the examining table with her shoulders and head slightly elevated and her knees slightly bent. Fundal heights may vary as much as 3.8 centimeters (1 ½ inches) in different women, depending on their height, weight, and build. The amount of amniotic fluid, the fetal size and attitude, and multiple gestation will also influence fundal height. The measurement reliability and evaluation will be greatly increased if the same person examines the woman at each of her prenatal visits. If this is not possible, all examiners should follow the same protocol for measuring fundal height. It is difficult to palpate the uterus abdominally before the 16th week of gestation. A bimanual examination should be performed on all prenatal clients at the time of their first prenatal visit. At that time, careful attention should be given to determining the size of the uterus of less than 20 weeks' gestation. Before the 20th week, it is nearly impossible to ascertain the lie, presentation, and position of the fetus. However, before the 36th week of gestation, the fetus is so active that this information may

TABLE 1-1
Introduction to the Abdominal Examination

Materials needed	Nursing actions	Purpose
Tape measure (in centimeters). Fetoscope or a Doppler device.	Ensure privacy and good lighting. Have the woman empty her bladder. Explain what is going to be done and why. Perform the examination. Assess the findings and share them with the woman. Develop a problem list. Develop a plan.	To measure the height of the fundus and determine its relationship to the number of weeks of gestation. To evaluate abdominal muscle tone. To determine fetal lie, presentation, position, and degree of descent. To detect fetal movement and uterine contractions. To auscultate fetal heart tones.

have little meaning for labor and delivery management. The fetal parts can be palpated at about the 20th week. The fetal heart tones can be heard with a fetoscope by the 20th week, and a Doppler device can pick up fetal heart tones as early as the 10th week. If at any time during the abdominal examination the woman becomes pale and/or her skin becomes clammy, or she expresses that she feels faint, the nurse should turn her onto her left side to relieve supine hypotension syndrome.

Abdominal inspection

1. Observe the abdominal skin and check for lesions, rashes, surgical scars, striae, and linea nigra.
2. Observe the contour and size of the uterus and note any departure from the norm, such as overdistention secondary to hydramnios or multiple gestation, and transverse ovoid contour instead of longitudinal ovoid (indicative of transverse lie).
3. Assess the abdominal muscle tone, which will vary according to parity.
   Primigravida: Usually has good muscle tone. The abdomen appears to be more ovoid and, therefore, has a long contour. When the primigravida stands, her abdominal muscles keep her uterus close to her body.
   Multipara: Muscle tone usually decreases with increasing parity. The abdomen has a broad contour. When the multipara stands, her abdominal muscles allow the uterus to assume a forward and downward position.
4. Observe for fetal movement and note sudden shifting and/or upward poking from within the uterus (*see* Chapter 3).

Determination of fundal height

Standing at the woman's right side (if the examiner is right-handed) and facing the woman's head, the examiner should place the palmar surfaces of his or her fingers on each lateral side of the uterus midway between the symphysis pubis and the fundus. Using gentle pressure, the examiner should move the uterus between his or her hands (being sure to stay on the lateral portion) and palpate up to the fundus. Near the top of the uterus, the examiner's hands will begin to come together, and they will meet at the top of the fundus.

Method 1: Fingerbreadths. A time-honored method of measuring fundal height combines a knowledge of where to expect the fundal height to be at various weeks of gestation in relation to the woman's symphysis pubis, umbilicus, and tip of the xiphoid process and the use of the examiner's fingerbreadths as the measuring tool. Although there is considerable variation in the width of different examiners' fingers (and, therefore, in their findings), a general rule is that, after 20 to 22 weeks of gestation, 1 fingerbreadth corresponds to 2 weeks of gestational growth. This is a useful method if a tape measure is not readily available. It also provides a guide for establishing general expectations that can be used as a base line against which to compare tape measurements (Fig. 1-2).

Method 2: Tape measure.   The most frequently used method for obtaining an exact measurement of the fundal height is with a pliable measuring tape (with centimeter markings). After 20 weeks of gestation, the height (in centimeters) of the uterine fundus above the symphysis pubis generally approximates the number of weeks of gestation. Correct estimations within 1 to 2 weeks of the date of delivery should be common in normal, singleton pregnancies. The abdominal midline is used as the line of measurement, and the zero line of a centimeter measuring tape is placed on the superior border of the symphysis pubis. The tape measure is stretched over the contour of the abdomen to the top of the fundus, and the number of centimeters at the top of the fundus is read (Table 1-2). (General rule: Approximately 1 cm/wk after 20 to 22 weeks of gestation is normal. The fundal height is abnormal if it is ±4 centimeters from the week of gestation.)

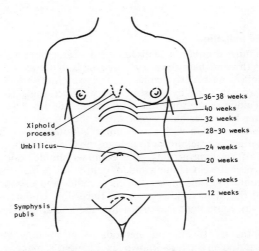

Figure 1-2.   Normal location of the height of the fundus during pregnancy. *Adapted from* Varney, H. Nurse Midwifery. Blackwell Scientific Publications, Inc., Boston. 1980. p. 499.

TABLE 1-2
*Expected Location of Fundal Height at
Various Weeks of Gestation*

Gestation	Location of fundal height	Height above symphysis pubis
wk		*cm*
12	Level of the symphysis pubis.	
16	Halfway between symphysis pubis and umbilicus.	
20	0-1 fingerbreadths below umbilicus.	20
24	1-2 fingerbreadths above umbilicus.	24
28-30	One third of the way between umbilicus and xiphoid process (3 fingerbreadths above umbilicus).	28-30
32	Two-thirds of the way between umbilicus and xiphoid process (3-4 fingerbreadths below xiphoid process).	32
36-38	1 fingerbreadth below xiphoid process.	36-38
40	2-3 fingerbreadths below xiphoid process if lightening occurs.	≤ 40

Adapted from Varney, H. Nurse Midwifery. Blackwell Scientific Publications, Inc., Boston. 1980. p. 499.

Abdominal palpation

The examiner should not be discouraged by an inability to perform this task with immediate accuracy. The goal is to determine and consistently follow an orderly sequence. The examiner should help the pregnant woman relax by assisting her with breathing techniques, which will aid in relaxation of her abdominal muscles. The examiner should place his or her hands *lightly* over the woman's abdomen to familiarize the woman with the examiner's touch, to avoid stimulating a uterine contraction, or to palpate the intensity, duration, and frequency of her contractions. The examiner should wait until the uterus relaxes before beginning and/or continuing palpation. The examiner should keep his or her fingers together and use the palmar surfaces of the fingers rather than the fingertips. Undue poking or pressure may cause contractions of the abdominal muscles and/or uterus.

One of the most common methods of performing abdominal palpation is the procedure known as Leopold's maneuvers. The procedure, findings, and significance of these findings are listed in Table 1-3, and the procedure itself is illustrated in Figure 1-3.

TABLE 1-3
Leopold's Maneuvers

Procedure	Findings	Significance
Step 1 Facing the woman's head, place the palmar surfaces of both hands over the fundus and gently palpate for the consistency, shape, size, and mobility of the fetal part in the fundus. Is it round, hard, smooth, and ballottable (as in a vertex), or softer, irregular in contour, and not ballottable (as in a breech)?	1.1 Fetal part feels round and hard, is readily movable, and can be ballotted between the thumb and a finger of one hand. 1.2 Fetal part feels irregular, larger/bulkier, and less firm than a head. It cannot be well delineated, readily moved, or ballotted. 1.3 Neither of the above is felt in the fundus.	1.1 Indicative of the fetal head. The mobility is a result of the head's being able to move independently of the trunk. The lie is longitudinal. 1.2 Indicative of the fetal breech, which cannot move independently of the trunk. The lie is longitudinal. 1.3 Indicative of a transverse lie.
Step 2 Continue to face the woman's head. Slide hands down from the top of the uterus over both sides equidistant from the midline. Stabilize the uterus with one examining hand and gently — but with deep pressure and rotary movement — palpate the other side for smoothness, resistance, convexity, and/or knobby irregular	2.1 A firm, convex, continuously smooth, and resistant mass extends from the breech to the neck. 2.2 Small, knobby, irregular masses. May move when pressed on, or may kick or hit the examiner's hand. 2.3 (*See* 1.1 and 1.2 above.) The head or breech is palpated on either	2.1 Indicative of the fetal back. The location of the back on the left or right side of the woman's abdomen indicates the position in a longitudinal lie. 2.2 Indicative of the fetal small parts, e.g., hands, feet, knees, and elbows. They should be on the opposite side of the woman than the fetal back.

Procedure	Findings	Significance
masses. Repeat this procedure for examination of the other side of the uterus.	side instead of in the fundus or at the symphysis pubis.	2.3 Indicative of a transverse lie.
Step 3 The *Pawlick grip* confirms fetal lie and presentation. Continue to face the woman's head. It is essential that she have her knees slightly bent in order to avoid discomfort during this maneuver and the next (*see below*). Grasp the presenting part between the fingers and the thumb of the right hand and grasp the part in the fundus with the other hand. It will be necessary to gently but firmly press into the abdomen in order to feel the presenting part below and between the fingers and thumb. As in the first step, palpate for size, shape, consistency, and mobility of the fetal part in the upper and lower pole of the uterus. Compare simultaneously what is in the two poles.	3.1 If the presenting part is the head, it will feel round and hard. It may not be readily movable if it is engaged. If the head is above the pelvic brim, it is readily movable and ballottable as described for the first maneuver. 3.2 Fetal part feels irregular, larger/bulkier, and less firm than a head. 3.3 Neither of the above is palpated.	3.1 Confirmation of longitudinal lie and cephalic presentation. 3.2 Confirmation of longitudinal lie and breech presentation. 3.3 Confirmation of transverse lie.

Step 4

This step will be used to determine the descent of the presenting part. Face the woman's feet. Place two hands gently on either side of the lower abdomen just below the level of the umbilicus and lower the fingers slowly on each side of the symphysis pubis. Note the contour, size, and mobility of the presenting part.

4.1 The examining hands converge around the presenting part with the fingertips touching in the abdominal midline. If the presenting part is the head, it will be readily movable. If the presenting part is the breech, it will move along with the trunk of the fetus.

4.2 The examining hands diverge from the presenting part and the abdominal midline. There is no mobility of the presenting part.

4.3 There is complete absence of any presenting part.

4.1 Indicative of unengaged presenting part floating at or above the pelvic inlet as determined by being at or above the symphysis pubis.

4.2 Indicative of either dipping or engaged presenting part. Dipping occurs when the presenting part has entered the pelvic inlet but has not yet descended to the point of engagement.

4.3 Indicative of a transverse lie.

Step 5

Finally, share the findings with the woman and offer to help her feel and identify various fetal parts.

Adapted with permission from Varney, H. Nurse Midwifery. Blackwell Scientific Publications, Inc., Boston. 1980. p. 503-507.

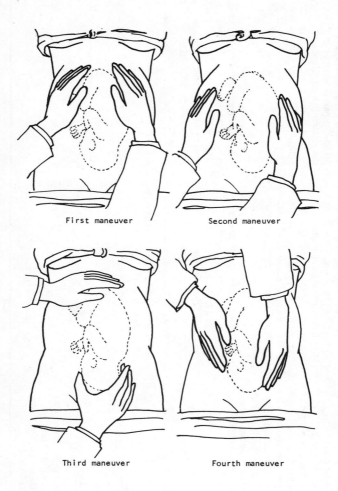

First maneuver

Second maneuver

Third maneuver

Fourth maneuver

Figure 1-3. Leopold's maneuvers. Used to determine the presentation, position, and lie of the fetus during abdominal palpation. (*See* Table 1-3 for the significance of the findings.) *Adapted from* Pritchard, J. A., and P. C. MacDonald. Williams Obstetrics. Appleton-Century-Crofts, East Norwalk, Conn. 1980. Sixteenth edition. p. 299.

Auscultation of fetal heart tones

Because fetal heart tones are transmitted best through the scapula and back of the fetus's shoulder in a vertex or breech presentation, it is important to determine the lie, presentation, and position of the fetus before attempting to locate fetal heart tones. The approximate locations of the fetal heart tones for specific fetal positions at term are shown in Table 1-4 and Figure 1-4.

The normal fetal heart rate is 120 to 160 beats/min. During a contraction the rate may drop to as low as 90 beats/min, but it quickly returns to normal during the rest period. Persistence of the low rate throughout the interval between contractions indicates that the fetus is in danger. This is especially true if the heartbeat also becomes irregular (*see* Chapter 18). Two fetal heart tones heard simultaneously in two different abdominal quadrants with a rate difference of at least 10 beats/min may be indicative of multiple gestation. Charting of the fetal heart tones should include the rate and location of maximum intensity. The location is usually spoken of in terms of four quadrants, which are determined by drawing vertical and horizontal lines that bisect each other at the area of the umbilicus (Fig. 1-5).

Failure to hear fetal heart tones may result from one of the following factors:

1. Less than 20 weeks of gestation
2. Maternal obesity
3. Hydramnios
4. Loud maternal or funic souffle
5. Defective fetoscope
6. Environmental noises
7. Fetal death

TABLE 1-4
Location of Fetal Heart Tones in Various Fetal Positions

Presentation/ position	Location
Cephalic	Midway between umbilicus and level of anterior superior iliac spine.
Breech	Level with or above umbilicus.
Anterior	Close to abdominal midline.
Transverse	In lateral abdominal area.
Posterior	In flank area or close to abdominal midline on other side of abdomen.

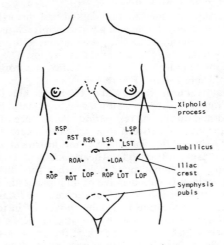

Figure 1-4. Illustration of the location of the point of maximum intensity of fetal heart tones for specific fetal positions. (*See* Table 1-5 for explanation of abbreviations.) *Adapted from* Varney, H. Nurse Midwifery. Blackwell Scientific Publications, Inc., Boston. 1980. p. 508.

THE FEMALE EXTERNAL AND
INTERNAL ORGANS OF REPRODUCTION

The external organs of reproduction include the following structures (Fig. 1-6):

1. Mons pubis
2. Labia majora
3. Labia minora
4. Prepuce
5. Clitoris
6. Frenulum
7. Vaginal vestibule
   a. Vaginal orifice
   b. Hymen/hymenal tags
   c. Bartholin's glands
8. Fourchette
9. Perineal body

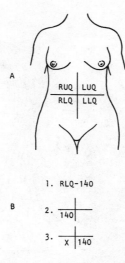

Figure 1-5. Charting the location of the fetal heart tones. (A) Chart depicting the four quadrants. (B) Three different methods of charting the fetal heart tones. In all three cases, the fetal heart rate is 140 beats/min, and it is best heard in the right lower quadrant (RLQ). LLQ, left lower quadrant; LUQ, left upper quadrant; RUQ, right upper quadrant. *Adapted from* Varney, H. Nurse Midwifery. Blackwell Scientific Publications, Inc., Boston. 1980. p. 508.

The internal organs of reproduction include the following structures (Figs. 1-7 and 1-8):

1. Vagina
2. Uterus
   a. Cervix
      External os
      Isthmus
      Internal os
   b. Corpus
   c. Fundus
   d. Uterine cavity
3. Oviducts (fallopian tubes)
4. Ovaries
5. Uterine ligaments

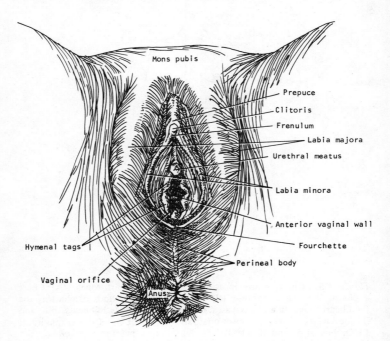

Figure 1-6.   External organs of reproduction. *Adapted from* Pritchard, J. A., and P. C. MacDonald. Williams Obstetrics. Appleton-Century-Crofts, East Norwalk, Conn. 1980. Sixteenth edition. p. 12.

THE BONY PELVIS

There are four basic pelvic types, which are primarily determined by the shape of the inlet. The **gynecoid** pelvis is round, with the transverse diameter slightly greater than or about the same as the anterior-posterior diameter. The **anthropoid** pelvis is oval, with the anterior-posterior diameter greater than the transverse diameter. The **platypelloid** pelvis is oval, with the transverse diameter greater than the anterior-posterior diameter. The **android** pelvis is heart-shaped. The majority of women display some combination of these four types (Fig. 1-9). The pelvic type that most readily facilitates delivery is the gynecoid pelvis. The other types *may* result in malposition, malpresentation, prolonged labor, or prolapse of the umbilical cord.

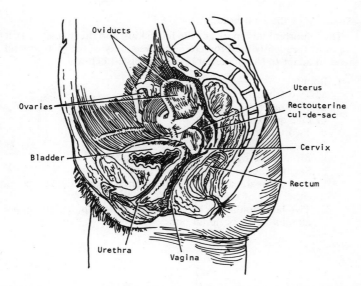

Figure 1-7.   Cross section of female pelvis illustrating relationships of pelvic viscera. *Adapted from* Pritchard, J. A., and P. C. MacDonald. Williams Obstetrics. Appleton-Century-Crofts, East Norwalk, Conn. 1980. Sixteenth edition. p. 16.

Pelvimetry is the measurement of the dimensions and capacity of the pelvis. These are most accurately measured by roentgenographic studies known as x-ray pelvimetry. It is a procedure that is usually not performed until labor has begun, and then only in special situations to determine the adequacy of the pelvis for the passage of the infant. Clinical pelvimetry is the estimated measurements of the critical diameters of the pelvis by means of the premeasured reach of the examiner's fingers and fist. A clinical evaluation of the pelvis is usually part of the initial antepartal examination and is repeated again at the time of the initial intrapartal pelvic examination.

THE FETAL HEAD AND CATEGORIES OF PRESENTATION AND POSITION

Obstetrically, the head is a most important part of the fetus because an essential feature of labor is the ability of the fetal head to adapt to the maternal pelvis.

Anatomy of the fetal head

The important landmarks of the fetal skull, and the diameters that are most frequently used to determine the ability of the mature fetal head to adapt to the maternal pelvis, are listed below:

1. Bones
   a. Two frontal.
   b. Two parietal.
   c. One occipital.
   d. Two temporal.
2. Sutures
   a. Frontal: between two frontal bones.
   b. Sagittal: between two parietal bones.
   c. Two coronal: each between the frontal and parietal bones on either side of the head.
   d. Two lambdoidal: each between the parietal bones and upper margin of the occipital bone.

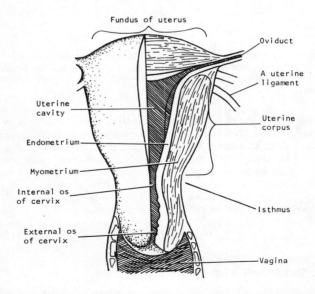

Figure 1-8. Anatomy of the uterus. *Adapted from* Olds, S. B., M. L. London, P. A. Ladewig, and S. V. Davidson. Obstetric Nursing. Addison-Wesley Publishing Co., Inc., Menlo Park, Calif. 1980. p. 91.

3. Fontanels
   a. Anterior: the shape of a diamond formed by the meeting of the frontal, sagittal, and two coronal sutures.
   b. Posterior: the shape of a triangle (much smaller than the anterior fontanel) formed by the meeting of the sagittal and two lambdoidal sutures (Fig. 1-10).
4. Diameters and approximate lengths
   a. Occipitofrontal: extending from a point just above the roof of the nose to the most prominent portion of the occipital bone. Approximately 11.75 centimeters.
   b. Biparietal: the greatest transverse diameter of the head, extending from one parietal boss to the other. Approximately 9.5 centimeters.
   c. Occipitomental: extending from the chin to the most prominent portion of the occiput. Approximately 13.5 centimeters.

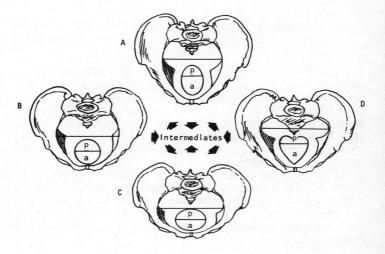

Figure 1-9. The four main pelvic types. (A) Anthropoid, (B) gynecoid, (C) platypelloid, and (D) android. Note that there may be intermediate variations on the four main types. The line passing through the widest transverse diameter divides the inlet into posterior (p) and anterior (a) segments. *Adapted from* Pritchard, J. A., and P. C. MacDonald. Williams Obstetrics. Appleton-Century-Crofts, East Norwalk, Conn. 1980. Sixteenth edition. p. 12.

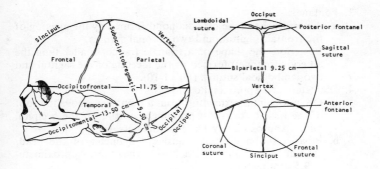

Figure 1-10. Illustration of the bones, sutures, fontanels, and diameters of the fetal head. *Adapted from* Ross Laboratories. Clinical Education Aids. Number 13. Ross Laboratories, Columbus, Ohio. 1979.

    d. Suboccipitobregmatic: extending from the middle of the anterior fontanel to the undersurface of the occipital bone. Approximately 9.5 centimeters.

The smaller the diameter that presents (as in a well-flexed vertex presentation in which the suboccipitobregmatic diameter presents), the easier the passage through the maternal pelvis.

There is mobility at the sutures of the skull and, therefore, fetal heads differ appreciably in their ability to adapt to the maternal pelvis by molding. Molding is the change in the shape of the head as a result of overriding or overlapping of the soft skull bones because they are not yet firmly united.

During labor, caput succedaneum (an edematous swelling of the fetal scalp) may develop on the most dependent part of the fetus's head as a result of pressure against the cervix and bony pelvis. Caput succedaneum is diffuse edema that crosses suture lines, and it resolves spontaneously a few days after birth. It must be differentiated from cephalhematoma (*see* Chapter 21).

Fetal presentation and position

Presentation and position are determined through careful abdominal palpation and confirmed on vaginal examination. The presenting part is the first portion of the fetus to enter the pelvic inlet. There are three possible presentations: cephalic, breech, and shoulder. The cephalic presentation is further subdivided into vertex (or occiput), sinciput, brow, and face. The breech presentation is further subdivided into frank, full (or complete), and footling, which can be single or double.

The position of the fetus indicates the relationship between an arbitrarily chosen point on the fetus (e.g., occiput, sacrum, mentum) and the maternal pelvis. Each position is described in relation to the left or right side of the mother's pelvis as well as the anterior, transverse, or posterior portion of her pelvis.

The categories of fetal presentation and position and their corresponding abbreviations are listed in Table 1-5 and illustrated in Figures 1-11 and 1-12.

TABLE 1-5
*Categories of Fetal Presentation and Position
with Their Abbreviations**

Presentation/position			Abbreviation
Cephalic			
	Vertex	Left occiput posterior	LOP
		Left occiput transverse	LOT
		Left occiput anterior	LOA
		Right occiput posterior	ROP
		Right occiput transverse	ROT
		Right occiput anterior	ROA
	Face	Left mentum posterior	LMP
		Left mentum transverse	LMT
		Left mentum anterior	LMA
		Right mentum posterior	RMP
		Right mentum transverse	RMT
		Right mentum anterior	RMA
Breech (Frank, full [or complete], and footling)		Left sacrum posterior	LSP
		Left sacrum transverse	LST
		Left sacrum anterior	LSA
		Right sacrum posterior	RSP
		Right sacrum transverse	RST
		Right sacrum anterior	RSA
Shoulder			
		Right acromion anterior	RAA
		Right acromion posterior	RAP
		Left acromion anterior	LAA
		Left acromion posterior	LAP

See also Figs. 1-3, 1-11, and 1-12.

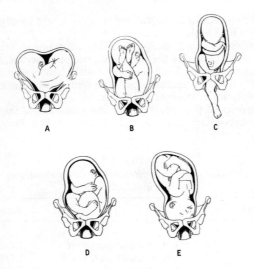

Figure 1-11. Categories of presentation. (A) Shoulder, (B) frank breech, (C) footling breech, (D) complete breech, and (E) brow. *Adapted from* Ross Laboratories. Clinical Education Aids. Number 18. Ross Laboratories, Columbus, Ohio. 1979.

THE VAGINAL EXAMINATION

The vaginal examination is an essential component of maternal care. The examination must be performed gently, thoroughly, and as quickly as possible. In addition, the number of vaginal examinations should be kept to a minimum in order to avoid unnecessary discomfort and increased risk of infection. The five indications for a vaginal examination are listed below:

1. To establish a base line and verify labor status upon admission to the labor and delivery suite.
2. To determine whether to give medication (and, if so, the type) when the need for medication is evident.
3. To rule out the possibility of a prolapsed cord after spontaneous rupture of the fetal membranes.
4. To verify a clinical impression of the progress in labor.
5. To verify complete dilation in order to be able to encourage or discourage maternal pushing efforts.

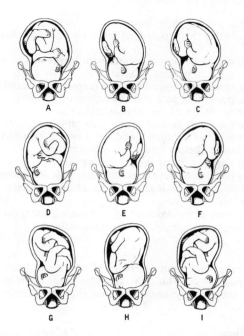

Figure 1-12. Categories of position. (A) Left occiput posterior (B) left occiput transverse, (C) left occiput anterior, (D) right occiput posterior, (E) right occiput transverse, (F) right occiput anterior, (G) left mentum anterior, (H) right mentum posterior, and (I) right mentum anterior. *Adapted from* Ross Laboratories. Clinical Education Aids. Number 18. Ross Laboratories, Columbus, Ohio. 1979.

The careful assessment of the woman's contraction pattern and observation of her behavior — the signs and symptoms of transition or her urge to push — provide a good idea of how labor is progressing. An increase in bloody show, in bulging, or in flattening of the perineum and anus, and the appearance of the fetal presenting part at the introitus are all signs of full dilation.

Purpose

The five basic purposes of the vaginal examination are listed below:

1. To diagnose labor.
2. To perform clinical pelvimetry when indicated.

3. To apply a fetal scalp electrode.
4. To determine the progress of labor by assessing the following factors:
   a. The degree of cervical effacement (expressed as a percentage, e.g., 50 percent effaced).
   b. The extent of cervical dilation (expressed in centimeters).
   c. The presenting part and the degree of molding.
   d. The condition of the fetal membranes.
   e. The degree of descent of the presenting part. The descent is expressed as "station" and described in centimeters above (minus) or below (plus) the ischial spines.
   f. The engagement of the presenting part.
   g. The position of the presenting part. This assessment requires the ability to distinguish landmarks on the fetal skull (*see* Fig. 1-10).
5. To diagnose abnormalities (e.g., prolapsed cord, shoulder presentation, anencephaly, and hydrocephalus).

Materials

The vaginal examination is performed with sterile lubricating jelly and examining gloves, which also must be sterile if the woman is in labor or if there is any possibility that the fetal membranes have ruptured.

Nursing actions

The woman should empty her bladder before the examination. The nurse should ensure privacy and good lighting and explain the procedure and its purpose to the woman. The woman should then be placed in the dorsal recumbent position and draped. The nurse should perform the examination in a systematic and thoughtful way, assess the findings, and share them with the woman and her family. The findings should then be recorded — plotting on a *Friedman curve* (*see* Fig. 9-1) is helpful in evaluating progress in labor — and reported to the physician and/or midwife.

General procedures

The following is a list of the procedures involved in the vaginal examination:

1. Assist the woman to assume a comfortable position and drape her properly. Help her to relax during the examination by reviewing relaxation and breathing techniques.
2. Wash hands and put on gloves, using aseptic technique.

3. Apply sterile lubricant to the index and middle fingers of the examining hand.

4. Spread the labia above the introitus with the thumb and index finger of the other hand.

5. Observe the introitus for any free flow of fluid and note its color (clear vs. meconium stained) and consistency (thick vs. thin meconium). **Remember:** Any vaginal bleeding must be distinguished from bloody show. Do *not* perform a vaginal examination if the woman is bleeding (*see* Chapter 17).

6. Gently insert the lubricated examining fingers (palmer surface downward) into the vagina and press downward as the fingers advance. Rotate the fingers upward as they continue to advance until the cervix or the presenting part is reached.

7. Avoid inadvertently touching the woman's clitoris and anus with the thumb of the examining hand: hold the thumb close to the palm.

The specific procedures and significant findings of the vaginal examination are listed and discussed in Table 1-6.

TABLE 1-6
The Vaginal Examination

Procedure	Significant findings
1. *Finding the cervix*. Locate the cervix with the examining fingers and feel for consistency, position, and size (length and width).	1.1 The cervix is soft, lies posteriorly, is about 2 to 3 cm long and 1 cm thick, and admits only a fingertip *before* labor begins.
2. *Determining cervical dilation*. Gently encircle the circumference of the cervical opening (os) with the examining fingers, moving them from side to side and forwards and backwards to estimate the diameter of the os. Form a mental image of the size. (The development of ability to assess the number of centimeters of dilation is facilitated by practice and comparison of the examiner's estimation with premeasured dilation models. It is also possible to practice with circular objects, such as assorted drinking glasses, circular containers, telephone dials, etc., by estimating their diameters in centimeters and then checking their actual measurements with a centimeter ruler.)	2.1 *Approximate width in fingerbreadths* / *Centimeters dilated (see* Fig. 1-13) Fingertip — 1 One large — 2 Two — 3 Three — 4-5 Four — 6-7 Five — 10 2.2 *A "rim" of cervix*. If the cervical tissue surrounding the presenting part is only palpable as ½ to 1 fingerbreadth, it is a "rim" of cervix; and regardless of the measurement of the dilated os, full dilation is imminent (*see* Fig. 1-14). 2.3 *Full dilation*. The cervix is said to be "fully dilated" when the diameter of the opening measures 10 cm, because the presenting part can usually pass through this space. Another important point is that when *no* cervix is felt surrounding the presenting part, the os is fully dilated and the second stage of labor has begun.

3. Determining effacement. The "obliteration" or "taking up" of the cervix is the shortening of the cervical canal from a structure approximately 2 to 3 cm long and 1 cm thick to one in which the canal is replaced by a circular orifice with almost paper-thin edges. The degree of effacement is expressed as a percentage. While carefully exploring the soft tissue that covers the presenting part, estimate its length and/or thickness. At term, the cervix is frequently 50 to 60% effaced as a result of myometrial activity called Braxton-Hicks's contractions. Effacement continues during the latent phase of labor.

3.1 See significant finding 1.1 (above) for a description of the "uneffaced" cervix.

3.2 Multipara's cervix at term. The cervix that is soft, directed forward in a midline position, about 1.0 to 1.5 cm in length or thickness, admits a finger easily, and is dilatable up to 3 to 4 cm is a "ripe" cervix (about 50% effaced).

3.3 Primigravida's cervix at term. The cervix feels very thin and is so close to the presenting part that it may feel fully dilated, until the os is found (more posteriorly and upward) to be only 1 cm dilated. This is a cervix that is 100% effaced. Effacement is often advanced in primigravidas at term before more than slight dilation occurs (see Fig. 1-15).

3.4 An edematous anterior lip of the cervix. This sometimes occurs toward the end of the first stage of labor. It may result when the cervix is compressed between the fetal head and the brim of the pelvis (e.g., in the occiput posterior position). It may also be caused by the woman's bearing down during the first stage of labor. It feels soft and spongy to the examining finger, is located anteriorly, and no other cervical tissue is found surrounding the rest of the circumference of the presenting part.

4. Touching the presenting part. Feel the presenting part either through the dilated cervical os or in the undilated cervix through the thin lower uterine segment. Confirm the findings of the abdominal palpation. It may help to move the fetus down to the examining fingers by applying some pressure on the fundus with the abdominal hand. Determine size, shape, and consistency of the presenting part.

4.1 Vertex presentation. This is hard and round to the touch. In approximately 95% of women, the vertex presents.

4.2 Frank breech. This is softer and less regular than the vertex. Male genitalia can sometimes be felt.

4.3 Footling breech or a hand. Either is distinctively small and moves when touched. A foot will move when touched or tickled but will not be able to pull away, as a hand will sometimes do.

Procedure	Significant findings
	4.4 *Face presentation or an anencephalic fetus.* This feels very soft and very irregular. In all cases where the vertex presentation is in doubt or underterminable, the obstetrician must be notified immediately.
5. *Determining the presence of intact membranes.* Without removing the examining fingers from the presenting part, wait for a uterine contraction and try to carefully reassess whether the membranes are intact. Correlate findings with the history that the woman has given.	**5.1** *Intact membranes.* The fetal scalp, when covered with mucus, has the same slippery feeling as the fetal membranes. Therefore, assessment during a contraction will be more accurate. During the contraction, the membranes become tense and/or bulge through the cervical os. They can be felt with the presenting part lying immediately behind them and fluid between them.
	5.2 *Ruptured membranes.* Fetal scalp hair is felt and amniotic fluid can sometimes be seen flowing over the examining hand. *If membranes are ruptured, vaginal examinations must be limited.*
6. *Determining the level of descent or station.* The woman's ischial spines are about halfway between the pelvic inlet and the pelvic outlet. Apply pressure along the right side wall of the vagina and sweep the examining fingers downward and inward at approximately the 8-o'clock level (if the left side wall is used, it may be located at the 4-o'clock level) and feel for a bony prominence. The ischial spines on a gynecoid pelvis are blunt and, therefore, sometimes difficult to palpate. (*Remember:* It is the bony prominence in a cephalic presentation and *not* the caput that is described in centimeters above or below the ischial spines.)	**6.1** *Station.* This is the relationship of the lowest portion of the presenting part to an imaginary line drawn between the ischial spines of the woman's pelvis. This imaginary line is referred to as the level of the ischial spines. Station is measured in terms of centimeters above (minus) or below (plus) the level of the ischial spines (*see* Fig. 1-16).
	6.2 *Floating presenting part.* This is a presenting part that *cannot* be felt even with a contraction or fundal pressure. Care must be taken *not* to inadvertently rupture the fetal membranes because rupture before engagement could predispose the fetus to a prolapsed cord (*see* Chapter 17).

6.3 *Progress in labor.* Descent of the presenting part is one of the mechanisms of labor and is an indication that labor is progressing (*see* Chapter 9).

6.4 *Designation of level of descent and engagement of the presenting part:*

Presenting part	Station
2 cm above the level of the ischial spines.	−2
Fixed low in the pelvis and easily felt at the level of the ischial spines. (Usually indicates that the head is engaged [*see* Figs. 1-17 and 1-18].)	0
2 cm below the level of the ischial spines with bulging of the perineum and flattening of the anus.	+2

6.5 *Delivery is imminent.* In the multipara, the presenting part is usually at the +2 station. In contrast, the primipara may push the presenting part to the +4 or +5 station. Imminent delivery is best estimated by the appearance of the presenting part at the vaginal outlet. In the vertex presentation, the vaginal outlet and the vulva are stretched further until they ultimately encircle the largest diameter of the fetus's head. This is known as crowning.

Procedure	Significant findings
7. *Determining fetal position.* (Example of vertex presentation only.) Wait until the cervix is at least 4 to 5 cm dilated, then slide the examining fingers gently over the lowest part of the presenting part and seek a linear indentation in the fetal skull. Decide the direction in which this indentation runs in the pelvis, follow it in both directions, and palpate both ends.	**7.1** *Fetal position.* The vaginal examination during labor after the cervix has begun to dilate will help to confirm abdominal examination findings regarding fetal position. This is because the fetal suture lines and fontanels can now be felt. Because the cephalic vertex presentations are the most common, it would be helpful to be well versed in the essential landmarks of the fetal skull (*see* Table 1-5 and Fig. 1-10).

The *sagittal* suture is perceived as a linear indentation or a shallow cleft in the fetal skull. Location of the sagittal suture confirms the presentation as vertex or brow.

To determine the location of the posterior fontanel, the examining fingers palpate a *triangle* of dense, thick, resistant *occipital bone*, which is often depressed below the two delicate overlapping parietal bones. The posterior fontanel is the point at which the sagittal suture ends or "forks" into the two lambdoidal sutures.

Position	Direction of the sagittal suture	Location of the occipital bone
LOA	Runs from 1-2 o'clock to 7-8 o'clock.	1-2 o'clock.
ROP	Same as above.	7-8 o'clock.
ROT	Runs from 3 o'clock to 9 o'clock.	9 o'clock.
LOT	Same as above.	3 o'clock.
ROA	Runs from 10-11 o'clock to 4-5 o'clock.	10-11 o'clock.
LOP	Same as above.	4-5 o'clock.

| OA | Runs from 12 o'clock to 6 o'clock. | 12 o'clock. |
| OP | Same as above. | 6 o'clock. |

When the posterior fontanel is recognized, it is unnecessary to search for the anterior fontanel. However, it is sometimes used to confirm the diagnosis. The bones in the region of the anterior fontanel recoil with palpation. A fourth suture — the frontal suture — is palpated beyond the anterior fontanel and is perceived as a continuation of the sagittal suture (see Figs. 1-19 and 1-20).

OA, occiput anterior; OP, occiput posterior.

Summary: The complete vaginal examination is an important skill that takes time and practice to acquire. The accuracy of the findings will require patience and concentration. Abbreviations may be used to chart findings. For example:

SVE: 8 cm - 100% - 0 Vtx, LOA.

Interpretation: Sterile vaginal examination: 8 cm dilated - 100 percent effaced - 0 station. Vertex presentation, left occiput anterior position.

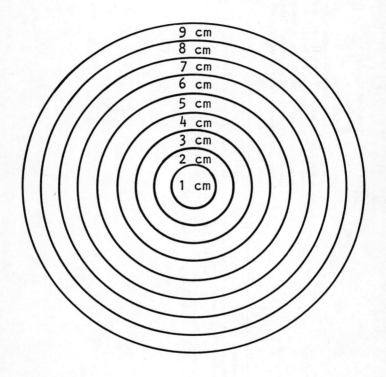

Figure 1-13. Diagrammatic representation of cervical dilation in centimeters (to scale). (*See* Table 1-6.)

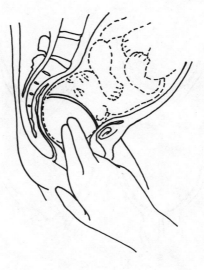

Figure 1-14. A ''rim.'' The cervix is almost fully dilated. (*See* Table 1-6.) *Adapted from* Myles, M. F. Textbook for Midwives. Churchill Livingstone, Inc., New York, 1981. Ninth edition. p. 250.

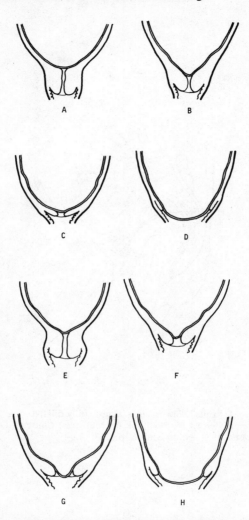

Figure 1-15.   Cervical effacement and dilation. Nullipara: (A) before labor, (B) early effacement, (C) complete effacement, and (D) complete dilation. Multipara: (E) before labor, (F) effacement and beginning dilation, (G) dilation, and (H) complete dilation. (*See* Table 1-6.) *Adapted from* Ross Laboratories. Clinical Education Aids. Number 13. Ross Laboratories, Columbus, Ohio. 1979.

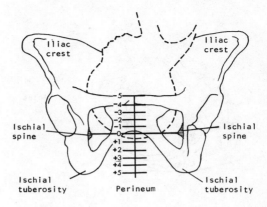

Figure 1-16. Station of presenting part (degree of engagement). Stations are expressed in centimeters above (minus) and below (plus) the level of the ischial spines. (*See* Table 1-6.) *Adapted from* Ross Laboratories. Clinical Education Aids. Number 13. Ross Laboratories, Columbus, Ohio. 1979.

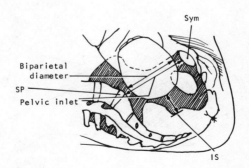

Figure 1-17. Descent and engagement of the presenting part. If the lowest portion of the fetal head is *above* the ischial spines, the biparietal diameter of the head probably has *not* passed through the pelvic inlet and, therefore, is not engaged (*see* Table 1-6). IS, ischial spine; SP, sacral promontory; Sym, symphysis pubis. *Adapted from* Pritchard, J. A., and P. C. MacDonald. Williams Obstetrics. Appleton-Century-Crofts, East Norwalk, Conn. 1980. Sixteenth edition. p. 282.

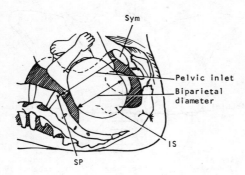

Figure 1-18.   Descent and engagement of the presenting part. If the lowest portion of the fetal head is *at or below* the ischial spines, it is probably engaged (*see* Table 1-6). IS, ischial spine; SP, sacral promontory; Sym, symphysis pubis. *Adapted from* Pritchard, J. A., and P. C. MacDonald. Williams Obstetrics. Appleton-Century-Crofts, East Norwalk, Conn. 1980. Sixteenth edition. p. 282.

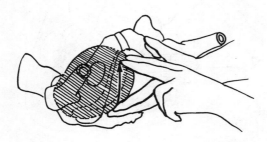

Figure 1-19.   Locating the sagittal suture during the vaginal examination (*see* Table 1-6). *Adapted from* Pritchard, J. A., and P. C. MacDonald. Williams Obstetrics. Appleton-Century-Crofts, East Norwalk, Conn. 1980. Sixteenth edition. p. 302.

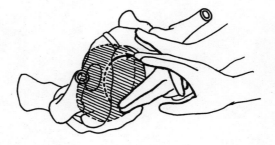

Figure 1-20. Differentiating the fontanels during the vaginal examination (*see* Table 1-6). *Adapted from* Pritchard, J. A., and P. C. MacDonald. Williams Obstetrics. Appleton-Century-Crofts, East Norwalk, Conn. 1980. Sixteenth edition. p. 302.

CHAPTER 2

DIAGNOSIS AND PHYSIOLOGY OF PREGNANCY

Barbara Decker

Prenatal care has been demonstrated to be the single most important factor in improving perinatal outcomes.[1] This chapter describes the methods and rationales for the diagnosis of pregnancy, and it provides the physiological bases for the provision of prenatal care.

DIAGNOSIS OF PREGNANCY

The diagnosis of pregnancy enables the caregivers and the client to (1) begin prental care, (2) promote maternal adaptation to pregnancy, (3) identify prenatal risk factors, and (4) identify the expected date of confinement. The signs of pregnancy that are used to establish the diagnosis of pregnancy are described in Table 2-1. Traditionally, these signs have been separated into **presumptive, probable,** and **positive** signs. Presumptive signs are considered the least reliable because they are subjective and may be related to many causes other than pregnancy. Although probable signs can often be objectively identified, they are susceptible to errors of measurement and they may be related to other causes. Positive signs are the most reliable because they are directly related to identification of the presence of the fetus. A diagnosis of pregnancy is most often made in the presence of a combination of the signs of pregnancy.

TABLE 2-1
Signs of Pregnancy

Sign of pregnancy	Time of appearance	Physiological basis	How elicited
Presumptive signs Cessation of menses	21-35 days after the last menstrual period (depending on individual menstrual pattern). Unreliable when periods are irregular or not established, when postpartum or postabortion, and when lactating or using oral contraceptives.	Conception inhibits menstruation because of the high levels of estrogen and progesterone produced by the functioning corpus luteum. (Nonmenstrual bleeding may mimic menses.)	Careful history will include onset of menses, menstrual pattern, date of last menstrual period, amount and duration of flow during last menstrual period, date of last normal menstrual period, obstetric history, contraceptive history, and history of deviations in reproductive health.
Breast changes	Variable. *Early weeks:* tenderness, tingling, feeling of fullness. *After 8 weeks:* gradual increase in size, increase in nodularity, appearance of blue veins under skin, enlargement and increased pigmentation of areola, appearance of tubercles of Montgomery. *After 12 weeks:* colostrum present in breasts.	Estrogen stimulates growth of mammary ducts and breast tissue. Progesterone stimulates alveolar and breast tissue development. Human placental lactogen is thought to contribute to breast development. Increased pigmentation is possibly due to high levels of melanocyte-stimulating hormone. Estrogen and progesterone may have similar effect.	Client may report breast growth, and/or tenderness. Inspection will reveal network of veins under skin, tubercles of Montgomery. Palpation will elicit breast tenderness and nodular breast tissue. Colostrum may be expressed after 12 weeks by gentle massage.

Nausea	6 weeks after last normal menstrual period, usually disappearing by 12 weeks. May be present with vomiting.	Unknown. Possible causes include high levels of HCG, psychological ambivalence, B vitamin deficiency, and orthostatic hypotension.	On interview, client often reports "morning sickness," but nausea and vomiting may occur at any time of day.
Urinary frequency	1st trimester of pregnancy. Reappears during 3rd trimester as fetal presenting part presses on the bladder.	The enlarging uterus competes with the bladder for space in the pelvis, reducing the bladder's capacity. Frequency related to this cause disappears when the uterus rises out of the pelvis after 12 weeks. It recurs at term when the fetal presenting part encroaches on the bladder.	Client reports frequent voidings of smaller than usual amounts of urine. "Physiological" frequency is not associated with signs and symptoms of urinary tract infection.
Fatigue	1st trimester.	Possible causes include rising progesterone levels or psychological ambivalence.	Client reports unusual sleepiness, desire for daytime naps, and loss of usual energy level.
Changes in skin pigmentation	Gradual during first trimester: A. Linea nigra: appearance of a dark line from symphysis pubis that fades above the umbilicus. B. Increase in nipple and areola pigmentation. C. Chloasma: appearance of brownish patches on face and neck.	Rising estrogen and progesterone levels stimulate high levels of melanocyte-stimulating hormone, which produces increased amounts of melanin in the skin.	History and inspection. Fair-skinned women will have light-brown linea nigra and dark-pink areolae. Dark-skinned women may have black linea nigra, and brown to black areolae. Changes that occur during a first pregnancy tend to persist; pigmentation changes are not reliable for diagnosis in subsequent pregnancies. Women taking oral contraceptives may also experience chloasma.

Sign of pregnancy	Time of appearance	Physiological basis	How elicited
Probable signs **Laboratory tests of pregnancy** Immunologic assays of HCG. Hemagglutination-inhibition tests (Pregnosticon Dri-Dot, UCG Test [2-hour tests])	Usually become positive 6-8 weeks after last normal menstrual period. Can become falsely negative by the 16th week of gestation due to lower levels of HCG. Thought to have lower false negative rate than latex-inhibition slide tests.	HCG is believed to be produced by the syntrophoblast. Production begins very early in pregnancy, reaching highest levels at between the 60th and 70th day of gestation (8-10 weeks). After that, in normal pregnancy, urinary and serum levels drop to a level that is then maintained throughout pregnancy. Hemagglutination-inhibition tests use sheep erythrocytes sensitized to HCG and an antiserum to HCG to provoke a reaction with a woman's urine.	The antiserum is mixed with urine, and sensitized erythrocytes are then added. If HCG is present in the urine, it will react with the antiserum. When the second reagent is added, there will be *no agglutination* of the cells added: a *positive* pregnancy test. If there is no HCG in the urine, the antiserum will react with the sensitized sheep cells by *agglutination* of the cells: a *negative* test.
Latex-inhibition slide tests (Pregnosticon Dri-Dot, UCG Slide Test, Gravindex, etc. [take only a few minutes])	Usually become positive 6-8 weeks after last normal menstrual period. Can become falsely negative by the 16th week of gestation due to lower levels of HCG.	Physiological basis is the same as above. HCG-coated latex particles are one reagent of this test; the other is a solution of HCG antibodies. This test also relies on an antibody response to HCG for its functioning. For both tests, there can be false positive and	A solution of HCG antibody is mixed with a drop of urine and then with the solution that contains HCG-coated latex particles. If HCG is present in the urine, it will combine with all the antibodies in the first solution and there will be *no agglutination* of latex particles:

false negative results.

False negative results are caused by:

1. Early testing: HCG levels are low.
2. Late testing: after approximately 16 weeks of gestation, levels are again low.
3. Threatened or imminent abortion: deficient trophoblast produces little HCG.

False positive results are caused by:

1. High levels of LH. A common cause of high LH levels is menopause, when menstrual periods are also likely to be irregular.
2. Proteinuria.

a *positive* test. Without HCG in the urine, the antibody solution will act on the latex particles to produce *agglutination: a negative* test.

Enlargement of the uterus

6 weeks: beginning enlargement detectable by experienced examiners on pelvic examination.
12 weeks: uterus rises out of pelvis, and by 16 weeks it is consistently measurable on abdominal palpation (*see* Chapter 1).

Estrogen causes stretching and enlargement of existing muscle cells. There is also an increase in elastic and fibrous tissue and a great increase in blood supply and lymphatic drainage. After the 3rd month, the growth of the fetus and the placenta and increased amounts of amniotic fluid contribute to the enlargement of the uterus.

Pelvic examination is necessary before 12-16 weeks. Abdominal palpation will show enlargement thereafter. Pelvic and abdominal palpation can be combined for more accurate assessment.

Sign of pregnancy	Time of appearance	Physiological basis	How elicited
Softening of cervix (Goodell's sign)	6-8 weeks.	Estrogen and progesterone cause increased vascularity and edema of the cervix and hypertrophy and hyperplasia of the cervical glands.	Palpation will reveal consistency of the cervix. In the nonpregnant state, it is firm, like the tip of the nose. During pregnancy, it becomes soft, like the lips.
Softening of the lower uterine segment (Hegar's sign)	6-8 weeks.	Estrogen and progesterone cause increased vascularity, congestion, and edema of the tissue.	Palpation will reveal the soft, compressible isthmus, felt between the firm cervix and the more muscular body of the uterus.
Blue discoloration of the vulva, vagina, and cervix (Chadwick's sign)	6-8 weeks.	Estrogen and progesterone cause increased vascularity, lymphatic supply, and, hence, increased congestion of pelvic tissues.	Inspection, either direct or with the aid of a vaginal speculum, will reveal color.
Enlargement of the abdomen	Gradual, after 16 weeks.	Enlarging uterus is accommodated by a gradual enlargement of the abdomen.	In a healthy woman, enlargement of the abdomen is a probable sign of pregnancy. However, careful inspection and palpation are required to rule out tumors, ascites, and other nonpregnancy-related causes of enlargement.

Palpation of the fetal outline	After 20 weeks.	Continued fetal growth permits palpation of the hard fetal head, smoothly curving back, firm rump, and angular arms and legs (*see* Chapter 1).	Although palpation may be difficult because of maternal obesity, excessive amniotic fluid, or myomas of the uterus; in general, it should become easier as pregnancy progresses.
Ballottement of the fetus	Approximately 18-20 weeks.	Volume of amniotic fluid is large in proportion to the size of the fetus, thereby permitting movement of the entire fetal body within the uterus.	Sudden pressure on the uterus will cause the fetus to float away and then softly rebound against the examining hand.
Braxton Hicks's contractions	3rd trimester.	Nonrhythmic, painless contractions of the uterus begin early in pregnancy and gradually increase in frequency and subjective intensity toward term. Physiological basis is not well understood: may be due to stretching of uterine muscle fibers and/or hormonally induced changes in muscle cell physiology.	A firming of the body of the uterus, followed by return to a relaxed state, may be palpated during the 3rd trimester. As pregnancy progresses, the mother becomes aware of these contractions and may report them as painful. At term, Braxton Hicks's contractions may be confused with contractions of labor (*see* Chapter 9).
Positive signs Fetal heart tones	Heard with stethoscope or fetoscope by the 20th week of gestation in nearly all pregnancies. The date the fetal	Blood begins to circulate in the fetus by the 6th week of gestation, but the sound produced by the closing of the	The fetal heart will be heard most easily when the stethoscope is placed on the abdomen over the area where

Sign of pregnancy	Time of appearance	Physiological basis	How elicited
	heart is first heard is often used to help validate duration of pregnancy. The fetal heart can be heard with portable ultrasound (Doppler device) or fetal monitor as early as 12 weeks.	fetal heart valves is not loud enough to be consistently heard until 20 weeks.	the fetal back lies. Often, a search over the entire uterus is necessary to locate it. A Doppler device or fetal monitor can be used when the fetal heart is inaudible because of maternal obesity, excessive amniotic fluid, or other reasons. The sounds of the fetal heart must be distinguished from other sounds: 1. Funic souffle: a whistling sound that has the same rate and rhythm as the fetal pulse. 2. Uterine souffle: a soft sound that beats to the rate and rhythm of the maternal pulse. 3. The maternal pulse. All except funic souffle may be identified by simultaneously palpating the client's radial pulse. Funic souffle must be differentiated from fetal heart tones by the quality of the sound: the souffle is a whistling sound, whereas the heart tones are clicking sounds.

Fetal movement	As early as 16 weeks, as felt by the client. 20 weeks, as felt by the examiner.	Fetal movements begin as early as the 12th week. By the 20th week they become strong enough to be felt outside the wall of the uterus.	Abdominal palpation of the uterus often stimulates fetal movement, or it may occur spontaneously. Fetal movements are best felt on the side of the uterus away from the back, where the limbs lie.
Sonographic recognition of the fetus	Gestational sac is apparent 6 weeks after the last normal menstrual period. Fetal heart action can be detected by a Doppler device or real-time ultrasonography after 11 weeks.	As soft tissue structures develop, they become recognizable on ultrasonogram.	Fetal soft parts reflect ultrasound waves, which can then be interpreted by a person skilled in this technology.
X-ray identification of the fetus	16 weeks.	Centers of ossification are identifiable as early as 14 weeks, but are usually not visualized on x-ray until 16 weeks.	Radiation from x-rays is considered a hazard to the fetus and, therefore, x-rays are contraindicated unless there is an overwhelming need for the information derived from them. In general, ultrasonography has replaced x-ray as a tool for the diagnosis of pregnancy.

HCG, human chorionic gonadotrophin; LH, luteinizing hormone.

PHYSIOLOGICAL ADAPTATIONS TO PREGNANCY

The physiological changes associated with maternal adaptation to pregnancy are complex. At no other time in life, except at birth, does the human body so extensively alter its functioning. The normal parameters of health often do not apply during pregnancy, and the physiological findings during pregnancy would often signal disease if they were found in the nonpregnant person.

In order to accurately assess the health status of the pregnant woman, and in order to assist her to participate fully in her own health care, it is important for the nurse to understand the basis for the physical changes that will occur. Although the following physiological changes are presented by organs and systems, it should be remembered that the changes are interrelated both physiologically and psychologically (*see* Chapter 6).

Adaptations in the organs of reproduction

Uterus. The uterus increases in size from an average prepregnant weight of 70 grams to 1,100 grams at term, and from 6 to 10 centimeters in length to a size large enough to accommodate the fetus and amniotic fluid at term (approximately 36 to 40 centimeters).

The nonpregnant uterus is pear-shaped. As it grows in size during pregnancy, it becomes globular. In a progressive manner, by about the 24th week of gestation, the uterine wall thins out and conforms to the shape of the fetus and other products of conception.[2]

The growth of the uterine muscle tissue is caused by increased levels of estrogen and progesterone. Muscle tissue grows primarily by hypertrophy and stretching of the individual muscle cells and, perhaps, by a slight increase in the number of cells.[3] There is also an increase in fibrous tissue, elastic tissue, connective tissue, blood supply, and nerve supply, further adding to the uterine mass. The greatest growth is in the fundus of the uterus, which is illustrated by the fact that the fallopian tubes insert near the top of the uterus early in pregnancy and, at term, insert slightly above the middle of the uterus. As the uterus rises out of the pelvis, it rotates slightly to the right (dextrorotation) as a result of the presence of the rectosigmoid colon in the left side of the pelvis.

The changes in the size and position of the uterus have important effects on the other organs of the pelvis and abdomen. The increasing size and dextrorotation lead to crowding of the right ureter and to encroachment on both ureters at the pelvic brim. These effects subsequently result in a tendency toward urinary stasis, especially on the right side, and an increased incidence of hydronephrosis and hydroureter. The uterus crowds the bladder in early and late pregnancy. Decreased bladder capacity is a common cause of urinary frequency in the first and third trimesters. (The growing uterus rises out of the pelvis during the second trimester, thereby alleviating pressure on the bladder.) The enlarging uterus displaces and crowds the stomach and intestines, contributing to a tendency to develop heartburn, constipation, and intolerance for large meals. Venous return from the pelvis and lower extremities is impeded by the large uterus, leading to a tendency to develop hemorrhoids, vulvar varicosities, and varicose veins. When the client is supine, the enlarged uterus rests on her inferior vena cava and aorta. Interference with venous return to the heart can cause syncope and/or transient anxious feelings. The rising uterus also leads to elevation of the diaphragm and changes in the position of the heart (*see* p. 50).

Cervix. During pregnancy there is an increased blood supply to the cervix, increased fluid in the extracellular compartment, and hypertrophy and hyperplasia of the cervical glands. These changes, caused by increased levels of estrogen and progesterone, have the effect of softening and discoloring the cervix to a bluish shade. The cervical glands proliferate and form a honeycomb, which is filled with thick mucus — the "mucous plug" that is normally expelled before or during early labor. The proliferation of glands and of the columnar epithelium of the cervical canal often leads to an eversion of the cervical canal epithelium outward to the vaginal portion of the cervix. This outgrowth can bleed easily (e.g., when a Papanicolaou [Pap] smear is obtained) and may be mistaken for an erosion.

Vagina. Increased levels of estrogen and progesterone cause increased vascularity in the vaginal tissues and a bluish discoloration of the walls. The walls become soft and greatly increased in length. Because of the lengthening and softening, pelvic examination during pregnancy is often much less uncomfortable for the client. For the examiner, locating the cervix during a speculum examination may be more difficult because of the increased relaxation and folding of the vaginal walls. Cervical and vaginal secretions are greatly increased during pregnancy and are generally more acidic. The increased secretions may be mistaken for a symptom of vaginal infection or, late in pregnancy, may be reported as a leakage of amniotic fluid. The increased acidity of the secretions is thought to control the growth of pathogenic bacteria in the vagina, but the increased quantity and glycogen content of the secretions may encourage the development of the monilial and trichomonadal infections that are common in pregnancy.

Ovaries. Ovulation does not occur in pregnancy because the high levels of estrogen and progesterone inhibit the production of follicle-stimulating hormone. The ovarian corpus luteum produces the estrogen and progesterone that are necessary to maintain the pregnancy until the placenta takes over that function shortly after implantation of the fertilized ovum.

Breasts. The breasts begin enlarging after approximately 2 months of pregnancy. Estrogen stimulates growth of the ducts and pigmentation of the nipples. Progesterone stimulates the development of the lobules and alveoli of the breast. After the first few months of pregnancy, colostrum — a thick, yellowish pre-milk substance — may be expressed by massaging the breasts. Clients may be advised that this is a normal change of pregnancy.

Other physiological adaptations

Gastrointestinal tract. Maternal gums become hyperemic and may become swollen. The interdental papillae may become hypertrophied (epulis), which may cause spontaneous bleeding of the gums or bleeding after brushing the teeth or eating. There is decreased tone and motility of the gastrointestinal tract as a result of the elevated progesterone levels. This detrimental relaxation and sluggishness is complicated by crowding and displacement of the stomach and intestines by the enlarging uterus. Delayed gastric emptying and diminished capacity lead to an inability to tolerate normal-sized meals. In conjunction with relaxation of the cardiac sphincter, this delay and diminished capacity also contribute to reflux of gastric acid into the esophagus (heartburn). Decreased motility contributes to constipation and accumulation of intestinal gas. The development of hemorrhoids may occur as a result of venous relaxation and pooling, pelvic congestion, and constipation.

Urinary tract. The maternal renal pelves and the ureters dilate and become more tortuous, especially on the right side. These effects may be a result of progesterone, and they are probably influenced by the pressure of the uterus on the pelvic brim. The result is a tendency toward hydronephrosis and hydroureter.

An increased glomerular filtration rate and renal plasma flow lead to lowered plasma levels of creatinine and urea. Because there is no concomitant increase in renal tubular reabsorption, there is greater excretion of nutrients (especially glucose) in the urine of pregnant women. Glycosuria during pregnancy is not necessarily indicative of diabetes mellitus, but it may contribute to the increased incidence of lower urinary tract infections. Water and sodium excretion have been demonstrated to be markedly affected by maternal posture.[4] There is decreased excretion during the day while the client is up and about, and leg and pedal edema often develop. There is also decreased excretion when the client is supine because of uterine pressure on the vena cava, ultimately leading to decreased renal plasma flow. Conversely, the lateral recumbent position increases water and sodium excretion by enhancing renal blood flow. This position is one cause of physiological nocturia during pregnancy.

The bladder lies adjacent to the uterus. Its capacity is decreased early in pregnancy while the uterus is still a pelvic organ, and again late in pregnancy when the fetal presenting part descends into the pelvis. The result is urinary frequency. The bladder becomes hyperemic during pregnancy, and, with increasing uterine crowding, it may become edematous and easily traumatized. These changes contribute to an increased incidence of urinary tract infection during pregnancy and the postpartum period and make the bladder more susceptible to injury during delivery.

Respiratory tract. Tidal volume, minute ventilatory volume, and minute oxygen uptake increase during pregnancy. The respiratory rate increases secondary to direct progesterone stimulation of the respiratory center in the brain. Progesterone also causes a reduction in pulmonary resistance and an increase in air conductance secondary to relaxation of the walls of the bronchial tree. The vital capacity and the maximum breathing capacity are not altered. The net effect is no diminution in respiratory function. In fact, because the number of circulating red blood cells is increased during pregnancy, the oxygen concentration in the blood is increased and carbon dioxide levels are decreased.

Late in pregnancy, the enlarging uterus encroaches on the diaphragm and may elevate it as much as 4 centimeters.[5] Although the rib cage circumference increases by as much as 6 centimeters because of the progesterone-mediated increased mobility of the thorax, it does not fully compensate for the loss of capacity secondary to elevation of the diaphragm.[5] This lack of compensation may account, in part, for the development of dyspnea during late pregnancy (*see* Chapter 6).

Cardiovascular system. Maternal blood volume increases markedly beginning in the first trimester, rising most rapidly during the second trimester, and increasing more slowly during the third trimester. The total plasma volume increase is often as much as 50 percent greater than prepregnancy levels.[6]

Although the rate of production of red blood cells also increases (with a total increase during pregnancy of about 30 percent), it cannot keep up with the blood volume increase during the second trimester.[7] This leads to a physiological decrease in the hematocrit level, and, consequently, a 2- to 4-point drop in hematocrit does not necessarily indicate anemia. .

Cardiac output, stroke volume, and pulse rate are increased during pregnancy. A normal cardiac change that may be confused with a pathological condition is that of rotation of the heart upward and to the left secondary to the progressive elevation of the diaphragm. On x-ray, this rotation produces a silhouette that is similar to that of cardiac enlargement. There is an increased incidence of benign heart murmurs in normal pregnant women — probably as a result of the change in cardiac position in conjunction with torsion of the large blood vessels and lowered viscosity of the blood.

Skin.   Very little is known about the causes of skin changes in pregnancy; however, estrogen and progesterone do stimulate the production of melanin, which probably accounts for the increased pigmentation of the areolae, the linea nigra, and the "mask of pregnancy" (chloasma). These changes regress, but may not totally disappear, after pregnancy.

Vascular nevi (minute red elevations of the skin) occur in approximately two-thirds of white and one tenth of black pregnant women.[8] Vascular nevi are thought to be caused by high levels of estrogen.[8] They are of no physiological significance and regress soon after the delivery.

Striae (stretch marks) frequently appear on the client's abdomen, breasts, and thighs during pregnancy. After pregnancy, their dark color fades, leaving a silvery line.

Endocrine system.   The placenta produces large amounts of estrogen, progesterone, chorionic gonadotrophin, and human placental lactogen (HPL). The functions of estrogen and progesterone have been described in relation to their effects on other body systems. Aside from its role in preserving the corpus luteum, the function of chorionic gonadotrophin is not well understood. HPL has metabolic effects that promote lipolysis to increase fatty acids to be used as a source of maternal energy. HPL also has an anti-insulin effect on maternal tissues, which diverts glucose to the fetus.

Carbohydrate metabolism is altered during pregnancy, but the roles of insulin and those agents that act to produce the changes are little understood. HPL acts to oppose insulin and promote the use of fats for maternal needs. Estrogen, progesterone, and cortisol appear to increase insulin production. The net result is a taxing of the insulin-producing capabilities of the client. Whereas normal women tolerate this stress well, women who are prediabetic or who have only chemical diabetes may not be able to adapt to this stress and may develop signs and symptoms of overt diabetes.

In addition, the thyroid enlarges during pregnancy. Although there is an increased secretion of thyroxine, there is no increase in the levels of effective hormone because the levels of thyroxine-binding plasma protein are also increased, thus rendering the increased hormone ineffective. The basal metabolic rate increases by as much as 25 percent, which is probably entirely accounted for by the metabolic activity of the products of conception and the growing maternal tissues.[9]

Musculoskeletal system.   There is increased mobility of the joints of the pelvis and lower back during pregnancy. This increased mobility is probably the result of the effects of relaxin, which is thought to be produced either by the ovaries or by the placenta, and which softens cartilage and connective tissue. The increasing weight of the fetus causes the maternal center of gravity to shift forward. The woman compensates by arching her back (lordosis) in order to thrust her shoulders backward. This compensation is more pronounced in women with weak abdominal muscles and in women who are carrying twins. The instability of the pelvic joint leads to the wide stance that is characteristic of pregnancy.

DEVELOPMENT OF THE FETUS

The following summary of fetal development is sufficient to provide the nurse with a basis for evaluating the status of the fetus and for teaching and counseling parents-to-be.[10] (Because it is a *summary*, it is simplified and does not describe some of the details that can be found in embryology texts.)

The developmental dates provided below are in *weeks after conception,* not in *weeks after the last normal menstrual period.* Two weeks (if the client has a 28-day menstrual cycle) should be added to these dates to correlate with the usual method of dating pregnancy, which is by weeks after the last normal menstrual period. (*See* Table 2-2 for information on the development of the embryo and the fetus. *See* Chapter 7 for detailed information on how to date the pregnancy and how to assess fetal status.)

Week 1.   Fertilization occurs within 12 hours of ovulation, normally in the ampulla — the outer third of the fallopian tube. Through cell division, the zygote (fertilized ovum) develops from the morula (ball of cells) to the blastocyst (hollow ball) stage. Inside the blastocyst is an inner cell mass, which will become the fetus. Around the outside of the blastocyst is the trophoblast, which will implant the blastocyst in the wall of the uterus by means of erosion of maternal cells. The blastocyst implants in the maternal endometrium on the sixth day, normally in the fundus of the uterus.

Week 2.   Implantation is completed and the blastocyst is completely buried in the endometrium. Primitive placental circulation

TABLE 2-2

Fetoplacental Growth and Development by Calendar Months, and Maternal Response

Weeks after conception*	Embryonic and fetal development	Uterine changes	Possible maternal signs and physiological changes in pregnancy
		Ovulation and fertilization	
Week 1	Unfertilized ovum to fertilized egg (zygote) to free blastocyst to implanting blastocyst.	Endometrial phase: progestational, secretory, or luteal.	Basal body temperature remains elevated.
		Implantation	
Week 2	Primitive villi formation; yolk sac prominent; digestive system forming; germ layers differentiated; primitive blood cells present.	Mucosa invaded by trophoblasts; endometrium becomes decidua.	Nausea, fatigue, and breasts tense and tingling from estrogen- and progesterone-induced engorgement.
		Amenorrhea	
Week 3	Embryonic stages begin 3 wk after ovulation; brain, nervous system, and heart forming and beginning to function; susceptible to teratogenic effect. Length: 3 mm (1/8 in).	HCG secreted in quantity by chorionic villi; HCG supports the corpus luteum.	Some painless bleeding (spotting) experienced by 25% of women — cause unknown; basal body temperature elevated and constant; blood glucose low; endocrine test for HCG positive.
Week 4	Circulation starts; susceptible to teratogenic effect. Length: 4-5 mm (3/16 in); weight 0.4 g.	Mild contractions start. Cervix blue: Chadwick's sign. Cervix soft: Goodell's sign. Lower uterine segment soft: Hegar's sign.	Pressure on bladder from enlarging uterus; turgescence of bladder and urethral walls from estrogen and progesterone stimulation causes urinary frequency and urgency.

Week			
Week 5	Reproductive system forming; facial features forming; arm and leg buds present; susceptible to teratogenic effect (e.g., thalidomide-produced phocomelia). Length: 14 mm (1/2 in).	Mucous plug forming in cervical canal.	Profuse, thick, and acidic vaginal secretions (leukorrhea); nausea subsiding; epulis may occur.
Week 6	Hands, feet, fingers, and toes forming; susceptible to teratogenic effect; becoming a fetus. Length: 22-24 mm (about 1 in); weight: about 1 g.		Breasts larger and nodular; tubercles of Montgomery appear.
Week 7	Eyelids forming; ossification of skeleton begins; tooth buds forming; genital ridge visible but sexless in character as yet. Length: 3 cm (1 ¼ in).	Placenta now secreting progesterone; corpus luteum decreasing in function.	
Week 8	Human appearance; respiratory activity evident; kidneys begin secretion; becomes a fetus at end of this week; subsequent development is primarily growth and maturation of existing tissues and structures. Length: 4 cm (1 ½ in); weight: 2 g.	Placenta covers one third of uterine wall.	
Week 9	Eyelids fused; external genitalia begin to differentiate; bile present in intestines.	FHTs may be heard by Doppler method in some women by weeks 9-10.	

Weeks after conception*	Embryonic and fetal development	Uterine changes	Possible maternal signs and physiological changes in pregnancy
Week 10	External genitals now show definite signs of male or female sex; fingernails and toenails forming. Length: 9 cm (3 ½ in); weight: 15 g.	Uterus is size of an orange; fundus is at level of SP.	Nausea and vomiting are now rare.
Week 11 (end of first trimester)	Muscles contract occasionally, weakly; period of organogenesis (organ differentiation and hyperplasia) ends; fetus less susceptible to teratogenic effect; maturation of organs and overall growth continue to term.	Uterus rising from pelvic cavity; becoming an abdominal organ.	Bladder pressure lessens; blood glucose elevated.
Week 12	Sex easily distinguishable; thyroid and liver functional; blood forming in bone marrow. Length: 10.0-11.5 cm (4 in); weight: 19 g.	Uterus is now an abdominal organ.	Blood volume starts to increase; cardiac output increases.
Week 13	Lanugo appearing: head hair forming.	Uterine contractions occur but are not externally palpable as yet.	Physiological anemia; free hydrochloric acid in gastric juice declines; colostrum may be expressed.

Week 14	Muscles contracting more vigorously; skin transparent; blood vessels visible. Length: 16 cm (6 ½ in); weight: about 100 g.	Fundal height: midway between SP and umbilicus, or 3-4 fingerbreadths above SP.
Week 15	Skeleton visible on anterior-posterior x-ray film (a positive sign of pregnancy).	Uterine souffle (bruit) heard.
Week 16	Vernix caseosa forming on skin; meconium collecting; FHTs may be heard with a fetoscope; fetal movements (quickening) felt by many women now. Length: 19 cm (7 in).	Uterine wall thin; fetal movements generally palpable to the examiner now.
Week 17	Onset of rapid growth; iron starts to be stored; enamel and dentine deposited.	Ballottement can be elicited by examiner during months 4-5.
Week 18	FHTs may be heard more easily with a stethoscope (a positive sign of pregnancy); downy lanugo covers almost entire body; some scalp hair. Length: 25 cm (10 in); weight: 300 g.	Fundal height: at umbilicus.
Week 19	Eyebrows and eyelashes visible; head hair forming.	Umbilicus flush with skin; relaxation of smooth muscle, vein walls, bladder, etc.

Pigmentation changes may occur after the 16th wk: chloasma, nipples, and areolas.

Decisive increase in blood volume starting; nitrogen storage increasing.

Secondary areola appear; internal ballottement may be felt.

Weeks after conception*	Embryonic and fetal development	Uterine changes	Possible maternal signs and physiological changes in pregnancy
Weeks 20-21	Skin less transparent and wrinkled; vernix caseosa accumulating.		Ureteral dilation marked; linea nigra; chloasma (facial melasma or mask of pregnancy) may appear.
Week 22	Skin wrinkled; if born, will attempt to breathe. Length: 30 cm (12 in); weight: 600 g.	Fundal height: 2 fingerbreadths above umbilicus.	Period of greatest weight gain starts (4-5 lb/mo).
Week 23	Skin red, shiny, and thin; face wrinkled ("old man" appearance).		Striae gravidarum may appear.
Week 24 (end of second trimester)	Fetal outline may be felt abdominally (a positive sign of pregnancy).		Period of greatest hemodilution and lowest hemoglobin concentration starts; iron therapy is begun now, if not started earlier.
Week 25	Much iron stored; storage of subcutaneous fat begins; testes begin to descend in the male.	Uterine wall soft and yielding; start of placental senility.	Weight gain continues (4 lb/mo).
Week 26	Thick, red skin covered with vernix caseosa; eyelids open; fingerprints set; if born, can move energetically and cry weakly; viable with appropriate environmental support. Length: 35-37 cm (14 in); weight: 1,000 g.	Fundal height: 4 fingerbreadths above umbilicus.	Period of lowest hemoglobin level continues.

Weeks 27-28	Weak cry; more rapid growth starts; start of considerable calcium deposit and storage.	Braxton Hicks's contractions palpable.	Marked protein storage; blood volume highest.
Week 29	Twice as much calcium deposited as retained by mother; considerable nitrogen stored.		Large amount of calcium lost to fetus.
Week 30	Presentation: usually vertex (3% breech); testicles may descend into scrotal sac. Length: 40-42 cm (16 in); weight: 1,700-1,800 g.	Fundal height: 6 fingerbreadths above umbilicus.	3-4 lb weight gain this month; striae gravidarum more evident; pelvic joints more relaxed.
Weeks 31-33	Storage of considerable iron, nitrogen, calcium, and other nutrients; subcutaneous fat storage continues; vernix covers body.	Braxton Hicks's contractions stronger.	Large amount of iron lost to the fetus; stomach flaccid on top of uterus; heartburn common.
Week 34	Skin thicker and less wrinkled as subcutaneous fat stores accumulate; if born, has excellent chance for survival. Length: 45-47 cm (18 in); weight: 2,000-2,500 g.	Fundal height: 8 fingerbreadths above umbilicus.	Umbilicus protrudes; shortness of breath; hemoglobin level starts to rise.
Weeks 35-36	High hemoglobin level; low PO_2 tension (cyanotic); body well formed (now considered full term); storage of maternal immunoglobulins to diseases she has had.	Fundal height: 3 fingerbreadths below xiphoid process.	

Weeks after conception*	Embryonic and fetal development	Uterine changes	Possible maternal signs and physiological changes in pregnancy
Weeks 37-38 (end of third trimester)	Lanugo shed, except for shoulders, generally; body contours plump; decreased amount of vernix; scalp hair 2-3 cm long; cartilage in nose and ears is well developed. Male: testes within well-wrinkled scrotum. Female: labia well developed and cover vestibule.	Fundal height: 3-4 fingerbreadths below xiphoid process (uterine height decreases when lightening occurs).	Lightening (nullipara); breathing easier; varicosities more pronounced; ankle edema; urinary frequency. Lightening with start of labor in parous woman; cervix generally soft, slightly patulous, and partially (para) or totally (nullipara) effaced.

FHTs, fetal heart tones; HCG, human chorionic gonadotrophin; SP, symphysis pubis.

*For embryonic/fetal age as calculated from last normal menstrual period, add 2 weeks after conception (e.g., week 1 postconception is week 3 after the last normal menstrual period).

Adapted from Jensen, M. D., R. C. Bensen, and I. M. Bobak. Maternity Care: The Nurse and the Family. C. V. Mosby Co., St. Louis. 1981. Second edition. p. 72-75.

begins through erosion of maternal capillaries and endometrial glands.

Week 3. The embryo has differentiated into endoderm, mesoderm, and ectoderm — the germ layers from which all organs and structures are derived. The fetal thyroid and heart begin to develop.

Week 4. The fetal heart begins to beat. The embryo assumes a folded position, and arm buds appear.

Weeks 5-8. Rapid growth of the fetal brain causes the head to become proportionately much larger than the body. Development continues in a cephalocaudal, proximodistal manner: structures of the head or nearest the head develop before those of the lower body, and structures closest to the vertical midline develop before those farther away. By the end of the 8-week embryonic period, the embryo has begun to develop all of the major organs of the body. This is the most crucial period of development — the one in which the fetus is most susceptible to harmful environmental influences, such as maternal drugs and viruses, x-rays, etc.

Weeks 9-12. Fetal growth is very rapid, and growth of the head slows. Sex can be clearly determined by the 12th week.

Weeks 13-16. Rapid fetal growth and maturation characterize this period. Centers of ossification of the skeleton are visible on x-ray by the 16th week.

Weeks 17-20. The client usually feels quickening (fetal movement) by the end of this period. The fetus is covered with vernix and lanugo. Eyebrows and hair on the fetal head also appear.

Weeks 21-25. Fetal weight gain continues. The fetal skin is wrinkled and red, with capillaries visible.

Weeks 26-29. At this point, the fetus has the potential to survive, if born, because it can direct rhythmic breathing and control body heat. The actual mortality rate is very high, however, because of the immaturity of the fetal lungs.

Weeks 30-38. The fetus assumes a plump appearance. Deposition of subcutaneous fat eliminates wrinkles and tones down the earlier red appearance.

SUMMARY

It is important for the nurse to understand the physiological basis for changes experienced by the client during pregnancy in order to identify the normal adaptations of pregnancy, to teach the client about the normal changes and common discomforts of pregnancy, and to identify deviations from the norm. Physical and psychosocial needs of the client (which will be discussed in Chapter 3) must also be

incorporated in the nursing care plan in order to meet the needs of
each client.

REFERENCES

1. Ryan et al.
2. Pritchard and MacDonald. 221-223.
3. Niswander. 41.
4. Davison. 295.
5. Pritchard and MacDonald. 240.
6. Niswander. 34.
7. Letsky. 48.
8. Pritchard and MacDonald. 269.
9. de Swiet. 89-90.
10. Moore.

CHAPTER 3

ANTEPARTUM CARE

Barbara Decker

Antepartum (or prenatal) care is a systematic plan of preventive and therapeutic care implemented through a schedule of visits between clients and health care team members. The goal of antepartum care is to enable the client, fetus, and family to enter the intrapartum period with all of their physical, emotional, and social resources maximized in order to yield the best possible outcome for the pregnancy.

The care that the nurse provides should be based on his or her understanding that pregnancy is a normal physiological event. Pregnancy is, however, a time of physiological stress, and complications may arise at any point. Most of prenatal care consists of assisting the client to maintain optimum health during the pregnancy while screening her for signs of complications. If complications arise, they must be treated while support for the normal aspects of the pregnancy continues.

The pregnant client is motivated to learn about the changes taking place in her body. She should be encouraged to learn about the normal process of pregnancy so that she is not alarmed by normal changes and so that she is able to identify deviations from the norm. Each client must accept a great deal of responsibility for her own health care because she makes only periodic visits to the health care provider. In addition, each client must be encouraged to contact her providers if she identifies any deviations from the norm.

During pregnancy the client is also highly motivated to change her health habits for the benefit of her unborn child. The nurse who recognizes this will be able to assist the client to establish sound health practices for herself and her entire family. The changes established during pregnancy will often become a permanent part of the health practices of that family.

The nurse must recognize that pregnancy occurs within a family system. The other members of the family are affected by the client's physical and emotional changes as well as by the inevitable changes in relationships when a new family member enters the family group. The nurse should encourage active participation in the pregnancy by all of the family members. The nurse should help them to understand the physical and emotional changes of pregnancy so that they can provide support to the client. The nurse can also help them prepare for the introduction of a new member into their family system.

The care that the nurse provides should be based on the nursing process. The nurse should first collect all pertinent information on which to base a complete and accurate assessment of the client's status. This data will consist of the client's psychosocial status, complete medical history, results of the physical examination, and laboratory findings. When all of the data is available, the nurse will be able to make a nursing diagnosis based on the client's current status (strengths, needs, and problems) and anticipated future status (strengths, needs, and problems). The nurse is then able to design, in collaboration with the client, a comprehensive plan of care, which is shared with other members of the health care team. The plan of care is then implemented and continually evaluated by the nurse and the client. Revisions in the plan of care are made whenever necessary. At any time, as new data become available, the assessment of client status may change, requiring a change in the plan of care.

The antepartum care plan includes a routine of initial and subsequent visits with standardized goals for each. The design is modified according to the individual client's needs, and additional visits may be scheduled in order to pursue such individualized needs (e.g., intensive nutrition counseling, special learning needs, family counseling, etc.).

THE INITIAL VISIT

A complete physical and psychosocial assessment of the client and her family should be performed to formulate an individualized plan of care for the pregnancy. Table 3-1 lists the components of the initial visit and their rationales.

In many settings, the nurse is responsible for taking all or part of the client's history. The history should always be taken in a quiet,

TABLE 3-1
Components of the Initial Visit

History	Rationale
Date of initial visit.	Base line for planning care for this pregnancy.
Psychosocial history.	Client identification.
Base-line data: Name, address, telephone number, date of birth, marital status, age, race, ethnic origin, religion, education, occupation.	
Family: Configuration of family, roles, communication patterns, satisfaction and/or problems with family life.	Factors that may affect risk status and adaptation to psychosocial demands of pregnancy.
Social system: Friends and supports outside family, economic problems, employment/student status, housing.	Base line for future nursing intervention, because pregnancy and childbirth require family adaptation of roles and behaviors.
Other concerns: Those identified by client or nurse.	Assessment of social resources. Evaluation of need for referral to social service.
Family medical and surgical history (members to be assessed: grandparents, parents, children, siblings, parents' siblings, and first cousins).	Complete identification of client's health care needs.
Factors: Tuberculosis, diabetes, cardiac disease, hypertension, anemia, cancer, kidney disease, epilepsy or other neurological disorders, mental	Identification of familial problems that have the potential to affect the course or outcome of this pregnancy.

History	Rationale
illness, inherited diseases or abnormalities, allergies, multiple pregnancies, obstetric problems, cesarean sections.	
Personal medical and surgical history.	Identification of problems that may affect this pregnancy (risk status). Base line for physical assessment and medical and nursing care plans.
Medical: Tuberculosis, respiratory disease, diabetes, cardiac disease, rheumatic fever, hypertension, cancer, anemia, kidney disease (including urinary tract infections), epilepsy or other neurological disorders, mental illness, inherited diseases or abnormalities, venereal disease, gynecologic disease, varicose veins, hemorrhoids, thromboembolic disorders, childhood diseases.	
Surgical: Operations (especially uterine), accidents, blood transfusions.	
Allergies: Medications (specifically antibiotics and anesthetics), foods, environmental substances.	
Habits: Smoking, alcohol intake, medications/drugs (including over-the-counter drugs and street drugs).	

Gynecologic/obstetric history.

Menstrual: Age at menarche; regular or irregular periods; interval between, duration of, and amount of flow and pain with periods; bleeding between periods; last normal menstrual period; last normal menstrual period; expected date of confinement (*see* Chapter 7).

Evaluation of reproductive health. Accurate identification of last normal menstrual period, estimated date of confinement, and current gestational age.

Previous pregnancies: Duration of pregnancy, date of termination, place of confinement, duration of labor, and type of delivery/termination. (Also note status, sex, and weight of infant at birth; maternal, fetal, or neonatal complications prenatally, at delivery, or postpartum; and present health status of child.)

Identification of maternal and fetal risk factors. Base line for plan of care for this pregnancy, birth, and postpartum period.

Contraceptive history: Method most recently used, when and why discontinued (planned pregnancy?), satisfaction with method, side effects. Previous methods used, satisfaction, side effects, when and why discontinued.

Further assessment of gestational age and estimated date of confinement (method may affect menstrual cycle). Base line for contraceptive counseling late in pregnancy and selection of postpartum method.

Sexual history: Frequency, number of partners, satisfaction, history of infertility, date client believes she became pregnant (if known).

Further assessment of gestational age (sexual patterns affect conception). Base line for sexual counseling during pregnancy.

History	Rationale
Current pregnancy.	
Base-line data: Weight at onset of pregnancy, exposure to teratogens (including medications and x-rays), infections and fever, date of quickening (if appropriate).	Base line for anticipated changes of normal pregnancy. Identification of additional risk factors.
Common complaints: Nausea, vomiting, round ligament pain, constipation, diarrhea, dizziness, visual problems, fatigue, depression, urinary frequency, vaginal discharge, breast tenderness, etc.	Identification of client's specific discomforts that require teaching and counseling (*see* Chapter 6).
Danger signs (those appropriate to gestational age [see Table 3-4]): Examples for early gestation include vaginal bleeding with or without pain, abdominal cramps, headaches with or without visual problems, evidence of rupture of membranes.	Identification of signs frequently associated with pregnancy at risk.
Psychological status and learning needs: Satisfaction with pregnancy; knowledge about pregnancy, nutrition, labor and delivery, and infant care.	Base line for preparation of nursing care plan.

private area so that the client will feel free to provide information that is frequently considered personal. The nurse should face the client, sit at the same level with her, and maintain eye contact. The nurse should remember that the client will be more likely to give complete and accurate information if open-ended questions are asked. The nurse should also be sensitive to cues that the client has more to say if given the encouragement to do so. The nurse should have sufficient time to obtain all of the information. The nurse should not act rushed. Finally, the nurse should be able to ask questions in language and terminology that the client is able to understand.

In different settings and in different types of nursing practice, the role of the nurse will include varying amounts of responsibility for assessment in each of the areas listed in Table 3-1. It is most important that health team members work together to achieve a total assessment.

Physical examination

At the initial visit, a physical examination is essential in order to completely evaluate the client's health status. The medical provider should perform a thorough evaluation, giving particular attention to vital signs; signs and symptoms of nutritional deficiency; and the examinations of the thyroid, heart, lung, breast, abdomen, extremities, and pelvis. (Table 2-1 lists the presumptive, probable, and positive signs of pregnancy.) Clients may be apprehensive at the prospect of the examination — particularly the pelvic examination. The nurse is usually responsible for preparing the client, having her undress, providing for privacy, and draping her (as the client desires) to prevent unnecessary exposure and chilling. Preparation for the pelvic examination includes the following nursing actions:

1. Make sure the client empties her bladder, if necessary, before the examination.
2. Explain all steps of the procedure to the client beforehand, taking care not to heighten her anxiety while doing so.
3. Show the client the vaginal speculum and explain how it works.
4. Explain the sensations that the client will experience during each portion of the examination. Ask her to tell you when she is experiencing pain or discomfort. Every effort should be made to prevent a hurried examination.
5. Teach the client techniques for relaxation, which may make the examination less uncomfortable (e.g., deep breathing, trying to relax the abdomen, and relaxing the muscles of the thighs to let the legs fall apart).
6. Make sure that the client is warm, comfortable, and free from

excessive distracting stimuli, with a pillow under her head and the stirrups at a comfortable position.

7. Provide encouragement and praise as each portion of the examination is completed. Clients should be helped to avoid feelings that they are "failing" the examination.

Clinical evaluation of the fetus

Abdominal and bimanual palpation (*see* Chapter 1) are always performed on an initial visit. The following list includes reasons for performing these examinations:

1. To evaluate the walls of the uterus for tone and surface characteristics.
2. To identify lie, presentation, position, and descent of the fetus.
3. To identify deviations from the norm that may indicate multiple gestation or pathology (e.g., pelvic tumor, inadequate pelvis, or abnormal fetus).
4. To estimate the size of the uterus and fetus in order to verify the estimated date of confinement that was determined from the history of the last normal menstrual period.

Estimation of fundal height and fetal size. The growth rate of the fetus is the single most important parameter used in evaluating fetal well-being. In the clinical situation, it is most common to measure the height of the uterine fundus as an indicator of fetal size. Practically speaking, this is all that can be measured outside the laboratory in early pregnancy. In late pregnancy, when the fetus can be easily felt, the height of the fundus is still used except when it clearly does not represent fetal size. Examples of situations in which fundal height does not correlate with fetal size include **hydramnios**, when fluid is responsible for unusual uterine distention, and **transverse lie**, when the true size of the fetus is not reflected by a longitudinal measurement. (Chapter 1 discusses in detail the various techniques of measurement.)

Fetal heart tones. The fetal heart rate is an important parameter of fetal health. It becomes audible by means of a stethoscope or fetoscope at approximately the 20th week of gestation. The date at which it is first heard is used in some clinics to validate gestational age. The fetal heart is best heard over the fetal back and is usually heard higher on the maternal abdomen than is usual during the intrapartum period. The normal range is 120 to 160 beats/min. Bradycardia or tachycardia indicates fetal distress and requires notification of the physician.

Fetal movements. The client should be asked to document the date of quickening, and she should be reminded at visits in the beginning of the second trimester of its importance. This date is used to validate gestational age. After quickening, daily fetal movement is an indicator of fetal health. The physician should be notified if the client reports a markedly lower frequency or a cessation of movement (*see* Chapter 7).

Laboratory studies

The laboratory tests that are considered routine vary somewhat from setting to setting. Table 3-2 lists a typical set of laboratory tests. (The reader is referred to Appendix B for normal values.)

Extra tests are often ordered at the initial visit. The rationale for more extensive testing may include identification or evaluation of a high-risk pregnancy (*see* Chapter 8), institutional protocols, or data collection for research studies. Examples of some of these extra laboratory tests are listed in Table 3-3.

SUBSEQUENT PRENATAL VISITS

At the initial visit, the client should be encouraged to return for subsequent prenatal visits. The frequency of prenatal revisits will depend on the health status of the client and her fetus. In a normal pregnancy, the client will be asked to return at least once a month during the first two trimesters, every 2 weeks until the 36th week of gestation, and every week thereafter. Clients who are at high risk (*see* Chapter 8) may be asked to return more frequently for adequate assessment, treatment, and evaluation.

At each revisit, the client should again be assessed by means of direct and indirect questions regarding her physical and mental status, with particular attention being paid to the interval since her last visit. In addition to questions about her general physical and psychosocial status, specific questions should be asked about her nutritional status and her preparations for the labor and delivery and the newborn. In addition, descriptions should be given about the common discomforts and danger signs of pregnancy (*see* Chapter 6).

Appropriate portions of the physical examination should be performed. Blood pressure, weight, and uterine growth should be assessed on every visit. After the 20th week of gestation, Leopold's maneuvers and fetal heart rate auscultation should be performed, and the client's hands, face, and lower legs should be checked for edema. Other portions of the physical examination will be determined by the client's history (e.g., assessment of costovertebral angle tenderness and deep tendon reflexes).

Laboratory tests should be performed as indicated. On every visit, urine should be checked for the presence of protein and glucose. The

TABLE 3-2
*Routine Screening Tests**

Test	Rationale
Papanicolaou (Pap) smear	Screen for cancer of the cervix and cervicitis.
Gonorrhea culture	Detect gonorrhea so that it can be treated and so that neonatal blindness can be prevented.
Tuberculin (tine) test or chest x-ray	Detect tuberculosis, which is medically hazardous to the client and to her baby after delivery.
Complete blood count	Identify anemia and screen for infection.
ABO blood type	Predict possible later ABO incompatibility and obtain type for possible transfusion in obstetric emergency.
Rh factor (and indirect Coombs's test if Rh-negative)	Identify fetus at risk for Rh incompatibility.
Serologic test for syphilis	Detect syphilis so that the client can be treated, thus preventing syphilitic congenital anomalies and neonatal infection.
Rubella titer	Identify the rubella-susceptible client and obtain a base-line titer for comparison if client is suspected of having contracted the disease.
Sickle cell prep‡	Screen for sickle cell trait.
Urinalysis	Screen for kidney disease, hypertensive disease, diabetes, and urinary tract infection.

*See Table 3-3 for a list of extra screening tests.
‡Hemoglobin electrophoresis is necessary to provide definite results if preparation is positive, or to screen for other hemoglobinopathies.

TABLE 3-3
Extra Screening Tests

Test	Rationale
Two-hour post-prandial urine and blood (or plasma) glucose test	Screen for diabetes. Pregnancy is diabetogenic. Medical and obstetric risks are increased if diabetes is present.
Ultrasonogram	Date pregnancy precisely when history makes expected date of confinement unclear or when premature delivery is likely. Identify fetal, placental, or uterine abnormalities.
Amniocentesis	Screen for Down's syndrome or other inherited genetic disorders.
Beta-hemolytic streptococcus vaginal culture	Identify fetus at risk for neonatal sepsis.
Urine culture	Screen for urinary tract infection or identify causative organisms for treatment of urinary tract infection.

hematocrit level should be checked periodically, the frequency depending upon previous results. Some tests — such as gonorrhea culture, serologic test for syphilis, and fasting blood sugars — may be performed routinely during revisits in some settings, and only upon indication in others. Table 3-4 lists the components of subsequent prenatal visits.

THE NURSING CARE PLAN

In the ambulatory setting, the nurse must act as teacher, counselor, and client advocate. The nurse's concern is with the whole person. Clinic settings vary widely in the extent to which they make use of the special abilities of the nurse. Nurses have a responsibility to organize the delivery of prenatal care in such a way that clients can efficiently use the entire range of services provided by the particular setting.

Obviously, if the nurse assumes a primary nurse role in the prenatal outpatient setting, he or she will have more data about the

TABLE 3-4
Components of Subsequent Prenatal Visits

Component	Rationale
History General.	
Any client questions, concerns, or problems since last visit.	Identification of client needs and priorities for health care.
Follow-up on any plan agreed on by client and nurse at previous visits.	Evaluation of previous care.
Fetal status.	
Fetal movement.	Indication of fetal well-being (after 20th week of gestation).
Common complaints.	Identification of client's specific complaints. (*See* Chapter 6 for physiological basis and nursing actions.)
Danger signs.	
Vaginal bleeding.	Possible indication of nidation bleeding, threatened abortion, premature labor, placenta previa, abruptio placentae. May also be related to friable cervix of pregnancy, cervicitis, or loss of mucous plug before labor.

Headaches, edema, visual disturbances, and/or epigastric pain.	Signs of preeclampsia. May also be due to more benign causes (e.g., indigestion, tension headaches, excessive standing, or need for eyeglasses).
Leg pain.	Possible sign of thromboembolic process.
Fever and/or chills.	Signs of infection, especially pyelonephritis.
Leakage of fluid.	Symptom of rupture of membranes, possible vaginitis, normal leukorrhea of pregnancy, or stress incontinence.
Abdominal pain.	Possible sign of ectopic pregnancy, threatened abortion, premature labor, abruptio placentae, or medical pathology such as appendicitis. May also be due to round ligament pain or Braxton Hicks's contractions.
Physical examination Blood pressure.	Screening for preeclampsia or hypertension.
Weight.	Assessment of nutritional status. Weight is also a measure of the amount of edema present.
Inspection and palpation of ankles, lower legs, hands, and face for edema.	Edema may be a sign of preeclampsia or physiological edema.
Fetal heart rate.	Assessment of fetal well-being. (Normal range: 120-160 beats/min with regular rhythm.)

Component	Rationale
Abdominal palpation: lie, presentation, position, descent, measurement of fundal height, and estimation of fetal weight.	Evaluation of gestational age and identification of fetal or uterine abnormalities.
Vaginal examination	Performed on indication for evaluation of vaginal discharge, rupture of membranes, labor status, or for performance of laboratory tests.
Laboratory tests	
Urine dipstick for protein, glucose, and acetone levels (every visit).	Screening for preeclampsia, urinary tract infection, diabetes, and metabolic problems leading to acidosis.
Gonorrhea culture (usually repeated at 34-36 weeks).	Diagnosis of gonorrhea for treatment before delivery to prevent gonorrheal ophthalmia neonatorum.
Hemoglobin/hematocrit (usually repeated in the 3rd trimester).	Evaluation of hematologic status.
Serologic test for syphilis (may be repeated in the 3rd trimester).	Diagnosis of syphilis for treatment before delivery.
Other laboratory work on indication.	Diagnosis, assessment, and evaluation of health needs.

client and a closer working relationship with her than any other member of the health care team. In most prenatal outpatient settings, nurses are able to work toward a meaningful relationship with the client in order to formulate and carry out a comprehensive nursing care plan.

The nurse must provide education for the client based on principles of the teaching-learning process. In some instances it may be appropriate to work with the client on a one-to-one basis, whereas at other times it will be appropriate to include her family members or a group of expectant mothers. It is important in all teaching situations to find out what the client knows in order to teach appropriate information at the right level. Because learning is facilitated by the involvement of several senses, the use of audiovisual aids, models, or demonstrations will probably increase learning. Appropriate literature may be suggested or provided to reinforce learning at a later time. Teaching should proceed from the basic to the complex, from the general to the specific. Learning is enhanced by repetition, but is hindered by the inclusion of too much information at one time or by the provision of facts without an organized structure. At the end of a teaching session, important points may be reviewed in order to reinforce learning through repetition. The client may be asked to provide feedback about the information presented in order to evaluate whether she learned from the session.

Pregnancy and birth provide a unique opportunity for nurses to exercise their professional talents. Families who are having babies have an extraordinary need for teaching, counseling, and support. Healthy families are often unaware of some of the basic processes of pregnancy and birth, and of the special attention that must be paid to maternal nutrition and to other daily activities during the pregnancy. They are also experiencing a major psychological life adjustment — acceptance of a new member into the family group — which will necessitate role adjustments by all members (*see* Chapter 4). High-risk families are even more in need of this assistance, and of assistance in adapting to the risk or stress of illness.

Table 3-5 outlines a basic plan of prenatal nursing care. All aspects of care will not be appropriate to the roles of all nurses in all settings. However, it is the responsibility of the nurse in each setting to see that the needs of the family are addressed. This sample basic plan is intended to be adapted to the needs of the client, the setting, and the capabilities and professional philosophy of the nurse.

TABLE 3-5

Prenatal Teaching and Counseling Guide*

Trimester	Needs/problems	Data Base	Teaching/counseling needs
First (up to 12 wk) (Initial visit)	Nursing care plan (general anticipatory guidance)	Review historical and current data obtained from nursing data sheet and the interview. Review chart and confer with physician. Derive nursing needs from complete assessment.	Explain findings of history and physical examination, including expected date of confinement. Explain functioning of the clinic as it affects client, anticipated schedule of visits, and routine procedures. Explain other resources available through the clinic (e.g., social service, prenatal classes, and/or WIC). Encourage father of baby to attend the clinic, if possible. Teach about, and prepare for, routine and special laboratory tests and procedures. Develop a comprehensive health care plan in conjunction with the client. Teach method and rationale for taking prescribed iron, vitamins, and any other medications. Provide anticipatory guidance regarding any deviations from the norm. Teach danger signals of preg-

		nancy: bleeding, cramps, fever, or other illness (see Table 3-4 and Fig. 3-1). Provide information about where to report if these signs or other problems develop between clinic visits.
Nutrition	Elicit diet history, including psychological and cultural factors that influence diet (see Chapter 5). Elicit client knowledge of sound nutritional principles and practice in pregnancy. Devise plan for meeting client's nutritional learning needs.	Teach client about increased nutritional requirements during pregnancy, especially the need for extra protein and calories. Help client develop a plan for meeting her nutritional needs. Provide anticipatory guidance about expected weight gain during pregnancy. Reinforce importance of taking iron and vitamins as prescribed. Provide nutritional guidance regarding variations in dietary patterns (e.g., pica, vegetarianism, etc.).
Common complaints (e.g., nausea, vomiting, fatigue, and urinary frequency)	Elicit data from chart and through careful client interview in order to determine presence and severity of symptom.	Explain the physiological basis and teach relief measures for specific complaints (see Chapter 6). Reassure client that these symptoms usually disappear by the 2nd trimester.

Trimester	Needs/problems	Data Base	Teaching/counseling needs
			Advise client to return to the clinic if symptoms worsen, or if fever or other signs of illness appear.
	Personal health and hygiene: 1. Use of drugs, alcohol, and/or cigarettes	Review with client her health and hygiene habits. Develop a plan for teaching the client additional self-care measures to be used during pregnancy.	1. Provide information about fetal hazards of drug use, and provide support to assist client to eliminate or decrease smoking, alcohol intake, and/or drug use (including over-the-counter drugs).
	2. Dental care		2. Teach toothbrushing and oral hygiene measures as necessary. Teach importance of dental care during pregnancy.
	3. Breast care		3. Explain the physiological basis of breast tenderness. Encourage the use of a well-fitting, supportive bra with wide, nonelastic straps.
	4. Activity/exercise		4. Explain the physiological basis for fatigue in the 1st trimester. Encourage adequate amounts of rest, including short periods of rest throughout the day. Reassure the client that she

may continue those activities and exercises that she was doing before the pregnancy, but advise her to stop if she gets tired. Advise her to check with her physician before engaging in strenuous sports such as skiing, diving, and horseback riding.

5. Employment

5. Determine with the client the possibility of exposure to fetotoxic substances in the work environment (e.g., x-rays or lead). Encourage her to stop working or seek transfer if exposed to such substances. Discuss the advantages and disadvantages of continuing to work during pregnancy (e.g., fatigue and inadequate daily rest periods vs. needed income and career opportunities).

6. Hygiene

6. Discuss the importance of daily bathing in relation to the normal increase in perspiration and leukorrhea. Reassure her that tub bathing is not harmful during pregnancy (although rubber mats or hand grips may be necessary late in pregnancy

Trimester	Needs/problems	Data Base	Teaching/counseling needs
			when her balance is altered). Reinforce that douching is contraindicated during pregnancy.
	7. Sex		7. Reassure client that changes in sexual desire are normal during pregnancy (see Chapter 4).
	8. Immunizations		8. Review risks and benefits of receiving specific immunizations during pregnancy (see Table 3-6).
	Psychological and emotional needs	Through interview, elicit each individual's psychological adjustment and coping styles, as well as common psychological changes specific to pregnancy.	Establish working rapport at initial visit. Provide atmosphere of privacy and trust to facilitate ongoing dialogue. Identify psychological and emotional needs and adequacy of family functioning. Provide anticipatory guidance concerning ambivalent feelings about the pregnancy and baby that are common in early pregnancy (see Chapter 4).
Second (13-27 wk)	Nursing care plan	Continue revision of nursing care plan according to medical needs of client. Review chart at each visit. Ongoing evaluation by client and nurse re-	Provide ongoing teaching, counseling, and coordination of services to support attainment of client's health care goals.

	garding her care and needs should lead to updating and revising of the plan.	
Nutrition	Continue evaluation of nutritional status, including weight gain, hemoglobin and hematocrit levels, dietary pattern, and pica.	Reinforce good nutritional practices. When nausea and vomiting subside, many women develop very hearty appetites.
Growth and development of fetus	Assess fetal growth, fetal heart tones, and fetal movement. Reassess client's perception of pregnancy. With quickening, the client's interest in her pregnancy and her desire to learn about the baby are heightened.	Teach about the growth and development of the fetus. Allow client to hear fetal heart beat and assist her to identify fetal parts by palpation. Discuss plans for childbirth education classes with client. Discuss plans for infant feeding with client. Provide literature as appropriate.
Common complaints (e.g., backache, constipation, round ligament pain, and varicosities)	Continue to question client about common complaints of pregnancy. Usually, clients will have very few complaints at this time. The 2nd trimester is characterized by feelings of well-being in a normal pregnancy.	Explain the physiological basis for her complaints. Teach specific relief measures for her complaints (see Chapter 6).
Personal health and hygiene:	Continue to evaluate personal health and hygiene needs of client through history and physical examination.	

Trimester	Needs/problems	Data Base	Teaching/counseling needs
	1. Clothing		1. a. Encourage client to wear comfortable, non-constricting clothing. Reinforce the fact that tight bands around legs or waist interfere with venous return. b. Encourage client to wear a well-fitting, supportive bra. c. Teach client to wear low-heeled shoes to minimize strain on the lower back and to avoid problems with maintaining balance. d. Encourage clients with varicose veins to wear support hose.
	2. Body mechanics		2. Teach client the pelvic rock exercises (Fig. 3-2) and to use proper body mechanics (Fig. 3-3).
	3. Sex		3. Encourage couple to discuss their sexual needs. Provide information as needed about alternative positions for intercourse and alternatives to vaginal intercourse (Fig. 3-4). Discuss normal

	4. Plans for contraception		changes in libido during pregnancy (see Chapter 4). 4. Discuss plans for future contraception, including tubal ligation.
	Psychological and emotional needs	Evaluate individual's psychological adjustments and coping techniques. (This is a time of great psychological change.) During this trimester, quickening occurs and the pregnancy becomes obvious to all who see the client. The client must come to grips with her anticipated new role.	Provide supportive atmosphere and opportunities to express feelings. Provide anticipatory guidance regarding changing roles and relationships during pregnancy, especially with her husband/partner and her mother. Reassure client that fantasies, dreams, and nightmares are normal during pregnancy.
Third (28-40 wk)	Nursing care plan	Continue revision of nursing care plan as medical needs change. Review chart at every visit. Ongoing evaluation by client and nurse regarding her care and needs should lead to updating and revising of the plan.	Provide teaching and anticipatory guidance about client's health care needs. Explain to client that she should expect increased maternal anxiety about the baby. Explain laboratory tests and procedures used in 3rd trimester as evaluation of the fetus intensifies. Review danger signs (e.g., bleeding, rupture of membranes, severe headaches, and signs of premature labor).

Trimester	Needs/problems	Data Base	Teaching/counseling needs
	Nutrition	Continue evaluation of nutritional status, including weight gain, hemoglobin and hematocrit levels, and dietary pattern.	Reinforce good nutritional habits. (Eating habits vary widely in the 3rd trimester: many women eat less because of crowding of the stomach and heartburn or to avoid becoming "fat," whereas others eat heartily.)
	Growth and development of fetus	Continue to assess fetal growth, estimated weight, fetal heart tones, and fetal movement.	Provide anticipatory guidance about fetal growth and development. Assist client to complete plans for care of baby, equipment, method of feeding, etc.
	Maternal expectations and preparations regarding labor and delivery	Determine the client's current knowledge, expectations, and anxiety regarding labor and delivery.	Encourage participation in childbirth classes (which usually begin at about the 32nd wk). Review signs and symptoms of labor; signs of true vs. false labor; timing of contractions; when to come to the hospital; what to bring to the hospital; permission, if necessary, for father to stay in labor and delivery room; and sibling visitation. Encourage hospital tour.

Common complaints (e.g., backache, Braxton Hicks's contractions, heartburn, constipation, flatulence, hemorrhoids, urinary frequency, pedal and hand edema, dyspnea, round ligament pain, leg cramps, and insomnia)

Continue to question client about common complaints of pregnancy. The many complaints of this trimester are chiefly due to the increasing size of the fetus.

If client does not attend childbirth classes, teach basics of usual course of labor; routine hospital procedures; maternal breathing, relaxation, and pain-relief techniques for labor and delivery; and events occurring in the delivery room concerning the mother, father, and baby.

Provide knowledgeable reinforcement of learning for parents who attend classes.

Review provision of care for other children, including plans for dealing with sibling rivalry.

Explain the physiological basis for her complaints and teach relief measures specific for her complaints (see Chapter 6).

Follow-up is important because, often, alternative measures must be tried before there is relief.

Provide the counseling and support needed to sustain the client through the increasing discomfort of the last weeks of pregnancy.

Anticipate the desire for early delivery, and distress if expected date of confinement is passed without delivery.

Trimester	Needs/problems	Data Base	Teaching/counseling needs
	Personal health and hygiene:	Continue to evaluate personal health and hygiene needs of client.	Reinforce earlier hygiene teaching.
	1. Preparation of the breasts for breast-feeding		1. a. Discuss techniques of breast preparation, including nipple-rolling and -toughening exercises and manual expression of milk (see Chapter 22).
			b. Encourage use of well-fitting, supportive bra.
	2. Activity and rest		2. a. Encourage client to avoid hazardous sports. Although the fetus is well protected, the client's coordination may be impaired.
			b. Discuss plans for termination and post-partum resumption of employment.
			c. Encourage frequent rest periods (lying on the left side during the day). This is especially important if edema, hypertension, or varicose veins are present.

3. Positions of comfort

3. Encourage left lateral or Sims's position (instead of supine) for rest. Pillows placed to support legs, arms, and back may increase comfort.

4. Sex

4. Encourage couple to discuss their sexual needs. Explore alternative positions for intercourse (see Fig. 3-4) and alternatives to intercourse. Reinforce that vaginal intercourse is contraindicated only in the presence of obstetric complications, such as bleeding, ruptured membranes, and threatened premature labor. Discuss the normal changes in libido (see Chapter 4).

5. Travel

5. a. Reinforce that travel during pregnancy is permissible; however, as term approaches, distant travel is discouraged so that the client does not commence labor far away from her home and care providers.
  b. Teach client to use seat

Trimester	Needs/problems	Data Base	Teaching/counseling needs
			belts positioned low (over the symphysis pubis). c. Discuss the need for frequent rest stops while traveling to prevent venous stasis in the lower extremities and to allow for emptying of the bladder.
	Psychological and emotional needs	Through interview, evaluate the individual's psychological adjustment and coping techniques. Assess development of maternal-fetal attachment (*see* Chapter 14).	Provide supportive atmosphere and opportunities to express feelings.

WIC, supplemental food program for women, infants, and children.
*This guide is intended to be adapted to the needs of the client, the setting, and the capabilities and professional philosophy of the nurse.

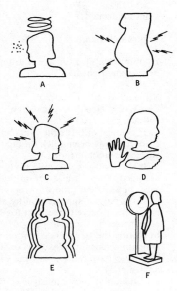

Figure 3-1.   Danger signs during pregnancy. (A) Dizziness, spots, or blurred vision; (B) stomach, back, or leg pains; (C) headaches; (D) edema of the hands, face, or feet; (E) sudden chills or fever; and (F) sudden weight gain. In addition, bleeding, discharge, or a sudden gush or steady leak of water from the vagina; daily vomiting; and/or small amounts of urine or burning on urination may indicate fetal or maternal complications.

TABLE 3-6

Immunizations during Pregnancy

Immunization	Comments
Tetanus-diphtheria	Administer if no primary booster or no booster within 10 years.
Mumps	Contraindicated.
Rubella	Contraindicated.
Influenza	Administer if client is at risk (same as for nonpregnant client).
Rabies	Same as for other persons. The World Health Organization recommends the following: 1. If contact with the rabid animal is indirect or if there has only been a lick on unabraided skin, no vaccine is recommended. 2. If the exposure was mild (only a lick on abraided skin or a bite *not* on the head, neck, face, or arm) the following apply: a. If the animal appears healthy at the time of exposure, observe the animal for 10 days. Do not administer the vaccine. b. During the 10-day observation period, if the animal is clinically suspicious or if the animal is proven to have rabies, start the vaccine immediately. c. If the animal has any signs of the disease at the time of the exposure, start the vaccine. Observe the animal and if no clinical or laboratory proof of disease is shown by the 5th day, discontinue the vaccine. If the animal is rabid, wild, dead, or if the status is unknown, administer a complete course of the vaccine. d. If there are multiple bites or any bites on the head, neck, face, or arm, the recommendations are the same as in number 2. (N. B. Some individuals may benefit from preexposure immunization in the postpartum period — veterinarians, metermaids, mail-carriers, laboratory personnel working with the virus, pet store or kennel personnel, etc.)

Immunization	Comments
Smallpox	Not necessary.
Hepatitis A	If exposed, or before travel in a high-risk area.
Yellow fever	Before travel in a high-risk area.
Cholera	Only if necessary to meet international travel requirements.

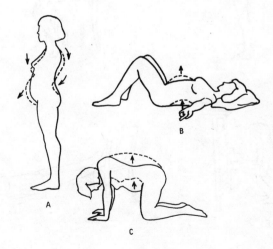

Figure 3-2. The pelvic rock exercises. (A) Standing position, (B) supine position, and (C) hands-and-knees position.

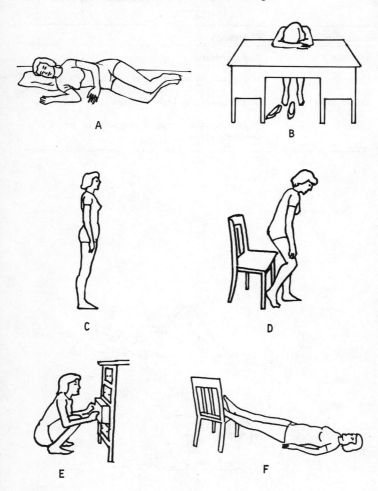

Figure 3-3. Proper body mechanics during pregnancy. (A) Turning on side before getting up from a supine position. (B) Relaxing at a desk with all muscles loose. (C) Erect posture with good head, neck, spine, hip, and leg alignment. (D) Using leg muscles to lower body into a chair. (E) Squatting — not bending — to reach low objects. (F) Resting with feet elevated to aid venous return.

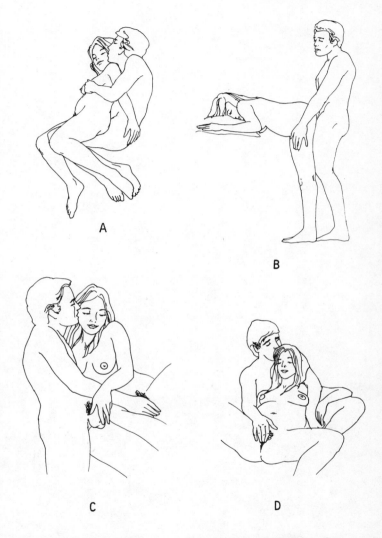

Figure 3-4. Alternative positions for, and alternatives to, sexual intercourse during pregnancy. (A) Side-lying and (B) rear entry positions. (C and D) Mutual masturbation as an alternative to sexual intercourse.

CHAPTER 4

EMOTIONAL CHANGES DURING PREGNANCY

Nancy J. Burton

Many social and emotional changes occur during the childbearing year that affect a pregnant woman and her family. The obstetric health care provider must be aware of these changes in order to provide counseling, support, and health education. The practitioner must be able to recognize emotional reactions that are within a normal range in order to reassure a patient and assist in a healthy adjustment to pregnancy. In addition, the practitioner must be able to detect reactions that deviate from the norm and that may require intervention. The purpose of this chapter is to acquaint the reader with expected changes that occur during pregnancy, with signals that may suggest a poor adaptation to pregnancy, and with methods of offering counseling and support.

FACTORS CONTRIBUTING TO EMOTIONAL CHANGES IN PREGNANCY

Many factors — physical, psychological, social, and cultural — can contribute to a woman's reaction and adjustment to pregnancy. Physiologically, many metabolic and endocrine changes occur in pregnancy (such as increased levels of ovarian hormones) that can affect a woman's emotional state. Bodily changes occur at various points in pregnancy and can affect a woman's mood and self-image. In addition, changes occur in the dynamics of her relationships with her partner and other people significant to her.

Social and cultural factors influence a woman's attitude toward her pregnancy. Whether or not the pregnancy was planned and/or desired, cultural background, age, career/work orientation, marital status, and the attitude of the woman's partner toward the pregnancy can all be contributing factors in the woman's adjustment to pregnancy. A woman's psychological state before pregnancy will also be of great importance in her adaptation to pregnancy and motherhood. Finally, a woman's role in life undergoes an adjustment, particularly with a first pregnancy, to allow for the role of motherhood.

FIRST TRIMESTER

Physical changes

For many women the initial physical symptoms of pregnancy can be unpleasant. Some of the earliest symptoms — nausea and vomiting, fatigue, and breast tenderness — can make a woman feel uncomfortable, ill, and depressed. It is important for the obstetrics practitioner to offer reassurance regarding the transient nature of these symptoms and to suggest comfort measures to help the client deal with the symptoms while they persist.

Ambivalence

A large majority of women experience some feelings of ambivalence when they learn of their pregnancy.[1-4] This ambivalence occurs even when a pregnancy is planned and strongly desired. The inconveniences and changes that will be brought about by a new baby almost universally cause women to pause and reconsider whether pregnancy at this particular time is desired. Ambivalence at the earlier stages of pregnancy should not be cause for alarm to either the woman or the practitioner. However, a woman who demonstrates a great deal of ambivalence or negative feelings toward the pregnancy should be observed for attitude later on. By midpregnancy, near the time of "quickening" (see below), most women have resolved their feelings of ambivalence and accepted the fact that they are having a baby. Ambivalence that continues beyond midpregnancy may be suggestive of potential problems in a woman's ability to mother her new baby. Obstetric and pediatric personnel should screen for indications of such problems.

Estrangement and introversion

If a woman does not have significant symptoms of early pregnancy, the pregnancy may seem unreal and she may forget for short periods of time that she is pregnant. Because there are not yet any outward signs of pregnancy, a woman may feel somewhat estranged from others and introverted. The initial hearing of the fetal heart beat (at 11 to 13 weeks of gestation with Doppler equipment) is often a profound experience for a woman — the first event that really convinces her of her pregnancy and a time when she begins to form her first attachment with the fetus.

Emotional lability, anxiety, and dependency

Beginning early in and continuing throughout the pregnancy, women tend to be more anxious and emotionally labile. Some of this is free-floating anxiety and some is related to distinct concerns that surface at different times during the childbearing year.[5,6] Childbearing women also often feel more dependent on their husbands, family members, friends, and health professionals.

Sexuality

Many women note changes in their libido during pregnancy. Some authors report a general trend toward decreasing interest in sex as pregnancy progresses,[7] whereas others find that most women note a decrease in interest in the first trimester, a resumption of interest in the second, and a decrease again in the third.[8] Although some women report increased sexual interest during pregnancy (often because birth control is no longer a concern), these women seem to be in the minority. The fatigue, nausea and vomiting, and endocrine changes probably all contribute to the decrease in libido that most women experience in the first trimester.

SECOND TRIMESTER

The second trimester has been referred to as the "happy trimester" because the unpleasant symptoms of early pregnancy have usually faded and the discomforts of late pregnancy have not yet begun.

Quickening

During the second trimester, as the pregnancy becomes visibly obvious, women first begin to feel fetal movement, which is known as "quickening." For most women this is an exciting time — a time when they can share the pregnancy with others and feel a strengthening attachment with the fetus. Couples usually begin to make concrete plans for the new baby by, for example, decorating nurseries, arranging for leaves of absence or termination of employment, and signing up for childbirth classes. (There are, however, cultural differences. For example, some cultures feel that activities such as setting up a nursery before the birth of the baby will bring bad luck.) Furthermore, couples begin to think seriously about parenting and how they want to raise their child.

Body image

In the past, pregnant women were thought of as unclean, and, in some cultures, they still are. Not too many generations ago it was considered improper for an obviously pregnant woman to be seen in public. A pregnant body is the antithesis of the ideal American female body: small hips, waist, and stomach. Body image is based on what others tell us, what we see, what we feel, and the attitude of our society. Moore found that nonpregnant women tend to rate their own appearance as less than the American ideal.[9] During pregnancy, the majority of women rate themselves as less attractive than nonpregnant women, and this rating decreases as the pregnancy progresses.

Pregnant women saw themselves as more ugly than beautiful and considered their bodies as more annoying than pleasing and more dirty than clean. They also viewed themselves as fatter, older, and slower than nonpregnant women. The increased perspiration and vaginal secretions and the decreased heat tolerance may contribute to the feeling of being dirty.[9] Despite all of these factors, there are many women who do enjoy looking pregnant and are proud of their protruding abdomen.

A woman may fluctuate between bliss and resentment or distress at her bodily changes.[10] Many factors may influence a woman's reaction to her body. Perhaps the most important is the reaction of her husband or male partner. Her degree of maturity, her comfort with her bodily functions, the importance that physical appearance has played in her life, and the degree of discomfort experienced are all factors that will affect how she feels about her changing body. A woman may also express concerns over the effect the pregnancy will have on her body and worry about sagging breasts, stretch marks, flabby abdomen, and slack vaginal muscles.[9]

Women often feel their bodies are no longer theirs and that they have been invaded by another being. At times they may feel estranged from their bodies and feel that they are nothing but vessels for their babies.[11] The frequent admonitions from family, friends, and health professionals to assume numerous responsibilities for the benefit of the baby reinforce this feeling. At other times, however, women feel joy at this close connection with their baby and maintain a two-way conversation between their baby and the rest of the world.[12]

Emotional lability and anxiety

Emotional lability and anxiety continue through the second trimester. Most women and their families are able to deal with these changes; indeed, they are often expected in pregnant women. Women also often begin to worry during this period about the health and normalness of the developing baby. Women vary in how much they worry about an abnormal baby. Some factors that may affect this are a personal or family history of abnormal children; an experience by friends or acquaintances with the birth (especially recent) of an abnormal infant; exposure to drugs, radiation, or environmental or occupational substances before or during pregnancy; stories told or warnings given by friends, acquaintances, or, occasionally, total strangers; and the number of previous pregnancies.

Fantasies and dreams

Pregnant women are prone to bizarre dreams and fantasies, which can begin in the first trimester and become quite vivid after quickening.[13,14] Many of the dreams and fantasies may center on the baby. For example, a woman may dream of delivering a monstrous baby or of carrying an animal.

Although women are usually able to deal with these fantasies, they do express relief when they learn that such fantasies are quite normal.

Sexuality

A couple's sexual activity and satisfaction can vary greatly during this time. Early in the second trimester some women are relieved to be feeling better, as the unpleasant symptoms of early pregnancy decrease, and find they have a renewed interest in sex. As the pregnancy progresses and the presence of the baby becomes obvious to both partners, either partner may become emotionally uncomfortable with sexual activity. One or both partners may be afraid of hurting the baby or may feel uncomfortable with the idea of sexual intercourse with the fetus so close. A man may be afraid to hurt his partner or to make too many demands on her and, therefore, refrain from initiating sexual activity. If the couple has not been able to communicate openly, the woman may interpret this apparent lack of interest as an indication that she is no longer attractive to her husband.

Some women find they are not very interested in sex throughout their pregnancy. Hormonal and other physical changes, the sex life before pregnancy, the ability of the couple to communicate openly, cultural background, and family teaching probably all play some part in the effect of pregnancy on a woman's libido. The woman's intellectual knowledge regarding this subject and her emotional reactions do not always coincide. If a pregnant woman achieves orgasm she will experience uterine contractions. Women need to be reassured that this is not harmful to the fetus.

THIRD TRIMESTER

During the third trimester, especially in the last month or two, the pregnancy may cause varying degrees of physical discomfort and difficulty with ambulation. Women often complain of feeling extremely bulky and state that their abdomen could not possibly stretch any further without bursting. The pregnant woman may again experience nausea, fatigue, and urinary frequency, and fetal movement may now be painful. Usually, women can physically cope with these changes; however, the changes often have some effect on their emotional outlook. Emotional lability continues to be a problem for many women, and it is not unusual for a woman to feel depressed at times during the final weeks of pregnancy as she waits impatiently for labor to begin.

Focus on labor and delivery

The focus of women's attention now becomes labor and delivery. Anxiety levels may be quite high, with fear of pain, physical damage, and an abnormal baby being the most prominent causes. Fantasies and dreams about death, mutilation, and monstrous infants are quite common.[5,15-17] Women also have strong fears regarding their performance. They often feel that they will "not do well" in labor. This is especially true since the advent of childbirth classes and prepared childbirth. Some women have come to feel that any use of medication and any loss of control will be a failure, and, therefore, they are very worried they will "fail."

Approximately 4 to 6 weeks before the expected due date, a woman often experiences a crisis: a failure of nerve. This is usually focused on labor and delivery, but may also be exhibited as a concern that she will not be a "good enough" mother. As the reality of the impending labor and birth dawns on the woman, she may feel that she had been overconfident. This crisis usually passes fairly quickly, and resolution is often aided by a gift or an evening out.[18]

Overprotective of the fetus

Women tend to become quite protective of their unborn child, and may be unusually anxious about safety in everyday situations. For example, a woman who has previously been comfortable with her husband's driving habits, may find herself finding fault with his driving ability and frequently expecting accidents to occur. If a woman is suddenly frightened, her first instinct may be to curl in such a position that would protect the fetus in her abdomen. It is not surprising that such instinctual actions begin before the birth of a child, because it is well known that mothers of all species are very protective of their young.

Finalization of plans

At this point, plans are finalized for labor and the introduction of the baby into the home and family unit. Nursery equipment is set up, baby-sitters for other children are arranged, ways of contacting the father or other support people when labor begins and transportation to the place where the birth will occur are all agreed upon. A woman may begin to wonder if she will ever have time alone with her husband or other children again.

ROLE CHANGE

Reva Rubin has described the steps that a woman goes through in adopting the role of "mother."[3] This is a continuous process but not a passive one. Women observe other women caring for their children. A pregnant woman will mimic those actions and begin to fantasize about how she will interact with her own child. Rubin describes a process of introjection, projection, and rejection, during which a woman takes in the actions of mothers and role of motherhood, projects herself into the situations she observes, then rejects those actions and attitudes that are incompatible with her own ideas of motherhood. Women vary greatly in their notions of which roles are compatible with motherhood. A woman will examine her professional and social life to decide how they will need to be altered to allow for the new role of mother. Individual and cultural ideas of womanhood and motherhood will play an important part in how each woman resolves these issues. A woman may grieve the loss of the old roles that she must forgo. This grieving process must be worked through before a woman can adapt to motherhood. The process may not be completely resolved until after the birth of the baby.

Today, when value systems and attitudes toward womanhood are undergoing close inspection and major changes, the process of role adjustment is often more complicated than it was in the past. Signs that a woman has assumed the role of motherhood are the use of the word "I" when speaking about motherhood and, after the birth of the child, the use of the present rather than the future tense.

SECOND AND SUBSEQUENT PREGNANCIES

Women often find the second pregnancy quite different from their first. Women are often concerned about the effect a new child will have on their relationship with the first child. Specifically, they may feel some resentment toward the impending intrusion of the new baby on the relationship with the first child. Women often express concern that they will not have enough love for another child and that they will never love the new child as much as the first. Many women feel guilty about these feelings and feel that something is wrong with them. By the second half of the pregnancy, women have usually worked through these feelings to a great extent, although there may be residual concern about dealing well with two children.

Women often find second pregnancies more uncomfortable than first pregnancies because of such signs and symptoms as pelvic pressure, lower backache, Braxton Hicks's contractions, and round ligament pain. Women are busier with taking care of their young child and have less time to think about themselves and dwell on the pregnancy. It is not uncommon for women to forget they are pregnant for short periods of time. If women are not aware that this is a normal reaction, they will often experience guilt feelings about their relative lack of involvement with this pregnancy as compared with the first.

Women sometimes worry more about the normalness of the second baby than they did with the first. It may be that people feel so lucky to have one healthy child that they are afraid they will not be so lucky again.

By the third and subsequent pregnancies, women seem to approach pregnancy in a more matter-of-fact manner. Physically, pregnancies often become more uncomfortable with increasing parity, and the discomforts associated with the latter months of pregnancy manifest themselves earlier.

Many factors affect reactions to second and subsequent pregnancies. Financial matters; spacing of children; whether a pregnancy is planned; previous experiences with pregnancy and labor and delivery; health of the other children; loss of a fetus, neonate, or child; remarriage; and age are all factors that can have great influence on adjustment to these pregnancies.

SPECIAL SITUATIONS AND HIGH-RISK PREGNANCIES

Multiple pregnancies

Although some women are excited and happy by news that they are carrying twins, most are stunned and overwhelmed when they are told. Women are usually most concerned with the practical, day-to-day aspects of caring for two infants and wonder if they will be able to handle the increased demands that twins will bring. They may also express concern about whether they will be able to give the babies individual attention, relate to them as two separate people, and have enough love for two infants. If there are other children in the family, women will often worry about the adjustment of these siblings to the twins.

Women will also need to adjust their expectations for care during the latter part of pregnancy and labor and delivery. If a woman's plans for delivery are not compatible with the demands of safe care for twins, she may initially grieve the loss of the experience she had hoped for. She need not, however, lose all control of her labor experience. Every attempt should be made to honor her wishes, and she should be reassured that this will be done.

Multigestations with more than twins are indeed very special situations. As much outside help as is available must be called on and organized. Pregnant women in this situation must learn to be comfortable in accepting help that they normally would not have asked for. This may be a difficult adjustment for women who have always been moderately self-sufficient. Pregnancies such as these are truly high risk and entail much special care. They usually result in premature neonates who often require prolonged periods of hospitalization and intensive care. Accepting this fact is likely to be difficult for most women.

It is a testimony to human adaptability that, if they know early enough before delivery, most women with multigestations are able to accept that they are having more than one baby and are able to make realistic plans for this event. One of the most difficult tasks in late pregnancy for these women is maintaining the bed rest that is often advised. This is especially true if there are other children at home. A woman may feel guilty if she does not rest as much as she thinks she should and subsequently delivers prematurely or has other complications. It is important that health care personnel explore with the woman the realities of her living situation and how likely it is that she will be able to maintain bed rest. The nurse should help the woman explore what support people she can call on for help at this time. Sometimes, home health aides can be brought into the home. (Some insurance plans cover part or all of the cost.) It is important that health personnel do not unthinkingly give a woman a set of instructions that she cannot possibly follow given her living situation.

High-risk pregnancies

There are many situations that will cause a pregnancy to be high risk. In situations where a mother's health and well-being are in jeopardy, anxiety levels may be high, and the client's physical needs may be constantly being weighed against the physical needs of the fetus. A woman may be reluctant to take medications necessary to maintain her health for fear of the possible effects on the fetus. If a woman's health begins to deteriorate as a result of the pregnancy, she may feel some resentment toward the pregnancy or the fetus, find it difficult to develop positive feelings toward the fetus, and feel guilty because of these feelings.[2]

A woman with a high-risk pregnancy enters a world of complex medical technology, often at the expense of her dignity and autonomy.[19] It is not unusual for the emotional and social aspects of pregnancy to be almost forgotten by the medical personnel concerned with maintaining the health of the client and fetus. Women in situations where the most emotional support is needed often find themselves in situations where the least support is available because everyone is so concerned with the medical problems.

Many high-risk pregnancies increase the possibility of premature delivery, cesarean section, and the need for neonatal intensive care. The woman in a high-risk situation needs to adjust to and prepare for such an outcome.

Adolescents

Adolescence is a period of growth and of physical, social, and emotional change. Adolescents often feel insecure as they struggle for their identity. When pregnancy occurs during adolescence, the girl, her partner, and her family have enormous tasks ahead of them. If the girl decides to carry the pregnancy to term, she must deal not only with her own psychological growth, but also with the role of motherhood or the emotional pain of giving up her baby for adoption. If a teenage girl decides to terminate her pregnancy, she may have feelings of guilt or ambivalence and may be afraid that an abortion will interfere with her ability to bear children in the future. It is important that every pregnant adolescent (for that matter, every pregnant woman) be allowed and encouraged to discuss her feelings and concerns and that all of her questions be answered completely and honestly. In addition, the health professional should be non-judgmental.

Adolescents are, by nature, crisis-oriented, and planning for their future is often not part of their daily lives. Pregnant adolescents have been found to have lower self-esteem than their nonpregnant counterparts. They are often from broken homes and low socio-economic groups, and they do not envision much hope for their future. They are less likely to have hobbies, an interest in sports, or academic outlets of self-expression.[20] Pregnancy and a young baby may give their lives meaning. The underlying patterns of their lives, however, remain unchanged. For a short time after the baby is born, they may still receive the attention they crave. However, as the child becomes older and more autonomous, an adolescent mother may feel frustrated and confused.

Ideally, care for pregnant adolescents should be multidisciplinary and continue after the birth of the baby. In addition to physical care, supportive emotional care during pregnancy, postpartum, and the early years of the child's life, and academic and vocational counseling are all integral parts of care for this group of young people.[21]

Older couples

Being in one's mid- to late thirties or early forties brings both positive and negative aspects to the pregnancy and the adjustment to child rearing. Couples of this age are often more secure emotionally and financially, and have marriages that are fairly stable. If it is the first child for the partners, they have usually had more opportunity to fulfill various interests and desires than a younger couple. They may, therefore, be more comfortable about the restrictions that child rearing places on life-style. Because they are more financially secure, they may not be as restricted as a younger couple would be. However, as people become older, they tend to become less flexible in their life-style, and they may find the adjustment to pregnancy and child rearing difficult to integrate into well-established patterns. Depending on their general physical condition, they may not have the physical stamina to deal with the discomforts of pregnancy or to keep up with a young child.[22]

A couple in their late thirties or early forties may express concern over the fact that they will be in their fifties or sixties when their children are adolescents. They may also face some disapproval from those around them because pregnancy at this age is often not considered acceptable.

FATHERS

Although relatively little has been written about the father's feelings about, and his adjustment to, pregnancy, the subject is finally gaining more attention. Adjustment by the father may be more difficult than that of the mother in at least one way: society offers little support to a "pregnant man." Women are expected to be more emotional during pregnancy, and they are usually offered support and understanding. For a man, however, the expectation is "business as usual." Whereas women often discuss their pregnancies and share their emotional concerns with each other, most men have not been brought up to discuss these feelings as openly with each other. Therefore, they may feel isolated in dealing with the stresses of such a major event. At the same time, they are often expected to be a source of support to the pregnant woman.

Initially, most men experience ambivalence toward a pregnancy, even if the pregnancy is planned.[23] They may think of many reasons why the present is not a good time for the pregnancy to occur. A man may be distressed by the changes he sees in his partner, and, if she is having a difficult first trimester, he may experience guilt feelings for having impregnated her.[23] Some men feel isolated if their partners become introverted and passive, and they find the increased dependency of their pregnant partners disconcerting. Others feel more needed by and protective of the woman.[23,24] Men sometimes find themselves somewhat in awe of their pregnant partner and jealous of the ability to bear a child — the ability to "create." Some men work through this by increasing their interest in areas such as music, art, or hobbies.[25,26]

Finances are often a man's primary concern when a new baby is about to become part of the family. Men often feel insecure about themselves as providers.[23,24,27] Even today, when sex roles are being reexamined, men are still considered the primary breadwinners in the family. A man may find fatherhood and the accompanying financial burdens a test of his manhood. It usually takes a man longer than a woman to feel involved with a pregnancy. For the first trimester and well into the second, the pregnancy may seem unreal and he may feel detached from it. With quickening, especially when the movement can be seen and felt externally, and with the obvious growth of the uterus, men tend to become gradually more involved. At this point, the man tends to become more protective of his partner and the fetus. Men may feel some jealousy and a sense of rivalry because of the attention their wives receive. Expectant fathers are not held in high esteem and have often been figures of ridicule in our society.[28]

A man may also be jealous of his mother-in-law and of his wife's strengthening relationship with her.[29]

As the third trimester begins, men become more involved with the pregnancy. There are now concrete things for them to do. Nurseries are prepared and childbirth classes begin. Childbirth classes often play a key role in getting men actively involved in the pregnancy and in helping them deal with the fact of the imminent birth. Like their partners, men focus a great deal of their attention on labor and delivery during the third trimester. They may be fearful for the health and well-being of their partner. If they plan on being present at the birth, they may have concerns over their role as the labor "coach" and fear they will not be "able to take it."[23] There is a great deal of variety, however, among individuals and cultures. In many cultures, childbearing and labor and delivery are very much within the province of womanhood and not something in which men are expected to get actively involved.

There is evidence that men, too, often have a decrease in their libido when their partners are pregnant; however, they often do not seem troubled by this.[30] Many men fear they will hurt their partner or the fetus, especially as the fetus gets bigger. They sometimes avoid initiating sexual relations because they do not want to make demands on their partner at this time. Whereas one man may find himself attracted to the physical changes in his wife, another may not be sexually aroused by his partner's changing body. A man's intellectual knowledge about sex in pregnancy may not always coincide with his basic emotional reaction.

At some point during the first pregnancy, a man usually begins to think about himself in the role of "father." He will think about his own experience as a child with his own father. Many men experience anxiety about what kind of fathers they will be, often having no role models to look back on, because men of previous generations often did little in the way of infant care.[31] Those with a poor or nonexistent relationship with their father may be quite fearful. Some men worry about how they will relate to and care for a girl.[32] They may be concerned about how a child will affect their relationship with their wife. Again, cultural differences are important in a man's view of and adjustment to the role of father.

The "couvade syndrome" is an interesting phenomenon that has been reported frequently.[23,26,30,33,34] A large number of men experience one or more of the symptoms that their wives experience in pregnancy, such as fatigue, nausea, vomiting, backache, or stomachache. Men have been known to experience wavelike backaches or stomachaches when their partners are in labor. In some cultures, while the women are in labor, their partners go through the actions and sounds and are attended to as though they were in labor.

SIBLINGS

Siblings often have a significant adjustment to make with the impending arrival of a new child. Although there are a multitude of variables that affect this adjustment, the age of a child may be the most important. Children who can articulate well enough to express themselves and who can understand more than the most basic general concepts often have an easier time dealing with a new sibling than toddlers, whose ability to verbally communicate is still quite limited. However, even toddlers seem to sense that a change is coming, although they may not know quite what the change will be. Young children, even those who are normally fairly calm and easygoing, often become unruly and more high-strung, and they cling more to their mothers in the last few weeks of pregnancy. Apparently, they sense tension and a change of attitudes in their parents. Older children may have an easier time adjusting, although this is not always true. A child who has been an only child for several years may find it quite hard to share the attention of his parents and other relatives with a sibling. If an older child's parents have been divorced or widowed, and the new child is the product of a remarriage, the older child may feel left out or resentful.

If the birth of a sibling coincides with another major adjustment for a child, it may cause problems with acceptance. For example, a 5- or 6-year-old child going to school and experiencing frequent separation from his mother for the first time, may find accepting a new sibling more difficult. For a more outgoing, independent child, who is looking forward to kindergarten, the beginning of school may help. A prepubescent or pubescent boy or girl, who has just begun to be in touch with his/her own sexuality, may find the sexual implications of a new pregnancy discomfiting.

ROLE OF THE HEALTH PROFESSIONAL

Importance of emotional support and anticipatory guidance in antepartum care

Health professionals must, first and foremost, acknowledge the importance of making emotional support, counseling, and education an essential, integral part of all obstetric care. It must not be viewed as "the icing on the cake," the "something extra" that is done if there is time. Instead, it must be considered as important as the physical aspects of prenatal care. Several studies have indicated that maternal attitude toward a pregnancy and high levels of anxiety are related to poor obstetric and neonatal outcomes.[6,35-39] It has been suggested that a woman's emotional needs must be met in pregnancy, so that she can later meet the needs of her infant.[40]

Pregnancy, labor and delivery, and the postpartum period are times of anxiety and stress, crisis periods in a woman's life and in a family's relationship. Marriages sometimes begin to fail with the stresses of childbearing and child rearing. The incidence of psychosis is decreased during pregnancy but is much higher in the postpartum period as compared with the incidence in the general female population.[41-43] Very often, women who have severe psychological problems in the postpartum period are described as normal on antepartum records.[44]

These facts illustrate the importance of emotional care and support during pregnancy, as well as of screening for those women who are at risk for psychiatric illness and postpartum maladaptation to pregnancy and motherhood.

Components of emotional and psychological care and anticipatory guidance

The following is a list of the components of emotional and psychological care that should be provided in any antepartum setting:[45]

1. Establish a relationship.
2. Encourage verbalization.
3. Provide teaching and anticipatory guidance.
4. Offer family-centered care.
5. Mobilize sources of support (family, professional, and community).
6. Be knowledgeable about community resources.
7. Accept the woman and her family as they are.
8. Allow dependency within reasonable limits.
9. Initiate motivation to obtain professional counseling or therapy when necessary.

Various health professionals can offer parts or all of this emotional and psychological care. However, the obstetric nurse, nurse practitioner, or nurse-midwife is often the ideal health professional to provide it.

Relationship.   It is obvious that a relationship must be established with a person for a professional to be able to offer support and guidance. The goal is for this relationship to be warm, open, and comfortable. The health professional must truly care for the emotional health of the clients in order to establish this type of relationship. Once a relationship such as this is established, a woman will feel more comfortable with bringing up problems or concerns. Continuity is important. A woman should have one person or a small group of people with whom she can relate.

Verbalization.   A health practitioner can encourage a client to verbalize her concerns, problems, or questions by inviting a woman and her family to ask questions and share concerns. A client should know that the practitioner will be available to her to answer questions and provide support during her pregnancy and the postpartum period. At each visit a woman should be asked if there are any questions or problems. Probing questions should be asked in a nonthreatening manner in order to encourage a woman to share what might be on her mind and to focus on issues of concern. Table 4-1 lists examples of questions that might be asked. Not all topics, however, can or should be addressed at each visit. Table 4-2 provides an outline of some of the general concerns and emotional changes that a woman may experience, with a time frame for their occurrence. The practitioner should bring up those topics that are known to be on a woman's mind during pregnancy. If the practitioner senses that

TABLE 4-1
Suggested Questions to Ask at Prenatal Visits

1. Was this pregnancy planned? A surprise?
2. How do you feel about being pregnant at this time?
3. How does your husband/boyfriend feel?
4. Do your other children know about the pregnancy? How are they reacting?
5. How do you think you'll like having a (two, three, etc.) child(ren)? Do you think the new baby will affect your relationship with your other child(ren)?
6. Have you experienced any changes in your sex life since becoming pregnant? Were there problems in your sex life before the pregnancy? Do you have any questions about sex?
7. Are you nervous about labor? Do you have any questions about labor? What are your preferences for labor and delivery?
8. Do you feel ready for parenthood?
9. How are you sleeping?
10. How are things at home?
11. Do you have any questions? Problems?

TABLE 4-2
Anticipatory Guidance: Time Framework

Trimester	Topics
First	Physical changes, e.g., fatigue, nausea, and vomiting Ambivalence *Emotional lability, anxiety, dependency *Introversion *Sexuality
Second	Body-image changes *Fantasies and dreams Plans for infant's arrival Role changes and/or conflicts Concerns regarding normalness of infant Adjustment of siblings to pregnancy
Third	Physical discomforts and body image Labor and delivery Crises, e.g., lack of confidence 4 to 6 wk before due date Adjustments to and expectations of postpartum period Helping siblings adjust to and accept new baby Preparation of siblings for labor and delivery (as needed)

*Discussion of these issues is likely to arise at any point during pregnancy.

something in particular is bothering the woman, the woman should be asked about it specifically. Often, a woman may feel guilty or embarrassed about certain feelings and therefore not share them. For example, a woman expecting her second child and feeling some resentment toward this baby for possible interference with her relationship with the first child, may feel quite guilty about her feelings and may not share them with anyone. If the subject is brought up by the professional, and the woman learns that her feelings are normal, she will usually feel a great sense of relief. This type of communication also benefits the practitioner. Much can be learned from women and their families about the changes they have experienced and how they have dealt with them. Some of this information can often be used later to help in counseling other families.

Teaching. Throughout the pregnancy and during the postpartum period, health professionals should be consistently teaching the woman and her family members about the physical and emotional changes she is experiencing. A woman should be taught how to take care of herself and the baby she is carrying. Pregnancy is an excellent time for health education, a time when a person is often highly motivated to improve her health practices. Women and their families should be told of future emotional and physical changes they may experience and of methods for dealing with these changes. To offer this anticipatory guidance, a practitioner must be knowledgeable about the emotional and physical changes of pregnancy and be able to differentiate the normal from the abnormal.

Family-centered care. All care provided should be family centered to the extent that the woman and family desire and within the bounds of medical safety. Practitioners should invite women to bring the father of the baby, siblings, or other family members to prenatal visits. *Their* questions and concerns should also be addressed. Children of all ages should be allowed to be a part of the care, and their interest in the pregnancy should be encouraged. This early involvement, in addition to early sibling contact during hospital postpartum visits, greatly assists children in adjusting to their new sibling. By including the family in visits, the practitioner is able to see the woman as part of a family and to have a better understanding of the whole person. Fathers should have an opportunity to express their concerns and receive the support they may need. A health professional is often able to facilitate open communication between a couple at a time when they are feeling stressed, and discord in the relationship may thereby be greatly decreased.

Support systems. If a woman is having problems adjusting to pregnancy, or if she is having other social problems, the practitioner should attempt to help her mobilize support systems. There may also be times when the practitioner must mobilize these supports. By offering family-centered care, a practitioner may have a better idea of what family supports do and do not exist for a woman. A practitioner should attempt to help a woman think about, explore, and organize reasonable supports to help her through pregnancy and the early postpartum period. A practitioner may also need to call on other health care providers, such as social workers, counselors, psychiatric personnel, and public health nurses.

Community resources. Professionals in health care should be aware of available community resources. In some areas there are prenatal classes that continue with postpartum support groups. YWCAs may have exercise classes for women with new babies, where a new mother can make friends with women in her own situation. La Leche League has groups all over the country. Women should be encouraged to explore church and community groups in their own town. In the care of pregnant adolescents, contact with school nurses, guidance counselors, or work counselors can be important. In some communities, special high schools have been established for pregnant adolescents.

Acceptance. A practitioner must also accept a woman and her family within their own belief systems. Individual families and cultures have different ideas of parenthood and the roles of father and mother. For example, attitudes toward health care, labor and delivery, and breast-feeding versus bottle-feeding will vary from one couple to another. Although a practitioner should encourage change from those practices that are unhealthy, no attempt should be made to change basic belief systems. The practitioner should respect and work within them. Personality traits will vary from individual to individual, and major personality changes should not be expected. If a woman is generally a nervous, high-strung person who is afraid of pain, she should not be expected to be relaxed and confident about labor. In such an instance, the practitioner should work with the woman to strengthen her coping abilities. The practitioner should attempt to decrease the woman's anxiety about her "performance" in labor by letting her know that those caring for her do not have expected behavior patterns for labor to which she must conform.

Dependency. As stated above, a woman's emotional needs must be met during pregnancy so that she can meet the needs of her infant later. Increased dependency is a normal occurrence in pregnancy and should be allowed within reasonable limits. It is difficult, however, to define "reasonable limits." Women should be encouraged to talk about their feelings and concerns. The practitioner should nevertheless remember that the relationship with the woman and her family is a professional one. The practitioner is not a member of that family or a close family friend, and, consequently, should not usurp the role of the husband or other family members. The goal is for the woman and her family to be a healthily functioning unit within a community. The practitioner must remember that the involvement with a family has a time limit and that the family must continue after professional contact with them has ended. A professional should also set realistic limits on the level of sustainable involvement. If a practitioner overextends herself, "burns out," and then pulls back support, the family has not been helped.

Counseling. If the support a woman needs becomes overwhelming or if there appear to be some severe long-term psychiatric problems, counseling or psychiatric therapy should be considered and referrals made as appropriate. Women have been found to be more open to psychiatric therapy during pregnancy. Memories and repressed conflicts from childhood emerge to consciousness and women have higher integrative ability during this period.[46-48]

Screening for risk of postpartum depression and maladaptation to pregnancy

The following is a list of some specific factors and situations that have been found to increase the risk of poor adaptation to pregnancy and/or postpartum depression:[2,49]

1. Postpartum depression with a previous birth.
2. Previous manic, depressive, or schizophrenic episode.
3. Parents or siblings who have had a manic, depressive, or schizophrenic episode.
4. Conflicts and/or defects in support systems.
5. A disordered relationship with her own mother or the loss of her mother before puberty with inadequate mother surrogate.
6. An alcoholic or aggressively antisocial father.
7. Loss of a parent through death or divorce during childhood.
8. An unhappy childhood resulting from an unfeeling or abusive parent.
9. Chronic marital discord.
10. A neurotic personality structure.
11. An unwanted pregnancy.
12. Adverse prior experience with childbearing or child rearing.
13. A long or difficult labor or complicated birth.
14. Feelings of being degraded or deceived by actions of professionals during labor.
15. Giving birth to a premature, ill, or defective baby.
16. Inadequate preparation for childbearing or child rearing.
17. Maternal health condition that may be adversely affected by pregnancy.
18. A recent move, especially to a new neighborhood, where people previously depended on are now unavailable.

Table 4-3 lists examples of questions that can be asked to screen for these factors. Other factors can be identified as part of an initial medical history. It must be realized that many women exhibiting some of these factors will still adjust well to pregnancy and the new baby. However, women who fall into this group should be observed for adjustment problems and offered support as necessary. Women with long-term, severe psychiatric problems should be cared for jointly by psychiatric, social work, and obstetric personnel.

TABLE 4-3

Questions Used in Screening for Risk of
Maladaptation to Pregnancy and/or Risk of Postpartum Depression

1. Is this pregnancy planned? A surprise?
2. How do you feel about the pregnancy?
3. Has anything happened (to you) in the past (or during this pregnancy) that might affect the baby or cause you concern for your own well-being?
4. Do you plan to raise your child(ren) any differently from the way you were raised?
5. Is the baby's father involved with the pregnancy? Is he of much help to you?
6. Do you plan to take prenatal classes? Will the baby's father be attending with you? If not, will someone else be going with you?
7. How much experience did you have with taking care of children while you were growing up?
8. Will anyone be available to help you in the first few postpartum days/weeks with the baby? Is your mother coming to stay with you? How do you think this will work out?
9. Do you have any condition(s) that you think may be aggravated by your pregnancy?

Adapted from Cohen, R. L. Maladaptation to pregnancy. *Seminars in Perinatology* (January 1979). 15-24.

One factor that is often overlooked by obstetric personnel, but that can have a great effect on a woman's adjustment, is her relationship with her own mother. A woman who is overdependent on her mother may have a great deal of trouble dealing with the needs of a newborn. She may still perceive herself in the role of "daughter" to her parents. An overdependent woman may, however, enjoy pregnancy and the attention she receives. She may be a very "obedient" patient, and may transfer her dependence to her midwife, nurse, or prenatal instructor. Such a woman may find labor a shattering experience, and may refuse to do anything for herself. With rigid control from the professional who is coaching her in labor, she may "perform" well, but the basic problem of overdependence still exists. A health professional may be unaware of such a dependence and unconsciously foster it. This may help a woman through pregnancy, labor, and delivery, but it ignores the basic problem. Professionals must remember that the goal is to wean a woman from dependence on them and to strengthen the woman's ability to deal with the stresses of child rearing.[50,51]

The following signs indicate that a woman is not adjusting well to her pregnancy and is at risk for problems once the child is born:[2,52-54]

1. Continued significant ambivalence beyond midpregnancy.
2. Failure to use the word "I" when speaking about mothering by the end of the pregnancy.
3. Denial of changes in body and appearance.
4. Constant overreaction to changes in body and appearance.
5. Preoccupation with vague emotional and/or physical complaints that cannot be remedied.
6. Appearance and actions at advanced stages of pregnancy that suggest denial of pregnancy.
7. Absent or minimal, disturbed, or distorted response to quickening.
8. Lack of nesting behavior in latter months of pregnancy.
9. Absence of fantasies about the baby, predominantly negative fantasies, or fantasies dealing only with later periods of life (e.g, toddler, school age, college age).
10. Display of solely intellectual attitude toward the fetus.
11. Overdependence on mother or intense need for mother's approval.
12. Need for precise instructions and external direction to guide her activities.

If time is allowed for questions and discussions at prenatal visits, if continuity of care is provided, and if a relationship has been established with the woman, these signs can usually be identified. Support should be available to such women during and after pregnancy. However, not all women who suffer postpartum depression will fall into this group, and women must still have an access to help after the child is born. One factor that has not been found to correlate with adjustment to motherhood is a woman's enjoyment of the actual pregnancy.[1,55] A woman may find pregnancy uncomfortable and annoying, but still feel strongly attached to her fetus and adapt very well to the demands of motherhood. On the other hand, a woman may enjoy pregnancy for the attention it brings her, but may not be able to accept the newborn as a separate being or handle the constant demands of motherhood.

STRESSES OF MODERN SOCIETY

Many changes that have recently occurred in society have added to the stress of pregnancy for women and families.

People today are highly mobile. Frequent moves can separate families and interfere with community integrity. Young couples with young children often find themselves fairly isolated, with few people geographically close that they can depend on and call on in time of need. The extended family system no longer exists for many, as it did a few generations ago. Pregnant women used to have many female relatives close by to help them and to answer their questions. In contrast with the present, most women had had experience caring for children before having their own.

Feminism has recently opened many new doors for women. For many women, however, it has also added to the stress of pregnancy. Conflicts between the demands of a profession and of motherhood are often difficult to resolve. Some women find themselves caught between two sets of expectations. On one hand a woman is expected to pursue a career as vigorously as a man, and in some circles she is looked down on if she does not keep up with her professional role. On the other hand, a woman is often still expected to keep up the home and fulfill the traditional role of motherhood. Some women find themselves struggling to meet both sets of expectations. Often, conflict arises between a man and a woman about roles and duties in the home. The business world has not yet become flexible enough to accommodate working couples with children.

The lack of extended family and community supports and the changing values of society require health professionals to take a more active role in the emotional support of women and their families during the major change of childbearing and child rearing.

REFERENCES

1. Caplan. 86.

2. Cohen.

3. Rubin.

4. Kitzinger. (1977) 89.

5. Westbrook.

6. Standley et al.

7. Falicov.

8. Masters and Johnson. 156-160.

9. Moore.

10. Jessner. (1966) 106.

11. Kitzinger. (1972) 56.

12. Kitzinger. (1977) 90.
13. Caplan. 78.
14. Coleman and Coleman. 22-23.
15. Our Bodies, Ourselves. 262.
16. Jessner. 113.
17. Caplan. 81-84.
18. Kitzinger. (1977) 91.
19. Reedy.
20. Curtis.
21. Burst.
22. Sheehy. 384.
23. Antle.
24. Kitzinger. (1972) 67.
25. Coleman and Coleman. 109.
26. Roehner.
27. Clausen et al. 417-419.
28. Jessner et al. (1970) 231.
29. Coleman and Coleman. 122.
30. Wapner.
31. Fein.
32. Coleman and Coleman. 113.
33. Trethowan and Colon.
34. Kitzinger. (1972) 66.
35. Newton et al.
36. Ascher.
37. Crandon. 109-111.
38. Crandon. 113-115.
39. Laukeran and vanden Berg.
40. Caplan. 76.
41. Coleman and Coleman. 146.
42. Melges.
43. Pugh et al.
44. Coleman and Coleman. 144.
45. Caplan. 163-184, 205-231.
46. Benedek. 248.
47. Coleman and Coleman. 32.

48. Caplan. 78.
49. Ciaramitaro. 116.
50. Kitzinger. (1977) 103.
51. Kitzinger. (1972) 106.
52. Caplan. 89-95.
53. Kitzinger. (1972) 55, 74.
54. Kitzinger. (1977) 103, 105, 106.
55. Kitzinger. (1977) 106.

CHAPTER 5

MATERNAL NUTRITION

Nancy Kulb

For many years, maternal nutrition has been viewed as an important factor in pregnancy outcome. In the last half of the 19th century, Prochownick advocated limiting the maternal diet in order to produce small babies that could be delivered easily. Limitation of maternal weight gain by dietary restriction was further popularized when it was noted that sudden weight gain preceded preeclampsia-eclampsia. It was hoped that by limiting weight gain, preeclampsia could be prevented.[1]

Medical advances in the 20th century have clarified the importance of good maternal nutrition, made delivery of the large infant less risky, clarified the disease process in preeclampsia, and invalidated the original reasons for limiting maternal intake.

MATERNAL AND INFANT WEIGHT

It has been found that neonatal morbidity and mortality are inversely related to weight at birth. Low-birth-weight babies have a high risk of death and an increased risk of neurological damage with possible mental retardation.[2] In general, the greater the infant birth weight, the lower the neonatal morbidity and mortality (up to 4,500 grams, above which diabetes and injuries from traumatic delivery influence outcome). Because weight is related to gestational age, this relationship generally holds not only for premature babies but also for most other infants (Fig. 5-1). Thus, birth weight is of crucial importance to pregnancy outcome.

Factors affecting birth weight

Numerous studies have been performed to determine which factors influence birth weight. Gestational age has been determined as the most important factor.[3] Although extensive research in obstetrics is currently focused on controlling prematurity, and although treatment of premature labor is becoming more sophisticated, prematurity still presents a major problem in terms of perinatal morbidity and mortality.

Other factors also influence birth weight. Cigarette smoking retards growth. On average, infants of smoking mothers weigh 6.1 ounces less than infants of nonsmoking mothers.[4] In general, birth weight is lower among lower socioeconomic classes, and birth weight of black babies is lower than that of white babies.[5] Certain maternal diseases, such as hypertension, may contribute to low birth weights, whereas others, such as diabetes mellitus, may contribute to excessively high birth weights. Fetal infections, such as rubella, are associated with low birth weights, as are certain congenital anomalies.[6] Increasing maternal age and parity are associated with greater birth weights.[5] The genetic potential of the baby also plays a part: a baby with small parents is likely to be small at birth, whereas a baby with large parents is likely to be large at birth.

The two factors other than gestational age that have the greatest relationship to birth weight are maternal prepregnancy weight and weight gain during pregnancy.[7] Fortunately, both factors are somewhat controllable. These two factors have effects on birth weight that are both additive and independent of each other. Table 5-1 shows desirable prepregnancy weights for women of various heights and frame sizes.

Components of weight gain during pregnancy

The components of weight gain during pregnancy can be thought of as the maternal component (e.g., blood volume expansion, growth of breasts and uterus, and extracellular fluid expansion) and the fetal component (i.e., fetus, placenta, and amniotic fluid). Table 5-2 shows the expected weight gain of each component by trimester. In addition to any special needs of the woman for growth or weight gain, the amount of weight required for the pregnancy is about 21 pounds (9.5 kilograms). Finally, approximately 5 pounds (2.7 kilograms) of fat is ''deposited'' in maternal stores to be used as a source

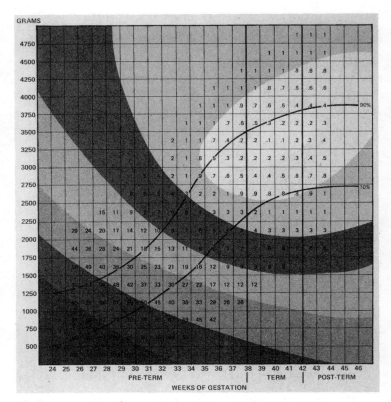

Figure 5-1. Newborn classification and neonatal mortality risk by birth weight and gestational age. *Reprinted with permission from* Lubchenco, L. O., D. T. Searls, and J. V. Brazie. Neonatal mortality rate: relationship to birth weight and gestational age. *Journal of Pediatrics* (October 1972). 819. (Courtesy of the authors; C. V. Mosby Co., St. Louis; and Mead Johnson & Co., Evansville, Ind.)

of calories during lactation. Technically, however, this is not required for the pregnancy.

Pattern of weight gain

It is recommended that most women gain 24 to 28 pounds (11 to 13 kilograms) over their pregravid weight during pregnancy. Normally,

TABLE 5-1

Desirable Weights for Women (Ages 25 and Over)

Height*	Small frame‡	Medium frame	Large frame
4′ 10″	92-98 (95)	96-107 (102)	104-119 (112)
4′ 11″	94-101 (98)	98-110 (104)	106-122 (114)
5′ 0″	96-104 (100)	101-113 (107)	109-125 (117)
5′ 1″	99-107 (103)	104-116 (110)	112-128 (120)
5′ 2″	102-110 (106)	107-119 (113)	115-131 (123)
5′ 3″	105-113 (109)	110-122 (116)	118-134 (126)
5′ 4″	108-116 (112)	113-126 (120)	121-138 (130)
5′ 5″	111-119 (115)	116-130 (123)	125-142 (134)
5′ 6″	114-123 (119)	120-135 (128)	129-146 (138)
5′ 7″	118-127 (123)	124-139 (132)	133-150 (142)
5′ 8″	122-131 (127)	128-143 (136)	137-154 (146)
5′ 9″	126-135 (131)	132-147 (140)	141-158 (150)
5′ 10″	130-140 (135)	136-151 (144)	145-163 (154)
5′ 11″	134-144 (139)	140-155 (148)	149-168 (159)
6′ 0″	138-148 (143)	144-159 (152)	153-173 (163)

*Heights given are with shoes on.
‡Weights given are with indoor clothing. For nude weights, subtract 2 to 4 pounds. For women between 18 and 25 years of age, subtract 1 pound for each year under 25.
Reprinted with permission from the Metropolitan Life Insurance Co., New York.

a weight gain of 2 to 3 pounds in the entire first trimester and about ¾ to 1 pound each week in the second and third trimesters is expected.

The pattern of weight gain is important. Weight loss or failure to gain weight may indicate a lack of available nutrients for the growing fetus. It may also indicate that maternal stores are being used to meet the needs for pregnancy. Acetonuria, as a result of maternal fat stores being broken down for energy, may be associated with low intelligence quotient (IQ) scores when the child reaches preschool age.[8] Thus, dieting during pregnancy is strongly discouraged. Women of low prepregnancy weight (less than 120 pounds [54.5 kilograms)] should be encouraged to eat as much as they want. If they have not gained 10 pounds by the 20th week of gestation, nutritional intervention should be instituted to help them to increase their weight gain for the remainder of the pregnancy.[7]

Sudden weight gain during pregnancy may also be a warning sign. It may indicate ingestion of excessive amounts of high-calorie foods

TABLE 5-2

*Average Components of Weight Gain in Pregnancy
(Cumulative Gain at End of Each Trimester)*

Component	First	Second	Third
Fetal	*kg*	*kg*	*kg*
Fetus	Negligible	1.0	3.4
Placenta	Negligible	0.3	0.6
Amniotic fluid	Negligible	0.4	1.0
Fetal subtotal		**1.7**	**5.0**
Maternal			
Increased uterine size	0.3	0.8	1.0
Increased breast size	0.1	0.3	0.5
Increased blood volume	0.3	1.3	1.5
Increased extracellular fluid	0.0	0.0	1.5
Maternal subtotal	**0.7**	**2.4**	**4.5**
Total gain accounted for	**0.7**	**4.1**	**9.5**

Reprinted with permission from the American College of Obstetricians and Gynecologists. 1972.

(many of which are low in nutrient value), or it may indicate retention of fluid (edema), which may be a symptom of preeclampsia, cardiac disease, or renal disease.

The prenatal weight-gain grid (Fig. 5-2) can be used to assess the status of the weight-gain pattern during pregnancy. The prepregnancy weight is plotted at the 0 point on the graph. As gestational age progresses (plotted along the horizontal axis), weight change above or below prepregnancy weight is plotted along the vertical axis. The average weight gain for a healthy woman during pregnancy is plotted for comparison. Variations in the normal pattern of weight gain are readily apparent when using this graph. It should be pointed out, however, that this graph represents an average for normal, healthy women. Some healthy women will gain more than 24 pounds, and some will gain less. Some women, such as adolescents or those who begin pregnancy underweight, may need to gain weight for themselves as well as for the pregnancy, and thus may need to gain significantly more than 24 pounds. Gravidas who begin pregnancy overweight may need to gain less than 24 pounds; however, they should be discouraged from dieting, and they probably need to gain at least 15 to 20 pounds (6.8 to 9.1 kilograms) to adequately provide for the fetus's needs.

To assess the weight-gain pattern, it is important for the nurse to use accurate measurements of weight. The following are some factors to consider when assessing a weight recording:

Was the same scale used previously?

Is the client dressed the same as for previous recordings (e.g., without purse, coat, or shoes)?

Has the client just eaten a large meal?

Nutrient requirements

Nutrient requirements vary from individual to individual and cannot be precisely determined. The recommended dietary allowances (RDAs) provide nutrient requirement guidelines for healthy populations of people rather than for individuals (Table 5-3). Most healthy people who consume the amounts of nutrients specified in the RDAs will have adequate amounts with an additional margin of safety. However, there may be a small percentage of people who will be lacking in one or more nutrients if they consume the amounts specified in the RDAs because the RDAs do not provide for extra nutrients that may be required for nonhealthy people. The RDAs are the best available guidelines for nutrient requirements for people in the United States. The major nutrients, their functions in the body, and their major food sources are listed in Table 5-4.

Protein. As can be seen in Table 5-3, certain nutrients are required in greater amounts during pregnancy and lactation in order to provide for the needs of both mother and baby. Because protein is the major material for building and repairing tissue, it is in great demand for the growth of maternal and fetal tissues during pregnancy. An additional 30 grams of protein above nonpregnant requirements is needed during pregnancy. For multiple gestation, even more protein is required: about 25 grams for each additional fetus.[9] Protein can only be used for building tissue if there are adequate calories for energy from other sources (i.e, fats and carbohydrates). Otherwise, the protein will be used for energy and will be unavailable for building and repairing tissue.

Calories. Energy requirements increase with the increased basal metabolic rate that is characteristic of pregnancy. Therefore, caloric requirements increase. Specific requirements for an individual (which are dependent on age, body size, basal metabolic rate, and activity levels), may change from day to day. It is not practical to calculate exact caloric requirements for an individual. As a general rule, however, caloric requirements increase by 300/day over nonpregnant requirements.[10] The total daily caloric requirement for most pregnant women is approximately 2,300 to 2,400 (more for women with multiple gestation). Because other nutrients are also in

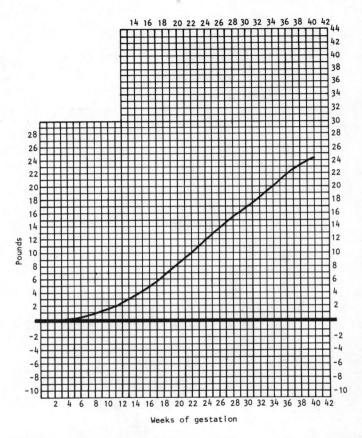

Figure 5-2. The prenatal weight-gain grid. This grid can be used to assess the status of the weight-gain pattern during pregnancy. Ideally, the same time of day and the same conditions (same scale, similar clothing weight, shoes, etc.) should be used for all weight measurements.

greater demand during pregnancy, women should be encouraged to meet caloric requirements with foods that provide other nutrients, rather than through foods that provide only calories.

Iron. Iron is required for production of hemoglobin, the oxygen-carrying molecule in red blood cells. Iron is found in liver and other

TABLE 5-3
Recommended Daily Dietary Allowances*

Age	Weight		Height		Protein	Fat-soluble vitamins			Water-soluble vitamins		
						Vitamin A	Vitamin D	Vitamin E	Vitamin C	Thiamin	Riboflavin
yr	*kg*	*lb*	*cm*	*in*	*g*	*μg RE‡*	*μg§*	*mg α-TE†*	*mg*	*mg*	*mg*
Infants											
0.0-0.5	6	13	60	24	kg × 2.2	420	10	3	35	0.3	0.4
0.5-1.0	9	20	71	28	kg × 2.0	400	10	4	35	0.5	0.6
Children											
1-3	13	29	90	35	23	400	10	5	45	0.7	0.8
4-6	20	44	112	44	30	500	10	6	45	0.9	1.0
7-10	28	62	132	52	34	700	10	7	45	1.2	1.4
Males											
11-14	45	99	157	62	45	1,000	10	8	50	1.4	1.6
15-18	66	145	176	69	56	1,000	10	10	60	1.4	1.7
19-22	70	154	177	70	56	1,000	7.5	10	60	1.5	1.7
23-50	70	154	178	70	56	1,000	5	10	60	1.4	1.6
51+	70	154	178	70	56	1,000	5	10	60	1.2	1.4
Females											
11-14	46	101	157	62	46	800	10	8	50	1.1	1.3
15-18	55	120	163	64	46	800	10	8	60	1.1	1.3
19-22	55	120	163	64	44	800	7.5	8	60	1.1	1.3
23-50	55	120	163	64	44	800	5	8	60	1.0	1.2
51+	55	120	163	64	44	800	5	8	60	1.0	1.2
Pregnant					+30	+200	+5	+2	+20	+0.4	+0.3
Lactating					+20	+400	+5	+3	+40	+0.5	+0.5

	Water-soluble vitamins				Minerals					
	Niacin	Vitamin B6	Folacin	Vitamin B12	Calcium	Phosphorus	Magnesium	Iron	Zinc	Iodine
	mg NE**	mg	µg	µg	mg	mg	mg	mg	mg	µg
Infants	6	0.3	30	0.5‡‡	360	240	50	10	3	40
	8	0.6	45	1.5	540	360	70	15	5	50
Children	9	0.9	100	2.0	800	800	150	15	10	70
	11	1.3	200	2.5	800	800	200	10	10	90
	16	1.6	300	3.0	800	800	250	10	10	120
Males	18	1.8	400	3.0	1,200	1,200	350	18	15	150
	18	2.0	400	3.0	1,200	1,200	400	18	15	150
	19	2.2	400	3.0	800	800	350	10	15	150
	18	2.2	400	3.0	800	800	350	10	15	150
	16	2.2	400	3.0	800	800	350	10	15	150
Females	15	1.8	400	3.0	1,200	1,200	300	18	15	150
	14	2.0	400	3.0	1,200	1,200	300	18	15	150
	14	2.0	400	3.0	800	800	300	18	15	150
	13	2.0	400	3.0	800	800	300	18	15	150
	13	2.0	400	3.0	800	800	300	10	15	150
Pregnant	+2	+0.6	+400	+1.0	+400	+400	+150	§§	+5	+25
Lactating	+5	+0.5	+100	+1.0	+400	+400	+150	§§	+10	+50

*The allowances are intended to provide for individual variations among most healthy persons in the United States. Diets should be based on a variety of common foods in order to provide other nutrients for which human requirements have been less well defined. See text for detailed discussion of allowances and nutrients.

†Retinol equivalents. 1 Retinol equivalent = 1 µg retinol or 6 µg β-carotene.

‡As cholecalciferol. 10 µg cholecalciferol = 400 IU vitamin D.

§α-Tocopherol equivalents. 1 mg d-α-tocopherol = 1 α-TE.

**Niacin equivalent. 1 NE is equal to 1 mg of niacin or 60 mg of dietary tryptophan.

‡‡The RDA for vitamin B12 in infants is based on average concentration of the vitamin in human milk. The allowances after weaning are based on energy intake (as recommended by the American Academy of Pediatrics) and consideration of other factors, such as intestinal absorption.

§§The increased requirement during pregnancy cannot be met by the iron content of habitual American diets nor by the existing iron stores of many women. Therefore the use of 30 to 60 mg of supplemental iron is recommended. Iron needs during lactation are not substantially different from those of nonpregnant women, but continued supplementation of the mother for 2 to 3 months after parturition is advisable in order to replenish stores depleted by pregnancy.

Reproduced from Recommended Dietary Allowances. National Academy Press, Washington, D. C. 1980. Ninth edition.

TABLE 5-4

Functions and Sources of Major Nutrients

Nutrient	Functions	Sources
Protein	Builds and repairs all tissues. Helps build blood, enzymes, hormones, and antibodies. Supplies energy: 4 calories per gram.	Meat, poultry, fish Eggs Milk and cheese Dried beans and peas Nuts Breads and cereals
Carbohydrate	Supplies energy: 4 calories per gram. Unrefined products supply fiber for regular elimination.	Breads and cereals Potatoes Dried beans and peas Corn Dried fruits (smaller amount in fresh fruit) Sugar, syrup, jelly, honey
Fat	Supplies energy: 9 calories per gram. Supplies essential fatty acids. Provides and carries fat-soluble vitamins A, D, E, and K.	Shortening, oil Butter, margarine, cream Salad dressing Sausage, bacon Fat in meat
Vitamin A	Assists formation and maintenance of skin and mucous membranes, thus increasing resistance to infection. Functions in visual processes, promotes healthy	Liver Dark-green and deep-yellow (orange) vegetables Deep-yellow (orange) fruits (e.g., peaches, cantaloupe)

Nutrient	Function	Food Sources
	eye tissue and eye adaptation in dim light. Helps control bone growth.	Butter, whole milk, cream Cheddar cheese Ice cream
Thiamin (Vitamin B1)	Promotes utilization of carbohydrate. Contributes to normal functioning of nervous system. Promotes normal appetite and digestion.	Pork and other meats Eggs Enriched or whole-grain breads and cereals Dried beans and peas Nuts Potatoes, broccoli, collard greens
Riboflavin (Vitamin B2)	Aids in utilization of oxygen and production of energy within body cells. Promotes healthy skin, eyes, tongue, and lips. Helps prevent scaly, greasy skin around mouth and nose.	Milk, cheese, ice cream Enriched or whole-grain breads and cereals Meat (especially liver) Eggs Green, leafy vegetables
Niacin	Aids in fat synthesis, tissue respiration, and utilization of carbohydrate. Promotes healthy nervous system. Promotes healthy skin, mouth, and tongue. Aids digestion and fosters normal appetite.	Peanuts, peanut butter Meat (especially liver) Milk Enriched or whole-grain breads and cereals Beans, peas
Pyridoxine (Vitamin B6)	Aids in metabolism of protein. Assists absorption of protein across intestinal wall.	Meat, poultry, fish Whole-grain products Legumes Potatoes, sweet potatoes Bananas
Vitamin B12	Assists in protein metabolism, including DNA synthesis and red blood cell formation. Functions in metabolism of fatty acids.	Meat, poultry, fish Small amounts in dairy products and eggs (Supplements are required for vegans)

Nutrient	Functions	Sources
Pantothenic acid	Aids in transmission of nerve impulses. Functions in production of energy. Aids in synthesis of fatty acids and cholesterol. Functions in the formation of hemoglobin.	Meat Milk, cheese, eggs Whole-grain products Legumes Peanuts Broccoli Mushrooms Corn Sweet potatoes
Biotin	Assists in protein and carbohydrate metabolism. Aids in synthesis of fatty acids.	Organ meat Egg yolk Legumes Peanuts Mushrooms
Folacin (Folic acid)	Assists in DNA synthesis. Aids transmission of nerve impulses. Assists in maturation of red blood cells.	Dark-green, leafy vegetables Meat (especially organ meat) Nuts Legumes Whole-grain products Yeast Asparagus
Vitamin C (Ascorbic acid)	Aids in production of cementing materials that hold cells together, thus strengthening blood vessel walls, hastening healing of wounds and	Citrus fruits Strawberries Cantaloupe

	broken bones, and increasing resistance to infection. Aids in utilization of iron. Helps regulate cholesterol level of blood.	Tomatoes Broccoli, green peppers Mango, papaya Raw or lightly cooked greens and cabbage
Vitamin D	Aids in absorption and utilization of calcium and phosphorus, both of which are required for normal bone mineralization, muscle contraction, and conduction of nerve impulses.	Fish liver oil Milk fortified with vitamin D Sunshine on skin (nondietary)
Vitamin E	Helps maintain integrity of cell membrane. "Spares" vitamins A and C.	Vegetable oils: corn, soybean, safflower, cottonseed
Vitamin K	Factor in blood coagulation.	Green, leafy vegetables Pork liver Eggs Vegetable oils
Calcium	Helps build bones and teeth. Assists in blood coagulation. Functions in normal muscle contraction and relaxation. Functions in normal nerve transmission. Helps regulate the use of other minerals in the body.	Milk Yogurt Cheese Sardines and salmon with bones Turnip, mustard, and collard greens Kale Broccoli
Phosphorus	Constituent of all body cells. Regulates transport of chemicals into and out of cells. Participates in energy production. Participates in regulation of acid-base balance. Aids in utilization of B vitamins.	Milk products Meat, poultry, fish Nuts Whole-grain products Legumes

Nutrient	Functions	Sources
Iron	Combines with protein to form hemoglobin. Functions as part of enzymes involved in tissue respiration. Increases resistance to infection.	Liver and other red meat Eggs Dried beans and peas Enriched or whole-grain breads and cereals Green, leafy vegetables
Sodium	Participates in regulation of water balance. Aids transportation of nutrients across cell membranes. Aids maintenance of acid-base balance. Participates in transmission of nerve impulses. Participates in muscle contraction.	Table salt Milk Meat, poultry, fish Eggs Green, leafy vegetables Carrots Swiss chard Celery
Potassium	Participates in regulation of water balance. Required for protein formation. Aids in converting glucose to glycogen. Aids in transmission of nerve impulses. Aids in muscle contraction.	Meat, poultry, fish Whole-grain products Legumes Prunes Leafy vegetables Bananas Oranges, grapefruits Tomatoes Potatoes

Adapted from Gazella, J. G. Nutrition for the Childbearing Year. Woodland Publishing Co., Inc., Wayzata, Minn. 1979; Green, M. L., and J. Harry. Nutrition in Contemporary Nursing Practice. John Wiley & Sons, Inc., New York. 1981; and National Dairy Council, Nutrition Source Book. National Dairy Council, Chicago. 1970.

red meats, egg yolks, enriched or whole-grain breads and cereals, and green, leafy vegetables. Foods cooked in iron pots and pans may absorb minute amounts of iron from the utensil that then become available for absorption. However, only about 10 percent of the available iron in animal sources and 4 percent of the available iron in plant sources is absorbed. Oxalic acid, which is present in green, leafy vegetables, interferes with the absorption of iron.

Nonpregnant females require 18 milligrams of iron per day. The amount of iron required for pregnancy, however, cannot be met by typical American diets. During pregnancy, an extra 300 milligrams of iron is needed for fetal red blood cell production, and an extra 500 milligrams is needed for maternal red blood cell production. Over the course of a normal 270-day pregnancy, this 800 milligrams breaks down to an additional 3 mg/day. In general, 18 mg/day can be obtained from a well-planned diet. The other 3 to 6 mg/day can be obtained by supplementation with at least 30 to 60 milligrams (10 percent of which is absorbed) of elemental iron per day.

Sodium.   Sodium requirements during pregnancy have been a source of great controversy. Because restriction of sodium is part of the management of nonpregnant hypertensive patients, it was once believed that restriction of sodium during pregnancy could prevent hypertension and edema, and thus prevent preeclampsia. Although American diets frequently contain excessive amounts of salt, the current recommendation for normal pregnancy is that the pregnant woman salt her food to taste. Sodium restriction and diuretic administration, which depletes sodium stores, are not recommended except for women with cardiovascular or renal disease.

Supplemental prenatal vitamins and iron.   Supplemental prenatal iron is administered routinely to pregnant clients by some clinical practitioners. The rationale for the use of supplemental iron is that most American women do not consume enough in their diets to meet the needs of pregnancy. Although there may be some women who consume an iron-rich diet, whose iron status can be monitored, who can get enough iron from their diets, and who do not need supplementation, those who do receive supplementation should be provided with the following information to maximize compliance with, and effectiveness of, the prescribed regimen:

1. Iron pills should be taken approximately 30 to 60 minutes after meals. Taking iron on an empty stomach may cause nausea or indigestion.
2. Iron may be constipating. This effect can be counteracted by drinking plenty of fluids (8 to 10 glasses of water a day); eating plenty of whole-grain breads and cereals, and fresh fruits and

vegetables for roughage; getting regular exercise; establishing regular bowel habits; and using natural laxative foods when necessary (e.g., prunes or prune juice, warm fluids, etc.).

3. Stools may turn dark or black: this is a normal side effect of iron supplementation.

4. Milk hinders iron absorption. Although milk is a very important part of the diet, iron pills should not be taken with milk products. Instead, iron pills should be taken with a vitamin C source (such as orange, grapefruit, or tomato juice) because vitamin C enhances iron absorption.

Supplemental vitamins are routinely administered by some clinical practitioners to ensure the ingestion of adequate amounts of all vitamins. Others believe that a client with a well-balanced diet, who is eating a wide variety of foods, is getting all the vitamins she needs from food sources.

ASSESSMENT OF NUTRITIONAL STATUS

Nutritional status is a difficult parameter to assess. The available methods of assessment include diet history, physical signs and symptoms of nutritional status, and laboratory measurements.

Diet history

There are many kinds of diet histories that can be used. Among the most common are the written 3-day history and the 24-hour diet recall.

The 24-hour diet recall consists of asking the client what she has consumed in the previous 24-hour period (Fig. 5-3). It is helpful to ask about amounts of food, times of eating, and what her activities were as she was eating, where she was, whom she was with, etc., because these questions may jog her memory regarding intake. They may also give a more complete picture of her dietary habits, which will be useful in counseling. In general, the client should be able to recall fairly accurately her intake for the previous 24 hours. Although this method is quick and easy to use, it does have several disadvantages. The previous 24-hour pattern may not have been typical for her — especially if it occurred on a weekend or a holiday or was unusual for her for any reason. She should be questioned as to whether the intake of the previous 24 hours is representative of her usual diet. Some clients may be reluctant or unable to give an accurate history. They may know what they should have eaten, and alter their recall accordingly. An explanation of the purpose of the recall and a nonjudgmental attitude will help to prevent unreliable histories.

TIME	PLACE	FOOD EATEN	AMOUNT	SUMMARY						
				Protein foods	Milk and Products	Grain Products	Vitamin C Products	Leafy Green	Other fruits & vegetables	
INFLUENCES ON DIET:			SUMMARY: Svgs. eaten							
			Svgs. needed	4	4	3	1	2	1	
			Difference							

Interviewer: _____

Patient's Name: _____   Date: _____

Figure 5-3. An example of a 24-hour diet intake recall chart.

A second type of diet history is the 3-day written record (Fig. 5-4). With this method, the client is instructed to take the form home and write down everything she eats for a 3-day period. It is helpful to have her include the amount eaten, the time, location, associated activities, and other circumstances in order to get a clear understanding of her dietary patterns and to help in providing relevant counseling. She should be instructed to bring the record to her next visit. The

FOOD RECORD

Name: _____

Date: _____

TIME	PLACE	FOOD EATEN	AMOUNT

Instructions:

1. Using the attached forms, list the foods you eat for 3 consecutive days. Begin each day with a new form.

2. Record everything you eat and drink in each 24-hour period.

3. Remember to write down when you ate or drank each food, and where this was.

4. Describe each food fully. Indicate whether it is raw or cooked. If cooked, tell how it was prepared (for example: fried, boiled) and how it was served (for example: with cream sauce, with Thousand Island dressing).

5. Record the amount of each food and beverage. If you are uncertain about the quantity, please estimate.

Example (excerpts from 24-hour period):

TIME	PLACE	FOOD EATEN	AMOUNT
9:30a.m.	Work	Glazed doughnut Coffee with sugar	1 1 cup/1 tsp.
11:30a.m.	Coffee shop	Tomato rice soup Sandwich made with: white bread turkey lettuce mayonnaise Ice water	1 cup 2 slices 3 thin slices 1 leaf light 1 large glass
1:15a.m.	Home	Warm milk	8 oz. glass

Figure 5-4.   An example of a 3-day written record of a diet history.

3-day written record has the advantages of providing a more realistic diet history and of being less subject to unusual circumstances than the 24-hour history. It requires motivation on the part of the client to remember to write down everything she eats. Keeping the diet history may alter her eating patterns: it is difficult to keep track of ingredients in condiments, sauces, and gravies, or of amounts of foods when mixed together (salads, vegetable mixtures, casseroles), so she may choose not to eat those foods. In addition, she may choose to forgo snacks she would ordinarily consume because of the difficulty of keeping the record.

Although diet histories have their limitations, they are useful in the assessment of nutritional status. After the record is obtained, the number of servings of foods eaten in each food group can be compared with the number of servings required each day (Fig. 5-5). Deficiencies or excesses can be readily spotted, and counseling specific to the needs of the client can be initiated.

Physical Parameters

The physical parameters of nutritional status consist of weight assessment (*see* p. 125) and assessment of physical signs of nutrient deficiencies. Table 5-5 lists symptoms of deficiencies by nutrient. Many of these symptoms are not specific to nutritional deficiency and must be differentiated from disease states.

Interviewer: _____

Patient's Name: _____ Date: _____

Food Group	Servings Eaten (3 days)	Daily Serving Average	Servings Needed	Suggested Changes
Protein foods (animal & vegetable)			4	
Milk & milk products			4	
Grain products			3	
Vitamin C rich fruits & vegetables			1	
Leafy green vegetables			2	
Other fruits & vegetables			1	

Comments and Follow-up:

Figure 5-5. Diet history evaluation sheet. This type of form provides quick, easy-to-read reference for the client's specific dietary deficiencies and excesses, and can aid greatly in client diet counseling.

TABLE 5-5

Symptoms of Nutrient Deficiency

Nutrient	Symptoms of Deficiency
Protein	Flaky dermatosis
	Hair easily plucked
	Mild wasting of fat and muscles
	Apathy
	Diarrhea
	Edema
	Mild anemia
Protein and calories	Hair easily plucked, sparse, dyspigmented
	Severe wasting of fat and muscles
	Impaired mental development
	Diarrhea
	Severe anemia
	Low body weight
	Flaky paint dermatosis, diffuse skin pigmentation
Vitamin A	Follicular hyperkeratosis, xerosis
	Eye abnormalities: night blindness, dryness of the conjunctiva, photophobia, swelling and redness of the lids, cloudy ulcerated cornea, blindness, Bitot's spots
Thiamine	Calf muscle tenderness
	Weakness, numbness, tingling of legs
	Loss of knee and/or ankle jerks
	Malaise

	Polyneuritis
	Loss of immediate memory
	Disorientation
	Ataxia
	Anorexia
	Nausea, vomiting
	Constipation
	Tachycardia, palpitations
	Edema of legs, trunk, face
	Hypertension
	Heart failure
	Dyspnea
Riboflavin	Cheilosis
	Angular fissures
	Seborrheic dermatitis
	Fatigue
	Neuropathy
	Photophobia
	Corneal inflammation, vascularization
	Soreness of mouth and tongue
	Glossitis
	Tongue: papillae hypertrophied, atrophied, or purple in color
Niacin	Dermatitis
	Mental apathy
	Depression, anxiety, disorientation, confusion
	Glossitis
	Anorexia

Nutrient	Symptoms of Deficiency
	Indigestion Weight loss Diarrhea Stomatitis Tongue: scarlet, raw, atrophy of papillae
Pyridoxine	Nausea In pregnancy, may be associated with toxemia, gestational diabetes, neurological symptoms, or mental retardation in the newborn
Vitamin B12	Megaloblastic anemia Central nervous system abnormalities
Folacin	Megaloblastic anemia In pregnancy, may be associated with toxemia and damage to the central nervous system of the fetus
Vitamin C	Dry, rough skin Petechiae, ecchymoses Inadequate wound healing Hemorrhages in muscles and joints Sunken chest Swollen, bleeding gums Anemia In pregnancy, may be a cause of spontaneous abortion and premature delivery

Vitamin D	Failure of calcification, skeletal abnormalities: head appears enlarged and flattened; bowed legs; knock-knees; knobbing at wrists; bowing of arms; rachitic rosary
	Decreased muscle tone
	Kyphosis
	Protruberant abdomen
Vitamin E	Deficiency in pregnancy has been associated with neonatal jaundice
Iron	Anemia
	Pallor of mucous membranes
	Koilonychia
	Atrophy of papillae of tongue
Iodine	Enlarged thyroid

Adapted from Gazella, J. G. Nutrition for the Childbearing Year. Woodland Publishing Co., Inc., Wayzata, Minn. 1979; and Green, M. L., and J. Harry. Nutrition in Contemporary Nursing Practice. John Wiley & Sons, Inc., New York. 1981.

Laboratory studies

Although there are laboratory studies available to assess the status of many nutrients in the body, few are commonly used for pregnant clients. Among those used are laboratory studies that assess for anemia: the indices of the complete blood count and the peripheral smear (both of which aid in the diagnosis of iron deficiency anemia or megaloblastic anemia), and serum iron, iron-binding capacity, and serum folate tests, all of which can determine the amount of iron or folic acid available in the blood (*see* Appendix B).

COUNSELING

Personal food choices

Eating behaviors are strongly ingrained and are not easy to change at any time. Pregnancy, however, is an ideal time to change behavior because of the client's motivation to give her child the best possible start in life.

Nutrition counseling must be consistent with the client's life-style: the client must be able to incorporate suggested changes into her eating patterns. Counseling must also be realistic: suggested changes must be acceptable to the client and must be of a kind to enable her to have a reasonable chance of success. If multiple changes are required, small, intermediate goals should be established for each visit. The following factors must be considered when providing nutritional counseling.

Economics. One of the main factors that influences eating behaviors is economics. It is of no use to suggest foods that the client cannot afford. One of the negotiable items in a family's budget is food: the rent must be paid and the bills must be paid, but it is possible to use cheap foods (regardless of nutritional value) to fill the stomach so that the money can be spent elsewhere. Although some inexpensive foods are nutritious, especially in combination with other inexpensive foods (e.g., beans and rice), it requires a great deal of knowledge and motivation to meet nutritional requirements on a low budget.

Culture/psychology. Food has different meanings for different people, and these must be considered when doing nutrition counseling. In the United States, people frequently think of milk as food for children, salads as foods for women, and meat and potatoes as food for men. Champagne and steak are foods for celebrations, sweet desserts are foods for reward, and chips or pretzels are foods for parties. Thus, foods have meanings that go far beyond their nutrient composition.

People tend to like familiar foods and to dislike unfamiliar foods (if they are even willing to try them). Foods that are characteristic of one's ethnic background may be more "comfortable" and can provide the nutrients required. Table 5-6 lists various foods that are characteristic of various ethnic groups.

Religion. Certain religious groups have dietary proscriptions. Some prohibit certain foods or foods in particular combinations. It is almost always possible to work within a client's religious constraints to achieve an adequate diet.

Vegetarianism. For a number of reasons — religious, ecological, economic, or personal — an increasing number of people are becoming vegetarians. Those who eat milk products and eggs (lacto-ovo-vegetarians) and those who eat milk products (lactovegetarians) are able (with careful planning) to meet most of their dietary requirements with the exception of iron, which requires a supplement. Diet planning must include the provision of complete protein. Most plant proteins are incomplete, i.e., they do not supply certain essential amino acids in adequate amounts for the body to synthesize the protein it requires. Consequently, the protein is used as energy and, therefore, is not available for functions that only protein can fulfill. Different plant proteins lack different amino acids, and they can be combined to provide the body with a complete set of amino acids for protein synthesis, or they can be used with animal proteins such as milk and eggs to provide complete protein. Table 5-7 gives a list of complementary plant protein combinations.

Vegans are vegetarians who consume neither milk products nor eggs. They have difficulty in meeting requirements for other nutrients that are found almost exclusively in animal products, such as vitamins D and B12. Vegans will need supplements of these vitamins and iron as well as careful meal planning to meet protein and calcium requirements.

Pica. Pica is the ingestion of nonfood substances such as clay, cornstarch, and refrigerator frost. The etiology of pica is not well understood, but it is frequently associated with iron deficiency anemia. Clients who have pica should be encouraged to substitute nutritious foods for nonfood substances they crave. Clients certainly should be encouraged to limit pica so it does not interfere with a good diet. Foods of similar taste or texture may help to satisfy the client's craving. Vitamin and mineral supplementation may be needed to treat deficiencies.

Personal preference. Personal preference plays an important role in dietary habits — both in foods consumed and in style of preparation. Personal preference must be considered if successful suggestions for dietary changes are to be made.

TABLE 5-6
Cultural Food Habits

Chinese

Milk. Considered luxury item, even disliked. Cheese rarely used. *Suggestions:* Encourage use of milk in cereals or steamed eggs (pudding). Encourage milk, cheese, ice cream, and bean curd.

Meat. Limited, mostly pork, fish, and eggs; some chicken, shellfish; sometimes excluded from diet of children. *Suggestions:* Encourage increased use of meat, fish, poultry, and eggs. Introduce "baby food meat" for children.

Vegetables and fruits. Spinach, broccoli, leeks, greens, bok toy (cabbage), carrots, pumpkin, sweet potatoes, mushrooms, soybeans, brussel sprouts, turnips, radishes, kohlrabi, white eggplant, yautia, eggplant, bamboo shoots, and snowpeas. Fruits considered a delicacy/snack food, some reserved for men. Common fruits: persimmons, peaches, plums, pears, large dates, apples, figs, winter melon, bananas, mango, red tangerines, papaya, pineapple, orange, litchee nuts, and small dates. *Suggestions:* Increased use of fruits or vegetables high in vitamin C as snack or "dessert."

Breads and cereals. Predominantly millet and rice; wheat products include noodles and steamed bread. *Suggestions:* Encourage use of brown rice.

Miscellaneous: Soybean oil, peanut oil, and lard are used. *Suggestions:* Affirm practice of limited use of fats but encourage liquid types.

Italian

Milk. Adults use little except in coffee. Seldom thought of as food. Children may or may not get recommended amounts. Cheese used frequently, and in preparation of cooked foods. *Suggestions:* Encourage use of milk for entire family. Greater use of dry skim milk and evaporated can be encouraged. Encourage wider use of cheeses at end of meal with fruit and in cooking.

Meat. Veal, beef, pork, and chicken are most popular. All parts are eaten, including organ meats. Highly seasoned meats are common. All kinds of fish, both fresh and canned, some fried in oil, used in stews or chowders. Eggs are liked, the most expensive grades preferred. Dried beans and peas are used in soups with pasta and served in salads. *Suggestions:* Encourage cooking methods other than frying. Discourage the use of highly seasoned fatty and fried meats for small children. Fish, eggs, dried peas and beans, and ricotta cheese make good meat substitutes.

Vegetables and fruits. Large quantities of escarole, swiss chard, mustard greens, dandelion greens, and broccoli are popular. Salads are part of most meals. Peppers and tomatoes are used in preparation of foods. Eggplant, zucchini, artichoke, mushrooms, and fava beans are favorites. Fruits liked: grapes, oranges, tangerines, figs, persimmons, and pomegranates. *Suggestions:* Less cooking time and less use of oil. Encourage use of canned tomatoes when fresh are out of season. Selection of fresh fruit in season and canned fruit juices when less expensive than fresh.

Breads and cereals. Pasta and rice are staples eaten each meal. Use of oatmeal and farina has increased. *Suggestions:* Encourage use of whole-grain bread.

Miscellaneous. Olive oil preferred for cooking. Lard and salt pork are flavoring for soups and tomato sauce. Butter preferred for baking. *Suggestions:* Urge families to use soybean, cottonseed, and corn oils.

Japanese

Milk. Fresh and canned milk is used in small amounts — in coffee and milk desserts (such as ice cream). Cheese is used in only small amounts. *Suggestions:* Encourage increased consumption of all forms of milk, including cheese.

Meat. Variety of salt and fresh water fish eaten, baked, boiled, and in soups. Raw fish consumed on occasion. Smoked, dried, and canned fish consumed. Beef, pork, and poultry preferred to lamb and veal, mixed with vegetables and seasoned with soy sauce. Eggs eaten raw, fried, boiled, scrambled, and in soups. *Suggestions:* Encourage use of highly nutritious variety of meats, hard and soft cheeses, and cottage cheese for protein. Discourage eating raw eggs. Use of pea and bean dishes as well as peanut butter can be encouraged.

Vegetables and fruits. Commonly used vegetables are spinach, broccoli, carrots, green beans, peas, cauliflower, tomatoes, cucumbers, eggplant, peppers, and squash. May be prepared with meat, fish, and chicken. Fruits eaten are oranges, tangerines, grapefruit, apples, pears, and melons. *Suggestions:* Encourage cooking procedures to preserve nutrients. Discourage par-cooking and draining of water. Emphasize use of fruits high in vitamin C.

Breads and cereals. Polished white rice is the staple. Consumption of wheat products is a post-World War II practice. *Suggestions.:* Encourage use of restored rice and discourage washing it before cooking. Suggest more frequent inclusion of potatoes cooked in skin in place of rice. Urge use of whole-grain breads and cereals.

Miscellaneous. Butter used in small amount. Fat used in food only for deep fat frying. Simple cakes and cookies of sugar and rice flour contain little or no fat. Seasonings are soy sauce or miso sauce. Pickles with high salt content eaten in variety. *Suggestions:* Seasonings and pickles should be used in moderation.

Jewish

Milk. Dietary laws prohibit using meat and milk at the same meal. (Six hours must elapse after a meat meal before dairy foods may be eaten; half an hour must elapse after a dairy food before meat may be eaten). Cheeses — American, muenster, and Swiss — well liked. Cottage cheese and pot cheese eaten plain or in blintzes and noodle puddings.

Suggestions: Encourage use of milk at breakfast and lunch times to ensure adequate milk intake. Explain that cream cheese is a fat, not a milk substitute and encourage cheeses high in protein and calcium.

Meat. Separate dishes and utensils must be used for preparing and serving meat and dairy products. Orthodox Jews use only the forequarters (rib section forward) of quadrupeds with a cloven hoof who chew their cud, i.e, cattle, sheep, goat, and deer. Animals and poultry must be slaughtered by a ritual slaughterer (shochet) according to specified regulations. Before cooking, meat is koshered by one of two methods: (1) soaking it in cold water for half an hour; salting it with coarse salt (koshering salt); and draining it to let blood run off. It is then thoroughly washed under cold running water and drained again before cooking. (2) Quick searing. Liver, for example, cannot be koshered by soaking and salting because of its high blood content. It is, therefore, rinsed, drained well, and broiled on a grill. It may then be fried, chopped, or combined with other foods. This second method is preferred for clients on salt-restricted diets. Meat is usually broiled, boiled, roasted, or stewed with vegetables added. Fish that have fins and scales may be used, such as whitefish (fresh and as gefilte fish), smoked sable, carp, lox (salmon), and caviar. Shellfish (such as oysters, crab, and lobster) and scavenger fish such as sturgeon and catfish are not allowed. Fish and eggs are considered "pareve" or neutral and may be eaten as dairy or meat. Eggs are eaten in abundance. An egg with a clot of blood must be discarded. Dried beans, peas, and lentils are eaten liberally, especially as soup. *Suggestions:* Discourage excessive use of delicatessen-type meats, such as corned beef, pastrami, and salami. Urge use of fish, cheese, and other sources of protein.

Vegetables and fruits. Greens, spinach, and sorrel leaves are used for soup (schav). Use is made of broccoli, carrots, chicory, sweet potatoes, and yams. Green peppers are often stuffed with meat or dairy mixture. Green cabbage is cooked slightly and stuffed with beef and raisin mixture with tomato sauce. Root vegetables and potatoes are liberally used. Noodles as a potato substitute are preferred to rice. Beets are used in soup (borscht). Orange or grapefruit is used for breakfast. Cooked dried fruits (prunes, raisins, apples, peaches, pears, and apricots) are commonly served with meat meals. *Suggestions:* Stress more variety in use of dark green, leafy and deep yellow vegetables. Their correct method of cooking is with small amount of water, covered pot, and short cooking time. Point out high caloric value of dried fruits.

Breads and cereals. Water rolls (bagel), rye bread, and pumpernickel are often used because they do not have milk or milk solids and, therefore, can be eaten with meat or dairy meals. They are considered "pareve." Matzoh, also "pareve," is the only bread product allowed during Passover, but is commonly used throughout the year. Whole grains such as oatmeal, barley, brown rice and buckwheat groats (kasha) are used. *Suggestions:* Encourage use of whole-wheat bread at dairy meals. Matzoh, crackers, and saltines are not enriched and make little contribution to diet, other than calories.

Miscellaneous. Sweet (unsalted) butter, usually whipped, is preferred to salted butter. Vegetable oils and shortenings are considered "pareve." Chicken fat is often the choice for browning meats and frying potato pancakes. Danish pastries, coffee cakes, and homemade cakes and cookies may be eaten in large quantities. Honey cakes are served for various holidays. There may be an overuse of relishes. Soup may be used at every meal. Soft drinks are served with meat meals when milk is forbidden. The code "U" on a package indicates it is permissible. If in doubt check with local rabbinical authorities. *Suggestions:* Encourage greater use of vegetable oils. Encourage desserts such as milk puddings, ice milk, and ice cream for dairy meals, and fruit with meat meals. Encourage soups high in daily nutrient needs. Discourage overuse of soft drinks.

Polish

Milk. Children drink fresh milk, whereas adults may prefer buttermilk. Sour cream is also popular and is used in soup, salad dressings, with berries, and raw vegetables. Cheese is well liked. Cottage cheese is well liked and may be served with sour cream. *Suggestions:* Encourage recommended intake of milk or milk products for whole family.

Meat. Meat commonly consumed: beef, pork, pigs' knuckles, sausages, smoked and cured pork, chicken, goose, duck, and variety meats (liver, tripe, tongue, brains). Small amounts used in soups and stews. Fish, fresh, smoked, dried, or pickled, is used. Eggs well liked and also used in pancakes, noodles, dumplings, and soups, along with legumes. *Suggestions:* For economy, greater use of meat substitutes and less expensive cuts of meats in the preparation of stews and soups. Greater amounts of meat may be desirable in mixed dishes.

Vegetables and fruits. Potatoes are a very important part of diet. Other popular vegetables include carrots, beets, turnips, cauliflower, kohlrabi, broccoli, sorrel, green pepper, peas, spinach, and green beans. Vitamin C-rich fruits are not traditionally popular, but citrus fruits may be used more today than in previous years. Dried fruits are liked. *Suggestions:* Encourage retention of vitamin A in use of broccoli, kale, sorrel, green peppers, raw cabbage, and fresh tomato in season. Canned and frozen citrus juices in off-season may be stressed for vitamin C. Encourage proper cooking methods for retention of vitamin C in vegetables. Stress use of root vegetables and fruits in season.

Breads and cereals. Bread eaten with each meal. Pumpernickel, sour rye bread, and white bread are well liked. Sweet buns are common. Oatmeal, rice, noodles, dumplings, cornmeal, porridge, and kasha are prominent. *Suggestions:* Encourage whole grains.

Miscellaneous: Wide variety of fats and oils are used. Fond of candy, sweet cakes, and other sweets such as honey. Coffee with cream and sugar is a favorite beverage. Tea is infrequent. Foods are highly salted and seasoned. *Suggestions:* More frequent use of fruits as desserts.

Puerto Rican

Milk. Milk may be used in insufficient quantities because of economic conditions rather than because it is not liked. Although milk may not be consumed as such, a cup of cafe con leche may contain 2 to 5 ounces of milk. The domestic American cheese is used in limited quantities. Native white cheese (resembling farmer cheese, but firmer and saltier) is used, but is expensive. *Suggestions:* Use of milk as a beverage and in cooking may need to be encouraged, including evaporated milk, nonfat dry milk, and in puddings and cereals. Greater emphasis can be placed on the use of cheese.

Meat. Chicken in combination with other foods is frequently eaten. Expensive cuts of pork and beef are usually fried. Ham butts and sausage are used to flavor different dishes. The intestine of the pig is eaten either fried (cuchifritos) or stewed with native vegetables (salcocho) and chick-peas. Fish is used in limited amounts. Salt codfish is common. Eggs used in cooking and fried and scrambled eggs are popular. Beans are eaten either cooked or served with rice daily. A sauce called "refrito" (green pepper, tomato, garlic, and lard) is served with beans and rice. Pigeon and chick-peas are popular. *Suggestions:* Variety meats may be used in increased amounts. Emphasize lean, tender, and lower cost cuts with slow-cooking methods. Suggest that use of cuchifritos be limited to holidays. Encourage larger quantities of vegetables and meat as well as peas in salcocho. More consumption of fresh, frozen, or canned fish. Greater use of eggs as a main dish and meat substitute. Suggest larger amounts of beans than rice. Milk, meat, chicken, cheese, or fish should be eaten with the bean meal for protein. Pigeon peas are more expensive than chick-peas, and chick-peas protein is almost as good as that of the soybean.

Vegetables and fruits. Expensive imported vegetables, such as yautia, apio, malanga, name, and plantain are frequently used. These viandas are high in starch and have fair amounts of B vitamins, iron, and vitamin C. Pumpkins, carrots, green pepper, tomatoes, and sweet potatoes are well liked. Pumpkin is used to thicken and flavor foods. Potatoes are eaten in small amounts in stews, soups, or are fried. Head lettuce, cabbage, fresh tomatoes, and onions are often salad ingredients. Long cooking of vegetables in stews is common. Imported fruits are used often. Fruit cocktail, canned pears, and peaches are liked. Peach, apricot, and pear nectar are commonly used. *Suggestions:* Encourage use of less expensive vegetables such as carrots, beets, yellow squash, and turnips. Root vegetables may be prepared and served in the same way as tubers (plantain, yautia, yucca, name). Urge the use of more cooked and raw green, leafy vegetables. Stress greater intake of other salad greens and cabbage. Emphasize correct cooking methods of vegetables: small amount of water, covered pot, and short time. Greater use of potatoes cooked in skin can be suggested. Greater amount of citrus juices, fresh, frozen, or canned can be used. Encourage use of bananas, pineapple, apples, and pears in season. Recommend use of fruits canned in light rather than heavy syrup.

Breads and cereals. Bread used in only small amounts. Plantain is often eaten in place of bread. French bread, rolls, and crackers are most frequent choices. Breakfast cereals — oatmeal, farina, cornmeal, and cornflakes — are increasing. Cereals are often cooked in milk instead of water. *Suggestions:* Encourage use of whole-grain breads and enriched or brown rice. Encourage cooking cereal in milk. Use of sugar-coated cereals should be discouraged.

Miscellaneous. Butter is used in small amounts on bread. Lard and salt pork are used for flavoring in large amounts. Olive oil is a favorite for salads. Sugar is liberally used in beverages and desserts. Cakes, pies, guava, orange and mango pastes, and boiled papaya preserves are favored between meals. Black malt beer is a favorite beverage, and is combined with beaten egg for convalescents and pregnant women. It contains a fair amount of iron and some B vitamins and is high in calories. Canned soups are often served as main dish. *Suggestions:* Suggest margarine in place of butter. Corn, cottonseed, or soybean oils in seasoning vegetables and other dishes rather than lard and salt pork. Encourage less frequent use of sugar. Recommend use of other nourishing beverages such as milk and fruit juices. Stress meal planning around a main dish made of a protein food rather than soups of low-protein value.

Southern United States

Milk. Limited amounts of milk are consumed. Buttermilk often preferred. Cheese is well liked in sandwiches and baked macaroni. *Suggestions:* Encourage use of evaporated and nonfat dry milk for both cooking and drinking, and greater use of cheese.

Meat. Chicken as "company" dish is enjoyed. Pork and variety meats are popular. Pigs' feet, hog jowls, ham hocks, cured ham, and heart are often eaten, stewed, boiled with vegetables, or fried. Spareribs are baked or barbecued. Lungs, kidneys, and brains are floured and fried. Chitterlings (intestines) are cut, dredged with cornmeal or flour, and fried crisp. Beef is used in hash or stewed with vegetables. Cured tongue is also eaten. Fish and shellfish, fresh, and canned, catfish dipped in cornmeal and fried, boiled shrimp, fried scallops, and fried, stewed, or raw oysters are popular. Game — rabbit, squirrel, opossum — are usually used in a stew. Eggs are usually fried. Legumes and nuts — dried black-eyed peas and beans cooked with salt pork — are a prominent part of meals. Peanuts and peanut butter are consumed. *Suggestions:* Emphasize the lean, economical cuts of meat and stress that salt pork and bacon are fats not meats. Encourage stewing, baking, roasting, and boiling as methods of cookery. Stress that white or brown eggs are equally nutritious, Grade B for cooking. Urge that milk or cheese be served with the "bean meal."

Vegetables and fruits. Vegetables are liked but few eaten raw. Leafy greens, turnips, greens, mustard greens, collards, cabbage, and green beans are cooked in water with bacon, ham hocks, or salt pork. The cooking liquid may be eaten with cornbread. Tomatoes, fresh and canned, white potatoes, sweet potatoes, fried, baked, or candied with syrup are popular.

Fruits, although little citrus fruit, may be eaten. Fruits in season are favorites in the summer. *Suggestions:* Discuss quick-cooking of vegetables in little water to save vitamins. Note that the addition of baking soda to water in which vegetables are cooked destroys the vitamins. Stress that cooked or raw vegetables should be served in addition to potatoes or legumes. Point out the value of fruits. For limited budgets, encourage serving citrus fruit or juice as well as cheaper grades of canned tomatoes, raw cabbage, "greens," and potatoes for vitamin C.

Breads and cereals. Few whole-grain cereals are used. Hominy grits with gravy, hot biscuits with molasses, and cornbread are eaten. White or polished rice cooked, combined with ham fat, tomatoes, onion, and okra is popular. Dumplings, pancakes, and hoecakes (originally baked on a hoe) are favorites. *Suggestions:* Teach the use of whole-grain breads and cereals. Stress the use of cooked cereals such as oatmeal. Emphasize inclusion of protein food such as meat or milk when casserole is served.

Miscellaneous. Bacon and salt pork are liberally used. Lard used for baking and frying. Butter for preparing desserts. Gravies are used generously. Sweets — cakes, cookies, pies, other pastries, and sweet breads — are popular. Molasses and cane syrup are employed as sweeteners. Ice cream, jams, and jellies are eaten. Soft drinks are consumed by children. *Suggestions:* Discourage the use of large amounts of bacon and salt pork where obesity and salt restrictions are factors. Suggest methods of cooking other than frying. Encourage the use of margarine and oil. Since rich desserts may tend to displace protective foods, especially in the low-income food budget, they should be used only in moderation. Excessive intake of sweets should be avoided, especially by small children.

Spanish American/Mexican

Milk. Milk use may be limited because of availability and economy. Limited amounts of cheese are used. *Suggestions:* Use various forms of milk in cooking, as a beverage — dried, evaporated, or fresh milk. Increase use of cheeses to improve quality of protein in diet.

Meat. Chicken, pork chops, weiners, cold cuts, and hamburgers usually used only once or twice a week. Eggs used, frequently fried. In rural areas, many have their own chickens. Beans are usually eaten with every meal, cooked, mashed, or refried with lard. *Suggestions:* Eggs are good meat substitute, and daily consumption is encouraged. Beans and lentils provide a good source of protein and calcium. Their protein is enhanced when eaten with animal proteins such as milk, meat, eggs, or cheese.

Vegetables and fruits. Fried potatoes are basic, maybe three times a day. Chilies from green and red peppers are popular each meal. These items are good sources of vitamin A even when dried. Green peppers are usually called "mangoes."

Fresh tomatoes are purchased all year and are the most popular vegetable. Occasionally, canned tomatoes are used. Pumpkin, corn, field greens, onions, and carrots are used frequently. Bananas, melons, peaches, and canned fruit cocktail are popular. Oranges and apples are used as snacks. *Suggestions:* Encourage wide variety of vegetables. Different cooking methods could be used. Encourage use of peppers but stress caution in home canning methods. Recommend a variety of fruit canned in light syrup as economical. Use of citrus fruits could be encouraged. Fruit drinks should not be substituted for fruit juices. Melons (cantaloupe in particular) are encouraged because of high vitamin C content.

Breads and cereals. Bread is a popular item. Tortillas from enriched wheat flour are made daily. Sweet rolls are purchased. Purchased bread for sandwiches in sack lunches is a status symbol. Breakfast cereals are usually the prepared type with emphasis on sugar. Occasionally, oatmeal is used. Fried macaroni is prepared and served with beans and potatoes. *Suggestions:* Continue use of enriched flour. In some sections where corn tortillas are used, encourage use of dried skim milk. Encourage whole-grain cereals. Cooked cereals are more economical. Encourage use of vegetables rather than excessive starch foods.

Miscellaneous. Lard, salt pork, and bacon fat are used liberally. Most foods are fried. Soft drinks, popsicles, and sweets of all kinds are used liberally. *Suggestions:* Encourage a variety of cooking procedures. Purchased cookies, soft drinks, and sweets are expensive and do not contribute to nutritional needs. Using more milk, ice cream, and juices would be helpful.

Reprinted with permission from Green, M. L., and J. Harry. Nutrition in Contemporary Nursing Practice. John Wiley & Sons, Inc., New York. 1981. p. 14-21.

TABLE 5-7

Complementary Plant Protein Sources

Food	Amino acids deficient	Complementary protein
Grains	Isoleucine Lysine	Rice + legumes Corn + legumes Wheat + legumes Wheat + peanut + milk Wheat + sesame + soybean Rice + sesame Rice + brewers' yeast
Legumes	Tryptophan Methionine	Legumes + rice Beans + wheat Beans + corn Soybeans + rice + wheat Soybeans + corn + milk Soybeans + wheat + sesame Soybeans + peanuts + sesame Soybeans + peanuts + wheat + rice
Nuts and seeds	Isoleucine Lysine	Peanuts + sesame + soybeans Sesame + beans Sesame + soybeans + wheat Peanuts + sunflower seeds
Vegetables	Isoleucine Methionine	Lima beans Green peas Brussel sprouts } + sesame seeds, brazil nuts, or mushrooms Cauliflower Broccoli Greens + millet or converted rice

Courtesy of the California Department of Health, Sacramento, Calif.

Discomforts of pregnancy. Three common discomforts of pregnancy may influence the amount and kinds of food ingested: nausea and vomiting, constipation, and heartburn. These discomforts must be considered when counseling a client about nutrition. (*See* Chapter 6 for specific dietary management of these problems.)

Family members. Most families share the same foods, regardless of whether meals are eaten together. The specific needs of other members of the family should be considered when making suggestions to the client. Pregnancy is an ideal time for improving the dietary habits of the mother. Frequently, the positive changes that she makes will influence the dietary habits of other members of the family.

Counseling methods

Counseling is an art in which there are many different methods and styles. One method or style that works for one client or clinician may not work for another. There are a number of educational materials available for nutrition assessment and counseling that may help some clients.

One frequently used method is based on food groups. Usually four food groups are used — dairy, meat, fruits/vegetables, and cereals/grains — although some clinicians subdivide these groups in an attempt to ensure that all nutrient requirements are accounted for. The client is advised to eat a specified number of servings from each of the food groups (*see* Fig. 5-5). She may need practice in determining particular foods belonging to each group and in devising menus that will meet the number of servings suggested. Charts showing foods contained in each group may be helpful for clients.

The food-groups method of counseling does have some drawbacks. A client who is not familiar with categorizing foods may make erroneous judgments about which foods belong in a group. It is possible for a client to make poor choices even though the number of servings in each group is met. For example, she could eat four servings of french fried potatoes as her vegetable requirement each day. It is important to stress that a wide variety of foods should be eaten in order to meet known requirements, and, perhaps, to meet some that are as yet unknown.

Another method of counseling, developed by Agnes Higgins, is being used successfully at the Montreal Diet Dispensary in Montreal, Canada. It is based on accurate assessment of the client's protein and calorie requirements (based on height, ideal weight, stage of gestation, nutritional intake, and identifiable high-risk factors) in comparison with her current protein and calorie intake. Intake is assessed by a very detailed and careful history, recorded in three parts to increase accuracy: client's sample meal pattern, average daily consumption of specific food items, and shopping habits. When need and intake are compared, specific corrections to the diet can be suggested that will meet the client's needs. The client is advised to "eat what you have always been eating, but add...." Frequent corrections include drinking a quart of milk a day, eating two eggs and an orange daily, and eating liver once a week. The client is informed of the need for protein for building both her own and the fetus's tissues, and of the need for calories to meet the energy requirements for growth and daily activities. She is reminded that she is eating for two and counseled to drink milk or eat certain foods for the fetus, since the fetus cannot yet eat for itself.

The Montreal Diet Dispensary method has been shown to be quite successful in terms of pregnancy outcome. Its major drawback is time — both the time required to learn the method and the time required for the careful assessment of needs and intake for each individual.

Various techniques for counseling may prove helpful. Some nutritionists have found that some clients respond to behavior-modification techniques, i.e., reward for success in changing habits. Others have used contracts, a similar concept, in which the client agrees to make specific changes for a specified time and, upon completion of the terms of the contract, she is given some reward. The reward may be something given by the clinic, or it may be something she gives herself (new shoes, a movie, etc.). Individual counseling usually allows more specific attention to an individual's needs, but some clients may respond better to a group situation in which they receive support from their peers. A combination of the two may be used.

Opportunities for nutrition education outside of specific counseling sessions may also be used. Some clinics or offices show films in the waiting room while clients are waiting to be seen. Others have educational posters on the walls or literature available in the waiting room. There is a large quantity of such materials available. (A partial listing is included at the end of this chapter.)

CLIENTS AT HIGH NUTRITIONAL RISK

A number of factors have been identified that place clients at high nutritional risk. Table 5-8 lists these factors, the nutritional problems they imply, and the suggested management for each.

RESOURCES

There are a number of resources available to help clients achieve good nutritional status during pregnancy: educational resources and resources for the provision of food. One of the biggest food resources is food stamps. Although the financial requirements for food

TABLE 5-8

Management of the Nutritionally High-Risk Client

Factor	Nutrition Problem	Management
Adolescence	Client is still growing, and therefore has high nutritional needs. Pregnancy superimposes additional nutritional demands. Many teenagers have poor dietary habits because of active life-style, habits of peers, or the desire to lose weight or stay slim. Studies show teenagers consistently have low intakes of iron, calcium, protein, and vitamin A.	Help client devise a diet plan that provides for demands of her own growth and that of the fetus. Use foods in the diet plan that are nutritious and acceptable to her peer group (e.g., milkshakes, hamburgers, and pizza).
Obesity	Client may have poor intake of certain nutrients because of ingestion of high-calorie, low-nutrient foods or because of an attempt to maintain or lose body weight during pregnancy through dietary restrictions.	Advise client to avoid attempts to lose or maintain weight during pregnancy. Use foods in the diet plan that supply other nutrients with calories. Avoid empty calories.
Poor obstetric history	Past obstetric history of abortions, pregnancy complications, low-birth-weight infants, or perinatal death may reflect poor nutritional status of the client. Poor obstetric history and/or close pregnancy spacing may serve to deplete the client's nutrient stores.	Develop a diet plan that provides extra protein, calories, and iron to replenish maternal stores as well as provide for herself and the fetus. (200 calories and 20 grams of protein in addition to normal pregnancy requirements are suggested by the Montreal Diet Dispensary).

Factor	Nutrition Problem	Management
Low income	A woman with low income may be unable to purchase enough foods of the right kinds to supply adequate nutrition for herself, her fetus, and the other members of her family.	Develop with the client a diet plan that uses low-cost, high-nutrient foods, such as peanut butter, organ meats, and fruits and vegetables in season. Provide referral or information regarding food stamps, WIC, or other food-assistance programs.
Underweight or insufficient weight gain in pregnancy	Inadequate weight gain and low prepregnancy weight have been associated with lowered birth weight, intrauterine growth retardation, and fetal/neonatal morbidity and mortality.	Encourage intake of adequate calories and other nutrients from the beginning of pregnancy, enough to compensate for underweight or failure to gain. Additional meals and/or nutritious snacks may be suggested.
Medical complications	Certain medical conditions may require dietary management that will affect the ingestion of specific nutrients: e.g., anemia, diabetes, hypertension, thyroid disorders, gastrointestinal disorders, liver or kidney disease, etc.	Encourage a diet that supplies adequate amounts of all the necessary nutrients for pregnancy. Compliance with requirements of the medical complication must be developed. Referral to a nutritionist may be helpful.
Dietary faddism	The client with unusual dietary regimens and/or pica may not be ingesting adequate nutrients.	Take time to plan for adequate nutrients within the restrictions of cultural or religious groups. Discourage dietary fads intended for

		weight loss. This is especially important during pregnancy. Discourage pica. Substituting nutritious foods of similar taste or texture may help. Any deficiencies (e.g., iron) should be treated.
Heavy smoking, drug addiction, or alcoholism	These habits cause physiological changes that may alter appetite and nutrient utilization. Interference with nutrition may result from failure to purchase and ingest nutritious foods.	Discourage use of drugs, tobacco, and alcohol during pregnancy. Referral to appropriate programs may help. Encourage a diet supplying adequate nutrients, eaten at regular intervals.
Psychological/ emotional stress	Stress may increase the need for certain nutrients: e.g., protein, calories, and B vitamins. Stress may also interfere with appetite, and thus result in reduced caloric and nutrient intake.	Encourage a diet supplying adequate nutrients, eaten at regular intervals. Additional protein, calories, and B vitamins may be required for severe stress.

WIC, supplemental food program for women, infants, and children.

stamps change annually, they can help low-income families. Food stamps have the advantage of allowing the client to select the foods she prefers. Social service departments can provide information on how to refer clients for food stamps in their local area.

The WIC (supplemental food program for women, infants, and children) program is a food-resource program sponsored by the United States Department of Agriculture. The program is administered by each state, so criteria and procedures vary from state to state. In general, the program provides specific foods for pregnant and lactating women, and for infants and children up to the age of 5 years. Foods include milk, eggs, orange juice, infant formula, and infant cereal. Eligibility criteria for the program include evidence of nutritional and economic need. The WIC program requires nutritional education of clients and continuing medical supervision. Some clients are motivated to seek or continue medical care in order to receive WIC program foods. It has been a widely used food resource program.

There are other food resources that may be available in each local community. Other government programs may supply food for some members of a family, which will allow the family to buy more food with their money. Two examples are the school lunch program for children and "Meals on Wheels" for elderly people. Frequently, churches or other groups will have food pantries to help families in crisis.

There are many educational resources available to help professionals and clients in nutrition assessment and counseling. A list of helpful materials is provided below. A much more extensive list may be found in Mary Lu Rang's "Bibliography for nutrition in pregnancy" (*[JOGN Nursing] Journal of Obstetric, Gynecologic and Neonatal Nursing* [1980]. 55-58.)

California Department of Health series: Nutrition for Pregnancy and Breastfeeding. California Department of Health, Sacramento.

Committee on Nutrition. 1974. Nutrition in Maternal Health Care. American College of Obstetricians and Gynecologists.

Luke, B. 1975. Nutrition during Pregnancy and Lactation. California Department of Health, Sacramento.

March of Dimes Birth Defects Foundation pamphlets:
Eating for Two
Be Good to Your Baby Before It Is Born
Nutrition and Pregnancy

Task Force on Nutrition. 1978. Assessment of Maternal Nutrition. American College of Obstetricians and Gynecologists.

U. S. Department of Agriculture. 1979. Food is More than Just Something to Eat. Bulletin No. 216. U. S. Department of Agriculture, Washington, D. C.

REFERENCES

1. Simpson et al.

2. Weiss and Jackson. 54-59.

3. Love and Kinch.

4. U. S. Department of Health, Education and Welfare. 1-24.

5. Papaevangelou et al.

6. Rosso and Winick.

7. Eastman and Jackson.

8. Churchill and Berendes. 30-35.

9. Varney. 127.

10. Beal. 153.

CHAPTER 6

COMMON DISCOMFORTS OF PREGNANCY

Kathleen Buckley

Complex maternal adaptations to pregnancy result in many new physical sensations, adjustments, and/or discomforts for most, if not all, pregnant women.[1] The client may perceive them on an emotional continuum that ranges from annoying to frightening. If not addressed by the health care team, these discomforts may ultimately result in an alteration of the client's self-image from that of a healthy woman experiencing a natural, joyous process to that of an ill woman with a "disease." For this reason it is crucial for the client to understand the etiology of any discomfort she may experience and to be aware of the relief measures that may alleviate it. Furthermore, it is important for the nurse to be able to differentiate a common discomfort from other associated pathologies that may develop or be exacerbated by pregnancy. This chapter, then, discusses the etiology, nursing relief measures, and associated pathologies of the most common discomforts of pregnancy. (The discomforts are listed in alphabetical order.)

BLEEDING GUMS

Etiology

During pregnancy, the blood flow to the gums and oral mucous membranes is increased. It is thought that increased estrogen and/or progesterone levels cause proliferation of small blood vessels in the corium of the interdental papillae.[2] In addition, elevated estrogen levels act on the adhesiveness of collagen fibers, resulting in "spongy" gums. Thus, the gums may bleed easily.

A highly vascular growth (epulis) may develop from hypertrophy of interdental papillae. These growths may bleed profusely or interfere with chewing. In rare cases, surgery may be necessary. However, epulis regresses spontaneously after delivery.

Nursing relief measures

1. Explain the cause of the discomfort to the client.
2. Reassure the client that this condition will completely regress after delivery.
3. Discuss dental care and hygiene measures:
    a. Brush teeth very gently with a *soft* brush.
    b. Avoid eating foods that traumatize the gums (e.g., apples and corn on the cob).
    c. Use dental floss or Water Pic regularly.

Associated pathology

The nurse should be aware of the client's dental history for pre-existing gum disease. A client with chronic gingivitis may need dental referral. The client's nutritional status should be assessed: a vitamin C deficiency predisposes the client to bleeding gums. In addition, the client's hematologic status should be assessed: in some clients, persistent, unexplained anemia is due solely to bleeding gums.

CONSTIPATION

Etiology

Increased progesterone levels act on the smooth muscle of the bowel and decrease peristalsis. In the second and third trimesters, the mechanical compression and displacement of the bowel by the uterus may also contribute to constipation. Prenatal iron therapy may exacerbate this problem for many women.

Nursing relief measures

1. Explain the possible causes of the discomfort to the client.
2. Evaluate the diet and advise the following measures:
    a. Increase fluid intake to eight glasses of water daily.
    b. Add sources of roughage and fiber to the diet (e.g., bran, whole-grain breads, fruit, celery, and lettuce).

    c. Add a natural laxative (prunes or a small glass of prune juice) to the diet daily.
3. Encourage daily exercise. Walking is probably the most effective muscle toner.
4. Discuss bowel habits and advise the following:
    a. Establish a regular time of day for having a bowel movement.
    b. Provide for privacy and a sufficient uninterrupted time for having the bowel movement.
    c. Never ignore the "urge" to have a bowel movement. Warm liquids (water or herb tea) may stimulate this sensation.
5. Ensure that mild laxatives, stool softeners, and/or suppositories are used only when natural methods have proven ineffective.
6. Evaluate iron therapy regimen. A modified iron supplement like Ferro-Sequels, which contains a stool softener, may be effective.

Associated pathology

The client should not use mineral oil as a laxative during pregnancy because it interferes with the absorption of fat-soluble vitamins.

DEPENDENT EDEMA

Etiology

As pregnancy progresses, the uterus presses on the pelvic veins and inhibits optimal venous return, which causes edema of the ankles and feet.

Nursing relief measures

1. Explain the cause of the discomfort to the client.
2. Instruct the client to elevate her legs periodically during the day (e.g., four times a day for 15 minutes) (Fig. 6-1).
3. Urge her to avoid sitting or standing for long periods of time. For the working client who is desk-bound, advise getting up to walk around her desk every hour. If the client needs to travel, advise frequent stops to walk and stretch. The client who must stand for long periods needs to sit down and elevate her legs.
4. Advise her to avoid constrictive clothing, especially knee-high stockings that bind just below the knee and inhibit venous return.
5. Suggest sleeping on her left side, which enhances renal blood flow and venous return.

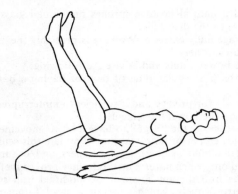

Figure 6-1. Position in which to reduce dependent edema and varicosities.

6. Emphasize that fluids and salt intake are *not* to be restricted. She should continue with eight glasses of water daily and she should salt to taste.

Associated pathology

The nurse should be aware of the difference between dependent edema and edema associated with pregnancy-induced hypertension (preeclampsia-eclampsia), cardiac disease, or renal disease (*see* Chapters 15 and 17). The nurse should also be aware of the client's nutritional status — specifically her protein intake: protein deficiency may manifest itself with edema.

DYSPAREUNIA

Etiology

Painful intercourse during pregnancy may have many psychological and/or physical origins. For example, couples may feel that they will somehow damage the growing fetus. Also, throughout pregnancy, women experience wide swings in libido. The resulting tensions may produce dyspareunia.

In the third trimester, the woman's inability to find a comfortable position may be the cause. Impaired venous return produces pelvic and vaginal congestion. Vulvar varicosities may also cause discomfort.

Nursing Relief Measures

1. Investigate the cause of dyspareunia.
2. Relief measures will depend on causative factors.
3. Emphasize the importance of communication between the couple.
4. Reassure the couple about the safety of coitus for the healthy pregnant woman.
5. Discuss alternative coital positions, such as the female superior, rear entry, or side-lying positions (*see* Fig. 3-4).
6. Explore alternatives to coitus, such as solitary or mutual masturbation, oral-genital sex, or anal intercourse.

Associated pathology

The nurse should be aware of the possibility of vaginitis as the cause of this discomfort.

DYSPNEA AND SHORTNESS OF BREATH

Etiology

Whereas the respiratory rate does not change during pregnancy, the volume of air inspired and/or expired with each normal breath (tidal volume) increases dramatically. This produces a state of "over breathing" or hyperventilation, which results in a lowered partial pressure of arterial carbon dioxide (30 to 32 mmHg). It is thought that progesterone may act directly on the respiratory centers to produce this physiological alteration.[3]

An increased awareness of the desire to breathe is common (70 percent) during pregnancy, and the client may interpret this as dyspnea.[4] Dyspnea may occur at any time during pregnancy. In many cases, it begins in the first trimester. Thus, it is not related to uterine size or activity. In the third trimester, the uterus may elevate the diaphragm as much as 4 centimeters. This, too, may cause a heightened consciousness of breathing or a slight shortness of breath because it may interfere with full expansion of the lungs.

Nursing relief measures

1. Explain the cause of the discomfort to the client.
2. Encourage good posture to allow for full expansion of the lungs (e.g., keep shoulders back and sit straight).
3. Emphasize continuation of normal activities of daily living and moderate exercise routines.

Associated pathology

Because asthma may have its initial onset during pregnancy, the nurse should be aware of the pulmonary status of the client who complains of dyspnea.

EPISTAXIS

Etiology

Blood flow to the nasal turbinates and septum is increased during pregnancy. Thus, epistaxis (nosebleed) is common. It is usually transient and harmless, involving rupture of small, superficial arteries. Epistaxis may be life-threatening, however, if the sphenopalatine branch of the internal maxillary artery is ruptured.

Nursing relief measures

1. Explain the cause of the discomfort to the client.
2. Emphasize that nasal passages should be cleared very gently by blowing passively into a tissue. One should never pick or poke the nasal mucous membranes.
3. In winter, the nasal passageways may become dry and brittle due to a lack of moisture in heated room air. Advise the use of a humidifier. A pan of water placed on top of a radiator will have the same effect.
4. If epistaxis occurs, advise the following measures:
   a. Apply pressure to both nares.
   b. Lower the head between the knees.
   c. Place an ice pack on the nape of the neck.
   d. Seek medical attention if the bleeding does not subside within 3 to 5 minutes.

Associated pathology

Frequent episodes of epistaxis may decrease iron stores. The nurse, therefore, should check the client's hematocrit level.

FATIGUE (FIRST TRIMESTER)

Etiology

Fatigue is a common problem during the first trimester. Although the causes are unknown, several theories have been proposed. Elevated levels of estrogen, progesterone, or human chorionic gonadotrophin may directly cause a sense of lethargy, or these hormones may produce the nausea and vomiting ("morning sickness") of the first trimester, which, then, affect general well-being.

In addition, ambivalence about pregnancy — a normal psychological response in the first trimester — may increase tension, which will, in turn, produce fatigue.

Nursing relief measures

1. Explain the possible causes of the fatigue to the client.
2. Explore her feelings concerning the pregnancy.
3. Explore the client's sleeping patterns. Advise her to maintain frequent rest periods during the day and get adequate sleep at night.
4. Reassure the client of the limited nature of this discomfort. (It usually abates by the beginning of the second trimester.)
5. Explain relief measures for morning sickness (*see* p. 175).

Associated Pathology

The psychosocial or economic status of the client may be the basis of her tension, strain, or depression. Consequently, the nurse should be aware of the need for social service counseling or psychiatric referral. Because poor nutritional status and/or anemia may also be the source of fatigue, the nurse should be aware of the client's nutritional status and check her hematocrit level.

FATIGUE/INSOMNIA (THIRD TRIMESTER)

Etiology

There are many causes of sleep disturbances in the third trimester. For example, the pregnant woman may not be able to find a comfortable position because of her enlarged abdomen. (Women who have habitually slept in a prone position are particularly uncomfortable.) In addition, fetal movements are notoriously nocturnal: as soon as the woman has settled down for the night, the baby begins to move. Nocturia may occur two or three times nightly. Late in pregnancy, many clients tend to decrease exercise and rest more. They may not be physically tired in the evening. Anticipation and anxiety about the impending labor and birth of the baby may also cause insomnia.

Nursing relief measures

1. Explore the possible causes of insomnia with the client.
2. Suggest a warm bath and/or a warm drink (e.g., milk or herb tea with honey) before bedtime.
3. Decrease the fluid intake after dinner for the client with

nocturia. (Counsel maintenance of adequate fluid intake during the day.)

4. Urge the client to maintain exercise and activity patterns of daily living. Walking is probably the best exercise late in pregnancy.

5. Teach the use of the side-lying (Sims's) position with a pillow propped between the legs, or have the client place two pillows under her head and one pillow under her knees (semi-Fowler's position).

Associated pathology

The nurse should explore the client's psychosocial milieu in order to understand the possible causes of her insomnia (which is a major symptom of depression).

FLATULENCE

Etiology

Flatulence, like constipation, is caused by the decreased peristalsis that results from increased progesterone levels, which relax smooth muscle in the bowel. In the second and third trimesters, the mechanical compression of the bowel by the growing uterus may contribute to this problem.

Nursing relief measures

1. Explain the cause of the problem to the client.
2. Explain relief measures for constipation (see p. 164).
3. Suggest avoidance of gas-forming foods.
4. Explore the client's activities of daily living. Sedentary clients are more prone to develop flatulence. Encourage some form of exercise and frequent position changes.

HEADACHE

Etiology

Pregnancy-related circulatory changes predispose the client to headaches. Vasodilation, increased blood volume, and/or increased cardiac output have been cited as the possible causes. The pain is described as dull, aching, or pounding.

The hyperemia and congestion of the nasal turbinates during pregnancy may produce discomfort similar to sinusitis. During pregnancy, subtle visual changes that result in eye strain also occur.

The most common form of headache at any time in the life cycle is that related to intermittent contraction of the muscles of the head and neck. A dull, bandlike, persistent pain is characteristic of "tension" headaches.

Nursing relief measures

1. Elicit the characteristics of the discomfort.
2. Relief measures depend on the type of discomfort:
   a. Vascular headache: encourage bed rest on her left side to enhance circulation.
   b. Sinusitis: advise a source of humidity in the client's home. In winter, a pan of water on a radiator in the bedroom is very effective. Warm, steamy showers may bring temporary relief.
   c. Eye strain: if the client has prescription glasses, urge her to wear them. She should not watch television in a dark room for long periods. Light in the room will reduce strain.
   d. Tension or muscle strain: investigate possible causes of tension and deal with specific problems. Advise rest in a quiet room with a warm glass of milk or herb tea with honey. Gentle effleurage may be helpful.
3. If necessary, prescribe acetaminophen, 325 to 650 milligrams orally every 6 hours.

Associated Pathology

Severe, continuous headache pain, with or without neurological signs, may be a symptom of many illnesses. The client with recurrent complaints of headache should be followed closely.

HEARTBURN

Etiology

Reflux of gastric contents into the esophagus produces heartburn — a common discomfort of pregnancy that occurs in perhaps 50 percent of all clients.[5] Symptoms usually begin in the second or third trimester.

Several physiological changes combine to overcome the normal barrier between the stomach and the esophagus, causing a gastroesophageal reflux. High circulating levels of progesterone reduce the tone of the esophageal sphincter. Progesterone also acts on the smooth muscle in the stomach, causing delayed emptying of stomach contents. The enlarged uterus encroaches on the stomach, upsetting the normal negative pressure gradient between the stomach and the esophagus.

Nursing relief measures

1. Explain the possible causes of the heartburn to the client.
2. Discuss the following dietary interventions:
   a. Eat six small meals daily, spaced over short time periods, rather than three large meals, which may overload the stomach.
   b. Drink a small glass of milk between meals and at bedtime to reduce acidity of the gastric contents.
   c. Avoid spicy, greasy, and fatty foods.
   d. Avoid orange juice, tomato juice, tomato paste, chocolate, and cigarette smoking because they decrease esophageal sphincter tone.
   e. Avoid large meals before bedtime.
3. Advise the client to avoid wearing clothing with a tight waist band.
4. Suggest that the client sleep with her head on two pillows to allow gravity to enhance esophageal functioning.
5. Teach a specific medication schedule for antacids (when appropriate).
6. Counsel the client to avoid Tums, Rolaids, and Alka-Seltzer because of their high sodium content.

Associated pathology

Esophagitis and hiatal hernia may also produce heartburn. Continuous use or an overdose of antacids may actually increase the amount of gastric acids. The client should be carefully instructed regarding the safe and effective dosage schedule for the specific antacid being used.

HEMORRHOIDS

Etiology

Hemorrhoids are dilated or varicose veins in the anal area. Progesterone causes relaxation or dilation of all vein walls, including those in the anal region, which encourages venous pooling. Hemorrhoids are also related to increased pressure in the hemorrhoidal veins secondary to obstruction of venous return by the enlarged uterus.[6] Another major cause of obstructed venous return is constipation.

Nursing relief measures

1. Explain the causes of hemorrhoids to the client.
2. Explain the relief measures for constipation (*see* p. 164).

3. Suggest using chilled witch hazel compresses to reduce the size and relieve the discomfort of hemorrhoids.
4. Urge avoidance of long periods of standing or sitting.
5. For moderate to severe hemorrhoids, teach the client to elevate her hips and lower extremities several times a day and at nighttime.
6. Suggest the use of topical anesthetics like Anusol.
7. Teach the client to replace internal hemorrhoids after each bowel movement.

Associated pathology

Bleeding from hemorrhoids may be sufficient to cause anemia. The nurse, consequently, should be aware of the client's hematologic status. Severe hemorrhoidal pain may indicate thrombosis of a hemorrhoidal vein.

LEG CRAMPS

Etiology

Muscle cramps of the thighs, calves, and feet are common during pregnancy. It is thought that a disturbance of the calcium:phosphorous ratio predisposes the client to muscle spasms. The pregnant uterus may also impede circulation or compress major nerves in the lower leg, especially in the sedentary client.

Nursing relief measures

1. Explain the possible causes of the discomfort to the client.
2. Advise the client to either increase or decrease her calcium and phosphorus intake to four servings of dairy products daily.
3. Review the client's diet history. A client with lactose intolerance (an allergy to dairy products, resulting in nausea or vomiting) may need a calcium supplement (e.g., calcium carbonate, 600 milligrams orally three times daily).
4. Teach the client to dorsiflex her foot if cramping occurs.
5. Urge daily exercise (e.g., walking or swimming) to improve circulation.

Associated pathology

The client should be evaluated for signs of thrombophlebitis: redness, heat, swelling, tenderness, or a positive Homans's sign requires careful assessment.

LEUKORRHEA

Etiology

Throughout the pregnancy, high estrogen levels cause increased production of cervical mucus, resulting in increased vaginal secretions (leukorrhea).

Nursing relief measures

1. Explain the cause of the discomfort to the client.
2. Teach the client vaginal hygiene measures:
   a. Wear cotton underwear and change them several times a day.
   b. Avoid washing too frequently; bathe or shower no more than once daily.
   c. Maintain clean, dry skin by using cornstarch.
   d. *Do not douche during pregnancy.*

Associated pathology

Increased vaginal secretions provide a medium for the growth of organisms that cause vaginitis. Complaints of itching, burning or malodorous discharge should be evaluated carefully.

LOW BACK PAIN

Etiology

Pain in the lumbosacral region of the spine is related to postural changes that compensate for the enlarged uterus. The added abdominal weight shifts the center of gravity backward, thereby causing a progressive lordosis. The spinal curvature stretches and strains the back muscles, resulting in backache.

Nursing relief measures

1. Explain the cause of the discomfort to the client.
2. Encourage good posture.
3. Teach body mechanics (*see* Fig. 3-3) (e.g., stoop, rather than bend, to lift objects; and, when arising from a supine position, turn on the side and push weight up with both hands instead of using back muscles to sit up).
4. Teach the client the pelvic rock exercises (*see* Fig. 3-2).
5. Instruct the client to wear supportive low-heeled shoes (high-heeled shoes exaggerate lordosis).
6. For sleeping, suggest the side-lying (Sims's) position with a

pillow propped between her knees. A firm mattress will give better support.

7. The multipara may have lax abdominal muscles, which exacerbate the postural changes. Suggest a source of external support (e.g, a maternity girdle).

Associated pathology

The onset of many back problems may be traced to pregnancy. To prevent back problems, the nurse must stress the importance of good posture and proper body mechanics during pregnancy (*see* Fig. 3-3). In addition, the client should be assessed for kidney disease and uterine contractions: back pain may be a sign of pyelonephritis or labor.

MORNING SICKNESS

Etiology

Although the causative factors of morning sickness are unknown, several theories have been advanced. These include hormonal changes in pregnancy, ambivalence about the pregnancy, a decrease in vitamin B complex, orthostatic vascular changes, and/or slowed intestinal peristalsis. Morning sickness is a common problem in the first trimester of pregnancy. Nausea, with or without vomiting, is most likely to occur when the stomach is empty — hence the name "morning sickness." It can occur, however, at any time during the day or night.

Nursing relief measures

1. Explain the possible cause of the discomfort to the client.
2. Reassure her about the limited nature of the discomfort.
3. Recommend the following dietary modifications:
   a. Take an adequate amount of vitamin B complex daily. (Prenatal vitamins provide 100 percent of the requirements.) Liver and other organ meats are important food sources of all B vitamins.
   b. Eat three or four dry crackers before sitting up in bed in the morning.
   c. Restrict fat in the diet.
   d. Avoid greasy, fatty, and spicy foods.
   e. Eat six small meals rather than three large meals daily.
   f. Have a bedtime snack. (Suggestion: herb tea with honey or a glass of warm milk with wheat toast and a small amount of jelly [no butter].)

4. Advise the client to arise from bed slowly in the morning to minimize orthostatic vascular changes. In addition, she should plan her morning so that she does not have to rush.

Associated pathology

Persistent nausea or vomiting beyond the first trimester may indicate hyperemesis gravidarum or hydatidiform mole. The client should be carefully assessed for serious complications, such as weight loss, ketosis, a drop in the hematocrit level, and electrolyte imbalance.

NASAL CONGESTION

Etiology

Increased blood flow to the nasal turbinates and septum not only increases the likelihood of epistaxis but also causes nasal congestion.

Nursing relief measures

1. Explain the cause of the discomfort to the client.
2. Advise the use of a humidifier — especially in winter, when heated room air tends to dry mucous membranes and exacerbate the feeling of nasal stuffiness. A pan of water placed on top of a radiator is an effective source of humidity.
3. Suggest a warm, steamy shower for temporary relief.
4. Urge the client to maintain hydration status.

Associated pathology

The client should be advised to avoid over-the-counter nasal sprays because they may *increase* nasal congestion if used incorrectly.

PRURITUS

Etiology

Pruritus, generalized itching without any eruptions, occurs in some pregnancies. Although the cause is unknown, it is thought to be the result of some alteration in liver or gallbladder functioning. Pruritus disappears after delivery.

Nursing relief measures

1. Explain the possible cause of pruritus to the client.
2. Reassure her about the limited nature of the condition.

3. Suggest a daily bath or shower with liberal applications of a moisturizing cream if her skin tends to be dry. The use of one half cup of baking soda or cornstarch in a warm bath may also provide relief.
4. Advise the following dietary regimen:
   a. Take prenatal vitamins daily.
   b. Drink four glasses of milk daily to maintain protein and calcium levels.
   c. Decrease fat in the diet.

Associated pathology

The client's liver function tests should be evaluated in order to rule out other forms of disease. In addition, this complaint should be differentiated from other dermatologic disorders.

PTYALISM

Etiology

True ptyalism is an unusual condition in which as much as 2 liters of saliva are produced each day. Mild versions of ptyalism are sometimes seen in normal pregnancy. The cause is unknown and the discomfort disappears after delivery.

Nursing relief measures

1. Reassure the client about the limited nature of the condition.
2. Advise her to use astringent mouthwashes and to suck on hard candies frequently during the day.

Associated pathology

The client should be assessed for the presence of nausea, vomiting, and weight loss — serious side effects of ptyalism. In addition, the client should be evaluated for pica habits: ingestion of large amounts of starch may produce excessive salivation.

ROUND LIGAMENT PAIN

Etiology

The body of the uterus is supported by round ligaments. The ligaments attach to the side of the uterus just below the fallopian tube, pass through the inguinal canal, and terminate in the labia majora.

As the uterus grows, the ligaments stretch. Round ligament pain is thought to be a result of this stretching. Clients may describe a "stitch in the side," which may be severe enough to cause discontinuation of activity. Typically, the pain radiates into the inguinal area.

Nursing relief measures

1. Explain the cause of the discomfort to the client.
2. Reassure her that this discomfort is a normal part of pregnancy.
3. Teach the client to bend toward the side that is painful. This may help relieve the stretching sensation in an acute attack.
4. Suggest the use of a warm bath or a heating pad to help relieve the feeling of soreness after an attack.

Associated pathology

The client should be assessed in order to rule out appendicitis or gallbladder disease.

SUPINE HYPOTENSION SYNDROME

Etiology

Supine hypotension syndrome is normally restricted to the third trimester. When the client assumes a supine position, the heavy, gravid uterus may cause occlusion of the venae cavae and aortic compression, thereby causing the client to complain of dizziness, nausea, or faintness.

Nursing relief measures

1. Explain the cause of the discomfort to the client.
2. Advise the client to turn on her side to relieve compression.

Associated pathology

If the condition is allowed to continue, blood flow to the uterus is decreased and fetal oxygenation is impaired. For this reason, in the third trimester and during labor, it is important for the nurse to minimize the amount of time that the client must be in the supine or the lithotomy position.

TINGLING AND NUMBNESS OF THE FINGERS

Etiology

Compression of the median nerve causes symptoms of numbness or tingling in the thumb, index, middle, and ring fingers (but not of the little finger). The cause of the compression is thought to be either edema in the wrist and hands or poor upper body posture, which places pressure on the nerve higher up in the arm. The discomfort disappears after delivery.

Nursing relief measures

1. Explain the possible causes of the discomfort to the client.
2. Reassure her that the symptoms will disappear after delivery.
3. Encourage good upper body posture (e.g., shoulders straight and head up).
4. Suggest raising the affected arm to the waist when walking or sitting. Flexing her fingers when her arms are at her side will enhance circulation.
5. Advise the client to avoid sleeping on the affected arm.

Associated pathology

Digital edema may be a sign of impending toxemia as well as of cardiac, renal, or hepatic disease. The nurse should observe the client carefully.

URINARY FREQUENCY/NOCTURIA

Etiology

Urinary frequency occurs most often in the first trimester and then again in the third trimester. In the first trimester, the small, but growing, uterus exerts direct pressure on the maternal bladder. As the uterus grows upward into the abdomen, this pressure is relieved. During the third trimester, the presenting part encroaches on the maternal bladder and diminishes its capacity.

In addition to these physiological causes of urinary frequency, there is also a physiological basis for nocturia. When a pregnant woman lies down, venous return from the lower extremities is facilitated and kidney perfusion is enhanced. Thus, urinary output is increased.

Nursing relief measures

1. Explain the cause of the discomfort to the client.
2. For nocturia, suggest decreasing fluids after dinner (while maintaining total fluid intake).

Associated pathology

The client should be carefully assessed in order to rule out urinary tract infection and/or stress incontinence (*see* Chapter 15).

VARICOSITIES

Etiology

Varicose veins tend to be a familial or a genetic trait. A woman is more likely to develop this problem if her mother or father also had it. Veins become engorged and dilated because the valve apparatus of the superficial venous system of the lower limbs is congenitally faulty or weak. Pregnancy aggravates the problem by impeding normal venous return from the legs because of the pressure of the gravid uterus on the pelvic veins (Fig. 6-2). In addition, high levels of progesterone cause further relaxation of vein walls and valves. Vulvar varicosities may cause discomfort during pregnancy. Although varicosities tend to decrease markedly or disappear after delivery, the damaged valves do not return to normal functioning.

Nursing relief measures

1. Explain the cause of the discomfort to the client.
2. Depending on the location and severity of the varices, the client must wear either maternity support hose, prescription elastic stockings, or thigh-high Ace bandages. Teach her to apply them

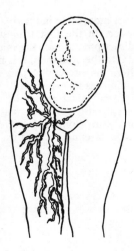

Figure 6-2. Pregnancy-aggravated varicose veins. The gravid uterus impedes normal venous return because of pressure on the pelvic veins. (*See* Fig. 6-1 for relief measure.)

before getting out of bed in the morning to enhance their effectiveness.
3. Urge the client to avoid the following:
   a. Crossing her legs.
   b. Long periods of sitting or standing.
   c. Constrictive hose or garters.
4. Encourage moderate exercise to enhance circulation.
5. Teach the client to elevate her legs several times during the day and to sit with her legs elevated. Whenever possible, the client with vulvar varicosities should also elevate her hips with a pillow.
6. Suggest the use of a sanitary napkin held in place by belt to support vulvar varicosities.
7. For severe varicosities, suggest the use of foot blocks to elevate the foot of her bed.

Associated pathology

Varicosities may rupture or become inflamed at any time during pregnancy. The client should be taught the signs and symptoms of thrombophlebitis, and she should return for medical attention if she suspects this problem.

REFERENCES

1. Jensen and Bobak. 1.
2. Burrow and Ferris. 277.
3. Pritchard and MacDonald. 240.
4. Burrow and Ferris. 557.
5. Burrow and Ferris. 294.
6. Pritchard and MacDonald. 324.

CHAPTER 7

DETERMINATION OF FETAL STATUS

Sister Rose Scalone

The United States has witnessed a sharp reduction in perinatal mortality since 1950. A few of the advances in the last decade that have contributed to the continued reduction of perinatal mortality are the introduction and acceptance of multifactorial risk assessment (*see* Chapter 8), biochemical and biophysical fetal monitoring, regionalization of perinatal care, and the increased availability of educational opportunities in perinatal nursing. The importance of the team approach for identification and management of those common problems that create risks for the perinate has been recognized and accepted by all perinatal specialists.

Determination of fetal status, including assessment of placental functioning, is an important part of prenatal care. Maternal and child health nurses, nurse-midwives, and perinatal nurse specialists play an active role in the clinical assessment of fetal status, in preparing the pregnant woman for specific tests, in assisting with some of these tests, in conducting tests such as the nonstress test (NST) and the contraction stress test (CST), in helping to interpret the results of these tests to the pregnant woman and her family, and in coordinating her plan of care based on the status of her fetus.

CLINICAL ASSESSMENT OF FETAL STATUS

First prenatal visit

The first prenatal visit is one of the most important visits for the pregnant woman because a historical, physical, and laboratory data base is established that will help in the determination and evaluation of the course of her pregnancy and the fetal status. Because there is so much information to be obtained, this is often the longest visit (1 to 2 hours). A more thorough discussion of the information obtained during this visit is detailed in Chapter 3.

Estimation of gestational age

The importance of obtaining a reliable estimate of the period of gestation during the first prenatal visit must be reiterated. The correct estimation of the period of gestation must be known before fetal status can be evaluated with any degree of accuracy. The earlier the woman seeks prenatal care, the more reliable the estimate of gestational age will be.

General factors to remember for estimating weeks of gestation

1. In the determination of the last *normal* menstrual period (LNMP), a menstrual history must be obtained, including the interval, duration, and amount of flow.
2. The number of weeks of gestation (according to specific dates) is most easily and quickly determined by using a gestational calculator (Fig. 7-1). The gestational calculator is usually based on a 28-day cycle. Therefore, correction must be made for those women whose cycles are shorter or longer than 28 days. Table 7-1 illustrates the procedure for the use of the gestational calculator.
3. The client's contraceptive history should also be charted (taking special care to note when oral contraceptives were discontinued).
4. The clinical evaluation should include the following information:
   a. date of the first positive pregnancy test,
   b. size of the uterus on bimanual examination,
   c. date of quickening, and
   d. date that the fetal heart tones are first heard with a fetoscope.
5. All of the above information should be recorded clearly and concisely (Fig. 7-2).
6. If the LNMP is unknown and/or there is a discrepancy of 3 weeks or more between the calculated gestational date and the clinical evaluation, an ultrasonogram should be considered for biparietal measurements between the 20th and 30th weeks of gestation.

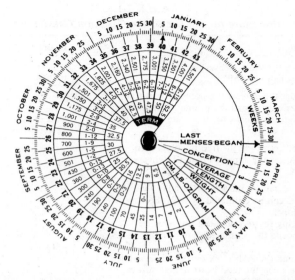

Figure 7-1. The gestational calculator. Refer to Table 7-1 for the procedure for its use. (Courtesy of Mead Johnson & Co., Evansville, Ind.)

Continued assessment of fetal status on revisits

During each subsequent prenatal visit, careful assessment should be focused on the pregnant woman's physical health (*see* Chapter 3) and on the fetal status. The latter is accomplished by careful abdominal examination, including auscultation of fetal heart tones (*see* Chapter 1), and by checking on the woman's continued perception of fetal movement. Through careful abdominal examination, conditions that need further follow-up assessment or care can be detected (Table 7-2).

Fetal movement

Fetal movement (FM) is a reliable test of fetal well-being and is also useful for determining when further evaluation is necessary (e.g., ultrasound, NST or CST, or a biophysical profile). Maternal perception of FM is subjective but usually quite accurate. All pregnant women should be taught how to count FMs, especially those women with high-risk pregnancies. The pregnant woman should be

TABLE 7-1

Procedure for the Use of the Gestation Calculator*

Procedure	Example
1. Place the "last menses" arrow at the *first* day of the LNMP.	LNMP = 4/1
2. Under the date of the prenatal visit (the outer edge), read the estimated number of gestational weeks for that date (found on the outer wheel).	Date of visit: 6/24 = 12 gestational weeks
3. The "term" arrow (red in color) then indicates the expected date of delivery or EDC.	1/6
4. If the date of the LNMP is unknown, the EDC can be estimated by the following actions: placing the second week on the wheel opposite the presumed date of conception, or	4/14
placing the 20th week on the wheel at the date when the fetal heart is first auscultated with a DeLee's fetoscope, or	
noting and recording the number of gestational weeks as calculated by the biparietal measurements determined by USG.	USG on 7/14 = 15 ± 2 wk
5. For a woman with a menstrual history of average cycles of every 40 days, ovulation usually occurs 14 days before the first day of menses: place the "last menses" arrow at the *first* day of the LNMP.	LNMP = 4/1
an average cycle of 40 days is 12 days longer than the 28-day cycle that the gestational wheel uses; therefore, the LNMP line is moved 12 days clockwise.	4/13
The "term" arrow indicates the EDC.	1/18

EDC, estimated date of confinement; LNMP, last normal menstrual period; USG, ultrasonogram.

*See Fig. 7-1. For a woman with a menstrual history of average cycles every 28 days.

GESTATIONAL AGE ESTIMATION

1. **Menstrual History**
   LNMP_____ (__certain,__uncertain)   LMP_____ PMP _____

   Menarche_____ Interval _____ Duration_____ Flow _____

2. History of Oral Contraceptives:___No ___Yes When stopped_____

3. **Clinical Evaluation**
   Pregnancy Test:
   DATE _____ GESTATION BY LNMP____Weeks   RESULT _____

   First Uterine Size Estimate:
   DATE _____ GESTATION BY LNMP____Weeks   SIZE BY EXAM____Weeks

   Quickening:
   DATE _____ GESTATION BY LNMP____Weeks

   FHTs First Heard:
   DATE_____ GESTATION BY LNMP____Weeks   GEST. AT PREV. VISIT _____

4. PREDICTED EDC _____ Based on _____

   Reliability of Predicted EDC:___Unreliable___Good___Excellent

Figure 7-2. Gestational dating form. All information about gestational age should be clearly indicated on this or a similar form. *Reprinted with permission from* Crane, J. P., J. P. Sauvage, and F. Arias. A high risk management protocol. *American Journal of Obstetrics and Gynecology* (May 15, 1976). 227-235.

asked to report any lessening or cessation of movement. She should also be informed that the number of FMs varies in individual cases. They are generally weak early in pregnancy and gradually become stronger and more frequent as pregnancy progresses. There is some decrease in FMs in the 2 weeks preceding labor in the full-term infant. Neldam suggests that if FM decreases to less than three movements in an hour and continues to be three or less movements in the next hour, the client should notify her obstetrician or the hospital prenatal clinic as soon as possible. This is considered to be a "movement alarm signal."[1]

For women who may be at risk for placental insufficiency (e.g., those with preeclampsia, diabetes, postdate pregnancy, or suspected intrauterine growth retardation), a "daily FM record" should be maintained (Figs. 7-3 and 7-4).

Most women are more aware of FMs when they are resting during the day and in bed at night. Therefore, women who have been instructed to lie in the left-lateral recumbent position or to rest periodically during the day can count FMs for periods of 1 hour three times a day (i.e., in the morning, afternoon, and evening). The sum total

TABLE 7-2
Conditions That Merit Further Follow-up Care

Condition	Example	Further evaluation for
Size of uterine growth does not correspond to gestation date.	Uterine size abnormally large for date.	Hydramnios. Multiple gestation. Macrosomia.
	Fundal height not progressively increasing, but remaining the same over a period of time (i.e., uterine size abnormally small for date).	Intrauterine growth retardation. Small-for-gestational-age fetus. Oligohydramnios. Fetal demise.
Inability to palpate fetal head in the lower abdomen.	Breech presentation.	Placenta previa. Uterine abnormality.
	Transverse lie.	
Inability to detect fetal heart tones by auscultation and/or Doppler device.	Not applicable.	Fetal demise. Maternal coagulation disorders.

of the 3 hours should be recorded. For other women it may be more convenient to use the Cardiff "count-to-ten" method devised by Pearson: starting at 9 a.m., they should count the number of FMs until the total equals 10.[2] They should then record the time of day that the 10th movement was perceived. Each woman should also be instructed that the "movement alarm signal" described above should be reported immediately.

Biophysical tests of fetal status

In the antepartum period, if there is any question of possible fetal jeopardy, specific tests may be performed to aid in the assessment and determination of placental function and fetal status. These include biophysical and biochemical evaluative tests and electronic fetal monitoring. No single test result is the sole criterion for termin-

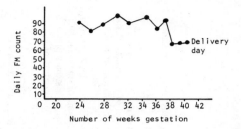

Figure 7-3. Daily fetal movement (FM) count graph. The daily FM count is the sum total of 3 hr/day. *Adapted from* Pearson, J. F., and J. B. Weaver. Fetal activity and fetal wellbeing: an evaluation. *British Medical Journal* (May 29, 1976). 1305-1307.

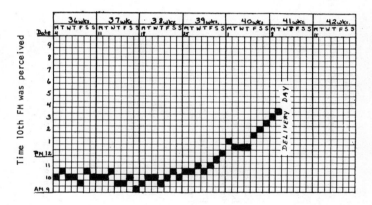

Figure 7-4. Example of "count-to-ten" fetal activity chart. FM, fetal movement. *Adapted from* Pearson's Cardiff "count-to-ten" fetal activity chart.

ating the pregnancy. When used with good clinical judgment, the proper application and interpretation of these tests can be extremely valuable in achieving the best possible outcome for both the client and her fetus. A summary of some of these tests is presented in Table 7-3.

Anticipatory guidance for women who are to have special tests during their pregnancy should include the following information:

1. Purpose of the test.
2. Where and when (the date and time) the test is scheduled.

TABLE 7-3

Summary of Specific Tests of Fetal Well-being*

Test	Results	Significance of findings
Biophysical monitoring tests		
Ultrasound		
A-mode	Biparietal diameter 8.7 cm.	GA 36 wk.
	Biparietal diameter >9.8 cm.	Term fetus.
	Biparietal diameter ≥1.5 cm of the normal GA chest diameter.	Small-for-GA fetus, IUGR, or cranial abnormalities.
B-mode	Presence of gestational sac.	Diagnosis of early pregnancy and GA.
	Uterine, tubal, or ovarian abnormalities.	Possible diagnosis of ovarian or uterine tumors, ectopic pregnancy, or molar pregnancy.
	Assessment of fetal lie, position, presenting part, and number of fetuses.	Possible diagnosis of multiple gestation, breech presentation, or transverse lie.
	Localization of placenta.	Possible diagnosis of placenta previa; location of area for insertion of amniocentesis needle.
	Fetal outline.	Possible diagnosis of fetal death or fetal abnormalities (e.g., anencephaly or hydrocephalus).
	Biparietal diameter (*see* A-mode).	GA (*see* A-mode).
	Amniotic fluid volume.	Possible diagnosis of hydramnios or oligohydramnios.

T-M-mode (Doppler device)	Fetal heart rate pattern.	Detection of fetal heart tones as early as the 10th week of gestation. Possible assessment of fetal jeopardy during the antepartum period (see below: NST, OCT, and CST) or during labor.
Real-time imaging	Same as A- and B-modes. Myocardial contraction. Fetal body movements: fetal limb movements, fetal breathing movements, and fetal tone.	Same as A- and B-modes. Detection of fetal heart tones. Possible diagnosis of cardiac anomalies. Development of a biophysical profile for aid in differentiating the normal fetus from the compromised fetus (Fig. 7-5).
Amnioscopy (color of fluid)	Clear or milky white. Meconium. Dark red or brownish.	Probable fetal well-being. Possible hypoxia or asphyxia (see Chapter 9). Possible fetal death.
Amniography	Soft-tissue silhouette of the fetus and fetal gastrointestinal tract.	Possible diagnosis of soft-tissue anomalies, including gastrointestinal tract abnormalities.
Fetography	Outline of the fetus with radiopaque agent.	Possible diagnosis of soft-tissue anomalies (e.g., fetal hydrops).
Fetoscopy	Direct visualization of the fetus. Sampling of fetal blood and skin.	Possible diagnosis of various morphological abnormalities. Possible diagnosis of hemoglobinopathies, coagulation abnormalities, or certain genetic disorders.

Test	Results	Significance of findings
Electronic fetal monitoring		
NST	Reactive.	General fetal well-being.
	Nonreactive.	Possible fetal jeopardy.
OCT or CST	Negative.	General fetal well-being.
	Positive.	Possible fetal jeopardy.
Biochemical monitoring tests		
Urine estriols*	High and rising levels.	Probable fetal well-being.
	Low and falling levels (i.e., day-to-day variation of >50%).	Possible fetal jeopardy.
Maternal blood		
Alpha fetoprotein	High levels at 12 wk postconception (>10 ng/ml) on two occasions.	Possible threatened abortion or neural tube defect.
Human chorionic gonadotrophin	Persistently high levels or rising levels beyond 100 days after the last normal menstrual period.	Hydatidiform mole.
Human placental lactogen	High levels.	Possible large, diabetic fetus or multiple gestation.
	Low levels (≤4μg/ml).	Possible threatened abortion, IUGR, or postmaturity.

Test	Value	Interpretation
Unconjugated and plasma estriol‡	High and rising levels. Low and falling levels (i.e., day-to-day variation of >50%).	Probable fetal well-being. Possible fetal jeopardy.
Oxytocinase	200 to 400 U at term. Low levels.	General fetal well-being. Possible fetal death, postmaturity, or IUGR.
Coombs's test	Titer of 1:8 and rising.	Significant Rh sensitization.
Amniocentesis (color of fluid)	Meconium.	Possible hypoxia or asphyxia.
Lung profile Shake test Phosphatidyl glycerol Polarization value Lecithin:sphingo-myelin ratio§	Complete ring of foam after 15 min. Present. <0.325. >2:1.	Probable fetal lung maturity, decreased incidence of respiratory distress syndrome.
Creatinine	>2.0/100 ml.	GA >36 wk.
Bilirubin (ΔOD 450)	<0.015. High levels (>0.15).	GA >36 wk: normal pregnancy. Fetal hemolytic disease in isoimmunized pregnancy with GA of ≥28 wk.
Lipid cells	>10%.	GA >35 wk.

Test	Results	Significance of findings
Alpha fetoprotein	High levels early in the first trimester: >4 to 5 standard deviations above the mean for the gestational week (12 wk postconception normal = <12 ng/ml).	Possible threatened abortion.
	High levels after 15 wk of gestation: >4 to 5 standard deviations above the mean for the gestational week.	Possible open neural tube defect.
Osmolality	Decline after 20 wk of gestation (11 mosmol/wk).	Advancing nonspecific GA.
Tests for genetic disorders: Sex linked Chromosomal Metabolic	Dependent on cultured cells for karyotype and enzymatic activity.	Possible genetic disorders.

CST, contraction stress test; GA, gestational age; IUGR, intrauterine growth retardation; NST, nonstress test; OCT, oxytocin challenge test; ΔOD, change in optical density.

*Results may be altered by certain medications, including ampicillin, methenamine mandelate (Mandelamine), phenolphthalein, and corticosteroids.

‡Results may be altered by diurnal variation.

§Results of this ratio may be altered by meconium or blood in the amniotic fluid. The ratio may be higher in the presence of preeclampsia, premature rupture of membranes, hypertension, heroin addiction, exogenous thyroid extract, poor nutrition, or exogenous cortisone.

Biophysical variables	Date_____ Score	Date_____ Score	Date_____ Score
Nonstress test			
Fetal breathing movements			
Fetal body movements			
Fetal tone			
Amniotic fluid volume			

Total Scores:

Figure 7-5. Charting the fetal biophysical profile. Variables are coded as 2 (normal) and 0 (abnormal). The lower the score, the greater the risk of perinatal mortality. *See* article by Manning et al. for definitions of normal and abnormal.

3. Special instructions for preparing for the test.
4. What she may expect (monitoring, who will conduct the test, length of time to complete the test, etc.),
5. What the results will indicate.

ANTEPARTUM HEART RATE TESTING PROTOCOLS

This section has been adapted from protocols that were developed by the Department of Obstetrics and Gynecology, Department of Nursing, Hospital of the University of Pennsylvania.[3]

Indications for use

Clients selected for these procedures are those believed to be at risk for uteroplacental insufficiency. The clients include pregnant women with the following conditions:

1. Hypertensive disorders.
2. Diabetes mellitus.
3. Cyanotic heart disease.
4. Other contributing diseases (e.g., sickle cell, renal, etc.)
5. History of a previous stillbirth.
6. Suspected intrauterine growth retardation.
7. Prolonged pregnancy.
8. Abnormal estriol levels.
9. Meconium in amniotic fluid on amniocentesis or amnioscopy.
10. Decreased fetal activity.

NST

Heart rate accelerations are observed in association with fetal activity in a normal fetus. The client is placed on an external monitor and, while the fetal heart rate is recorded, is asked to indicate each time FM occurs. A "reactive" NST shows fetal heart rate (FHR) accelerations with FM. Failure to demonstrate FM and/or failure to elicit accelerations, even after external manipulation, is considered a "nonreactive" NST.

Nursing responsibilities

1. Take the client to the antepartum testing unit.
2. Explain the procedure to the client, including the time involved. (The test itself requires an average of 30 minutes.)
3. Have the client change into a gown.
4. Place the client in a semi-Fowler's position at a 30- to 45-degree angle with a slight left tilt (which can be facilitated by a folded blanket or sheet).
5. Place the client on an external monitor and use an ultrasound transducer or a phonotransducer to record the FHR. A tokodynamometer should be used to document FM.
6. Record the client's blood pressure initially and at 5- to 10-minute intervals.
7. Instruct the client to indicate each time FM occurs by pressing the record button on the monitor.
8. Obtain a 20-minute graph of the FHR and FM.
9. Record all results and consultations on the client's prenatal chart.

Interpretation of data

Reactive.   Good base-line variability (6 to 10 beats/min) and two or more FHR accelerations of greater than 15 beats/min above the base line, which last 15 seconds or more with FM in a 20-minute period, indicate probable fetal health (lack of distress).

Nonreactive.   Very little base-line variability (less than 6 beats/min), no FM spontaneously or with stimulation, and no FHR changes with activity indicate probable fetal compromise.

Suspicious.   Three or fewer FMs in 40 minutes, accompanied by FHR accelerations of less than 15 beats/min above the base line that last less than 15 seconds, indicate possible fetal compromise.

Unsatisfactory.   Poor tracing quality means that no interpretation is possible.

CST

This test requires a period of either spontaneous or stimulated uterine contractions and simultaneous external monitoring of the FHR response to these contractions. Uterine contractions interfere with uteroplacental blood flow. In pregnancies with diminished fetoplacental reserve, the fetus may become hypoxic during contractions. This hypoxemia will be reflected in a monitor tracing demonstrating late decelerations.

Contraindications

1. High risk for premature labor (e.g., multiple pregnancy, history of prematurity, or history of cervical incompetence).
2. Conditions in which uterine contractions may be dangerous (e.g., placenta previa or previous uterine surgery).

Nursing responsibilities

1. Take the client to the antepartum testing unit.
2. Explain the testing procedure to the client, including the time involved (an average of about 90 minutes, but it is not uncommon for the procedure to last 3 hours).
3. Have the client change into a gown.
4. Place the client in a semi-Fowler's position at a 30- to 45-degree angle with a slight left tilt (which can be facilitated by a folded blanket or sheet).
5. Place the client on an external monitor. A phonotransducer or an ultrasound transducer is used to record the FHR, and a tokodynamometer is used to measure uterine contractions.
6. Record the client's blood pressure initially and at 5- to 10-minute intervals.
7. Obtain at least a 10-minute base-line recording of FHR and observe for spontaneous uterine contractions. The client may be taught to stimulate her breast nipples in an attempt to initiate spontaneous uterine activity. If spontaneous uterine contractions without late decelerations are noted at a frequency of fewer than three in 10 minutes, or if no spontaneous uterine activity is observed, proceed with oxytocin infusion.
8. Start an intravenous infusion of 500 milliliters of 5 percent dextrose in water as a primary line to keep the vein open.
9. Prepare an oxytocin infusion.
   a. Five units of oxytocin are added to 250 milliliters of normal saline (0.9 percent solution). This yields a solution with a

concentration of 20 milliunits of oxytocin per milliliter (*to be used with a Harvard pump*),

Or

2.5 units of oxytocin are added to 500 milliliters of normal saline (0.9 percent solution). This yields a solution with a concentration of 5 milliunits of oxytocin per milliliter (*to be used with an IMED or a 2620 Harvard pump*).

b. Prepare the infusion pump (IMED, 2620 Harvard pump, or Harvard pump).

c. Set the infusion pump according to the dosage of oxytocin ordered by the obstetrician.

d. Start the oxytocin infusion (secondary line) by inserting the needle into the connector of the primary line. Be sure to keep primary line running at a slow rate.

e. Start with 0.2 mU/min of oxytocin. The oxytocin infusion may be increased every 15 to 20 minutes.

Start infusion at 0.2 mU/min

0.4 mU/min

1 mU/min

2 mU/min

4 mU/min

8 mU/min

Hold at 10 mU/min

f. The client must be evaluated by the obstetrician when the dosage of oxytocin reaches 10 mU/min. If the oxytocin infusion is to be continued, the obstetrician must write on the client's order sheet to increase the dosage every 15 to 20 minutes until 20 mU/min is reached. The infusion should be increased as follows:

Continue to 12 mU/min

16 mU/min

Hold at 20 mU/min

10. Discontinue the oxytocin infusion if

a. adequate stress is achieved (three moderately firm uterine contractions in 10 minutes),

b. hyperstimulation occurs (i.e., uterine contractions lasting longer than 60 seconds or less than 2 minutes apart), or

c. definite repetitive late decelerations are seen with uterine contractions.

11. After the oxytocin infusion has been discontinued, continue monitoring until the

a. FHR returns to a stable base line, and

b. uterine contractions are decreased to the base-line level.

12. Review all results with the obstetrician and record them on the client's prenatal chart.

Interpretation of data

Negative. No late deceleration of FHR with uterine contractions (three contractions in 10 minutes) associated with good base-line FHR variability, *and/or* FHR accelerations with FM indicates adequate uteroplacental sufficiency.

Positive. Consistent and persistent late decelerations occurring repeatedly with most uterine contractions (even if less than three contractions in 10 minutes) *or* decreased variability and/or no accelerations with FM indicates probable uteroplacental insufficiency and/or fetal jeopardy.

Suspicious. Inconsistent, but definite, late decelerations that do not persist with continued uterine contractions *or* decreased variability and/or FM with accelerations is suggestive of uteroplacental insufficiency.

Hyperstimulation. Deceleration of FHR with excess uterine activity (contractions closer than every 2 minutes, duration greater than 90 seconds, or uterine hypertonia) is not necessarily indicative of uteroplacental insufficiency.

Unsatisfactory. Uterine contractions of less than three in 10 minutes *and/or* FHR tracing of poor quality are not useful for interpretation.

FOLLOW-UP CARE OF ANTEPARTUM FHR TESTING RESULTS

A summary of an antepartum FHR testing nursing protocol is illustrated in Figure 7-6. The following is a list of nursing actions for the follow-up period of an antepartum FHR test:

1. If the NST is reactive, reschedule for 1 week later.
2. If the NST is nonreactive, shake fetus and determine reactivity during the next 20 minutes.
3. If now reactive (two accelerations with FM during the next 20-minute period), reschedule for 1 week later.
4. If still nonreactive, schedule for CST.
5. If fetus becomes "reactive" (two accelerations in 20 minutes) during CST, the CST procedure may be terminated.
6. If NST is nonreactive and CST is negative, repeat NST 24 hours later.
7. If NST is nonreactive and CST is positive, notify obstetrician immediately to plan further evaluation.

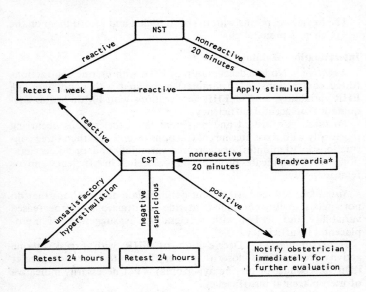

Figure 7-6. Summary of an antepartum fetal heart rate (FHR) testing nursing protocol. CST, contraction stress test; NST, nonstress test; *, FHR of 90 beats/min (or a reduction in FHR of 40 beats/min below the base line) for 60 seconds or greater.

8. If CST is negative, repeat NST 24 hours later (back to step 1).

Figure 7-7 illustrates a sample of a high-risk pregnancy management protocol that uses several of the quantitative tests of feto-placental function mentioned above. (Refer to the article by J. Crane et al. for a complete discussion of this protocol.[4])

SUMMARY

Any pregnancy that requires special tests for the monitoring of fetal status has a psychological, social, emotional, and economic impact on the woman and her family. The nurse must be available to allow for verbalization of fears and clarification of any misconceptions. The nurse must make an effort to alleviate the family's anxiety

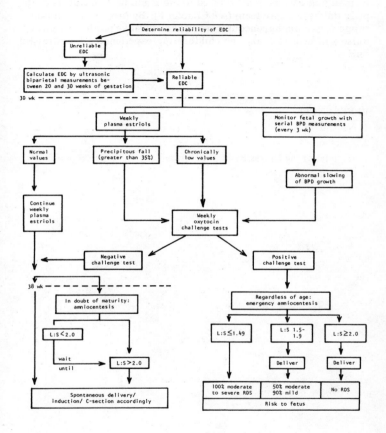

Figure 7-7. Sample of a high-risk pregnancy management protocol. BPD, biparietal diameter; C-section, cesarean section; EDC, estimated date of confinement; L:S, lecithin:sphingomyelin ratio; RDS, respiratory distress syndrome. *Adapted from* Crane, J. P., J. P. Sauvage, and F. Arias. A high risk management protocol. *American Journal of Obstetrics and Gynecology* (May 15, 1976). 227-235.

with regard to the pregnancy and serve as the coordinator of the woman's care as she is introduced to more and more members of the perinatal health care team (*see* Chapter 8). By providing continuous support, counseling, encouragement, and positive reinforcement, the nurse will help to make the childbearing experience a less stressful one.

REFERENCES
1. Neldam.
2. Pearson.
3. Hospital of the University of Pennsylvania.
4. Crane et al.

CHAPTER 8

SCREENING FOR HIGH-RISK PREGNANCY

Sister Rose Scalone

High-risk pregnancy is defined as a pregnancy in which some aspect of the maternal or fetal environment or of the past reproductive performance represents an increased chance of maternal and/or fetal morbidity and/or mortality. It is a pregnancy in which the prospects of optimal outcome for either the client or the fetus are reduced.

IDENTIFICATION OF HIGH-RISK PREGNANCY

Screening for high-risk pregnancies is a continuous process that begins on the first prenatal visit, continues throughout the pregnancy, and includes the intrapartum and postpartum appraisal of the client and her baby. Most perinatal deaths are associated with six obstetric complications: (1) preeclampsia-eclampsia, (2) multiple pregnancy, (3) breech presentation, (4) hydramnios, (5) abruptio placentae, and (6) pyelonephritis.[1] (*See* Chapters 15 and 16 for discussions of these complications.)

Each of these complications can be screened for during the prenatal period. Accurate diagnoses and careful management may help to prevent perinatal deaths.

CRITERIA FOR DIAGNOSIS OF HIGH-RISK PREGNANCY

The following is a list of those factors to be assessed and evaluated when screening for high-risk pregnancy. An in-depth discussion of the factors in the list is superfluous because it is self-evident that all of these factors predispose the client to potential problems and complications. The presence of any one or more of these factors indicates the need for further assessment and evaluation.

The initial prenatal screening

1. Biologic, genetic, and environmental maternal factors:
    a. Maternal age of 15 years or younger.
    b. Maternal age of 35 years or older.
    c. Family history of hereditary abnormality or congenital anomaly.
    d. Obesity (more than 20 percent over standard weight for height).
    e. Excessive thinness (less than 100 pounds or more than 10 percent under standard weight for height).
    f. Short stature (60 inches or less).
    g. Exposure to teratogenic substances:
       radiation,
       viral infection, or
       chemicals.
    h. Cigarette smoking (more than one half pack of cigarettes per day).
    i. Continual presence of stressful events or situations.
    j. Emotional and/or psychological problems.
2. Gynecologic history:
    a. History of infertility.
    b. Uterine or cervical abnormality:
       uterine malformation,
       leiomyomas (submucous or 5 centimeters or greater),
       ovarian mass,
       previous uterine or cervical surgery,
       incompetent cervix,
       cervical malformation,
       cervical cancer or abnormal cervical cytology, or
       history of endometriosis.
3. Obstetric history:
    a. Previous stillborn or neonatal loss.
    b. Two or more previous spontaneous abortions.
    c. Previous premature labors.

    d. Previous low-birth-weight infants (less than 2,500 grams).

    e. Grand multiparity (parity of five or greater).

    f. Close birth intervals (less than 1 year apart) or pregnancy occurring 3 months or less after past delivery.

    g. Previous macrosomatic infant (greater than 4,000 grams).

    h. Previous infant with isoimmunization or prior ABO blood group incompatibility.

    i. Previous infant with a congenital anomaly and/or known genetic disorder.

    j. Previous infant with need for special neonatal care.

    k. History of preeclampsia or eclampsia.

    l. Medical or obstetric indications for termination of previous pregnancy.

    m. Previous operative deliveries:
        midforceps delivery, or
        cesarean section.

    n. Border line or contracted pelvis.

    o. Prior fetal malpresentation.

    p. Previous severe postpartum depression.

4. Medical and surgical history:

    a. Chronic hypertension (nonpregnant blood pressure of at least 140/90).

    b. Heart disease:
        history of rheumatic heart disease or congenital heart disease,
        history of congestive heart failure or arrhythmia, or
        class II-IV heart disease.

    c. Renal disease.

    d. Pulmonary disease.

    e. Diabetes mellitus or strong family history of diabetes.

    f. Sickle cell disease or other hemoglobinopathies.

    g. Thyroid disease.

    h. Epilepsy.

    i. Malignancy.

    j. Drug addiction or alcoholism.

    k. Gastrointestinal or liver disease.

5. Socioeconomic factors:

    a. History of social problems:
        child abuse and neglect, or
        inadequate follow-up of health care.

    b. Current problems:
        poor housing,
        few or no support systems,

family management and parenting problems,
financial problems,
late registration for prenatal care, or
no prenatal care.

Screening on subsequent prenatal visits

1. Review of the above history, results of the initial physical examination, and the laboratory data.
2. Additional screening in early pregnancy:
   a. Suspected ectopic pregnancy.
   b. Suspected missed abortion.
   c. Vaginal bleeding.
   d. Anemia (hemoglobin less than 9 g/100 ml, or hematocrit less than 27 percent) not responsive to nutrition counseling and iron therapy.
   e. Positive serologic test for syphilis (STS).
   f. Positive gonorrhea culture.
   g. Hyperemesis gravidarum.
   h. Unresponsive urinary tract infection.
3. Late pregnancy:
   a. Vaginal bleeding, i.e., placenta previa or abruptio placentae.
   b. Preeclampsia-eclampsia.
   c. Rh isoimmunization.
   d. Hydramnios or oligohydramnios.
   e. Intrauterine fetal demise.
   f. Thromboembolic disease.
   g. Inappropriate fetal growth for gestational age:
      small for gestational age, or
      large for gestational age.
   h. Multiple pregnancy.
   i. Abnormal presentation or lie:
      breech, or
      transverse lie.
   j. Anemia (hemoglobin less than 9 g/100 ml).
   k. Chronic or acute pyelonephritis.
   l. Premature labor (gestation of 36 weeks or less).
   m. Premature rupture of membranes (gestation of 36 weeks or less).
   n. Prolonged rupture of membranes (longer than 24 hours) and/or evidence of amnionitis or sepsis at any time.
   o. Tumor or other obstruction of birth canal.

p. Suspected fetopelvic disproportion.

q. Postdate pregnancy (gestation of longer than 42 weeks).

r. Decreased fetal movement (less than three fetal movements per hour for 2 hours).

s. Abnormal oxytocin challenge test (OCT).

t. Falling estriol levels.

u. Inadequate weight gain.

(For screening in the intrapartum period, *see* Chapters 9 and 16. For postpartum appraisal of mother and baby, *see* Chapters 19 and 21.)

MULTIFACTORIAL RISK ASSESSMENT TOOLS

Advocates of the problem-oriented medical record have helped to devise multifactorial risk assessment tools for evaluating the risk status of a pregnancy. These tools are used to identify problems, provide direction in management of care, provide an educational experience, support clinical research, and satisfy audit directives.

In many institutions it is the nurse's responsibility to keep such tools up-to-date and complete. The conscientious nurse who is familiar with deviations from normal is often the first person to identify and report potential or actual high-risk factors. Figures 8-1, 8-2, and 8-3, three examples of multifactorial risk assessment tools, are included to help nurses become familiar with these tools and their use.

THE PERINATAL CENTER

All pregnant women whose pregnancies have been identified as being high risk should ideally be referred to a perinatal center for continued screening and care. The perinatal center should reflect the mutual interdependence of the high-risk obstetric unit and the neonatal intensive care unit. The personnel in the perinatal center include obstetricians, neonatologists, maternal and child health nurses, perinatal nurse specialists, nurse-midwives, nutritionists, social service workers, public health nurses, neighborhood outreach workers, and many other counselors and aides who work in an interdisciplinary manner with the pregnant woman and the neonate as their central focus. It is through the collaborative efforts of each member of the perinatal team that the woman and her family may be assured of optimal prenatal care and a safe pregnancy outcome for both the mother and her baby. (The flow of care in the perinatal center is illustrated in Figure 8-4).

Maternal-Child Health Care Index

Name: _____ Date: _____ EDC: _____ Hospital: _____

Number: _____

The scoring system below is an attempt to categorize the degree of maternal and fetal risk based on the information available at the initial history and physical upon registration in our obstetric clinics. Please circle the numbers under each of the 8 categories that you feel apply and, at the bottom of this sheet, add up these numbers and subtract from a perfect score of 100.

I. Maternal age:

Under 15	20
15-19	10
20-29	0
30-34	5
35-39	10
Over 40	20

II. Race and marital status:

White	0
Non-white	5
Single	5
Married	0

III. Parity:

0	10
1-3	0
4-7	5
Over 8	10

IV. Past obstetric history:

Abortions		Prematures		Fetal death		Neonatal death		Congenital anomaly		Damaged infants	
1	5	1	10	1	10	1	10	1	10	Physical	10
2	15	2+	20	2+	30	2+	30	2+	20	Neurological	20
3+	30										

V. Medical-obstetric disorders and nutrition:

Systemic illnesses		Specific infections		Diabetes		Chronic hypertension	
Acute, mild	5	Urinary:		Pre	20	Mild	15
Acute, serious	15	acute	5	Overt	30	Severe	30
Chronic, nondebilitating	5	chronic	25			Nephritis	30
Chronic, debilitating	20	Syphilis:		Heart disease			
		treated	0	Class I or II		10	
		untreated	20	Class III or IV		30	
		at term	30	History of prior failure		30	

Endocrine disorders

		Anemia	
Definite adrenal, pituitary, or thyroid problem	30	Hgb, 10-11 g	5
Recurrent menstrual dysfunction	10	Hgb, 9-10 g	10
Involuntary sterility: Less than 2 years	10	Hgb, less than 9 g	20
More than 2 years	20		

Rh problem		Nutrition	
Sensitized	30	Malnourished	20
Prior infant affected	30	Very obese	30
Prior ABO incompatibility	20	Inadequate diet but not malnourished	10

VI. Generative tract disorders:

Prior fetal malpresentations	10
Prior cesarean section	30
Known anomaly or incompetent cervix	20
Leiomyomas:	
Over 5 cm	20
Submucous	30
Contracted pelvis:	
Borderline	10
Any contracted plane	30
Ovarian masses:	
Over 6 cm	20
endometriosis	5

VII. Emotional survey (Grade 0-20 based on):

Fears, attitudes, biases, hostilities, motivations, and behavioral patterns; prior pregnancies without supervision; time of registration; standard of child care and responsibilities; family unit and marital relationship; and history of psychiatric illness in family

VIII. Social and economic survey (Grade 0-10 based on):

Employment: husband, patient; annual income adequacy; public assistance; education: husband, patient; housing: location, quality, facilities, and neighborhood environment.

Total score of all 8 categories _____

100 less above score equals MCHC Index _____

A STATEMENT ON THE SCOPE OF HIGH-RISK PERINATAL NURSING PRACTICE

The American Nurses' Association defines perinatal nursing and the scope of perinatal nursing practice as follows:[2]

Definition

High-risk perinatal nursing is a specialized area of maternal and child health nursing focused on providing perinatal care to childbearing families at risk. Maternal and child health nursing is a specialized area of nursing focusing on (1) health needs of women, their partners, and their families throughout their reproductive and childbearing years, and (2) children through adolescence. Perinatal care refers to care of the health needs of families during the childbearing continuum, through the fourth trimester [the first 3 months after birth]. High-risk perinatal care refers to care of the health needs of childbearing families who are at risk for increased maternal-fetal neonatal morbidity and mortality.

High-risk perinatal nursing focuses on acute and chronic psychosocial and physiological illness, with the goal of maintaining and restoring optimal levels of health attainable by the childbearing family.

Nursing care of the high-risk perinatal family takes place throughout the childbearing continuum. The role of nurses in providing this care is determined by nurses' specific knowledge, skills, and ability to make clinical judgments.

Scope of practice

High-risk perinatal nursing practice includes, but is not limited to, the following:

1. Assessment
   Assessing the psychosocial and physiological status of the high-risk childbearing family by differentiating levels of

---

Figure 8-1. Example of a maternal-child health care index form. This form is used prenatally to identify clients with potentially poor outcomes. The client's score can be determined by subtracting the sum of the factors from 100. A score of 70 or less indicates risk. The lower the score, the greater the risk. *Reprinted with permission from* Aubry, R. H., and J. C. Pennington. Identification and evaluation of high risk pregnancy: the perinatal concept. *Clinical Obstetrics and Gynecology* (March 1973). 13-27.

INTAKE DATE & INITIALS: **PAST PREGNANCIES**

OB INDEX						Preg-nan-cy No.	Termi-nation Date Mo. Yr.	EARLY LOSS <20 wks Spon	Ec-top	In-duced*	GA wks	Birth Wt	Sex	≥20 wks LIVE OR STILLBORN VAGINAL Living Y/N**	Spon Vtx	Br	For-ceps	CPD	C-SECTION Fetal Dis-tress	Abn Pres	Re-peat	Othe-r/Unk	ASSOCIATED PROBLEMS
Age	Term	Premi	Ab-Ectop	Living																			
						1																	
BIRTH CONTROL ☐ Yes						2																	
PILLS IN PAST YEAR ☐ No						3																	
MENSES **CYCLES**						4																	
Onset / 1st / Dur ☐ Regular						5																	
☐ Irregular																							
LMP: **EDC:**						6																	
☐ Normal						7																	
☐ Abnormal PMP:						8																	
POSITIVE PREGNANCY TEST																							

*D&C S(Suction) Sa(Saline) P(Prostaglandin) H(Hysterotomy) O(Other) U(Unknown) **S(Stillbirth) N(Neonatal) I(Infant) C(Childhood)

Date: Prob. No.	±	Risk Value	**HISTORICAL PROBLEMS**		**HEALTH STATUS INDICATORS**

HISTORICAL PROBLEMS

Prob. No.	Risk Value		
1	5		☐ AGE <17 ☐ AGE ≥ 35
2	5		**MULTIPARITY (5 or more ≥20 weeks)**
3	5		**INDUCED ABORTION**
4	10		**HABITUAL ABORTION (3 or more)**
5	10		**PREMATURE (≤37 weeks)** ☐ LGA
6	10	PREVIOUS INFANTS	**SGA (Small for Gestational Age)**
7	5		**BIRTH WEIGHT >4000 gms or 9 lbs**
8	10		**PERINATAL DEATH** ☐ Stillbirth ☐ Neonatal
9	5		**POST NEONATAL PROBLEM** ☐ Sudden Infant Death ☐ Neurologic Handicap ☐ Mental Retardation
10	10		**NEONATAL JAUNDICE** ☐ Rh ☐ ABO ☐ Physiologic ☐ Unknown ☐ Other:
11	5		**GENETIC DISEASE** ☐ Chromosomal ☐ CNS ☐ Inborn Errors of Metabolism ☐ Other: ☐ Structural Congenital Anomalies:
12	5		**HISTORY OF INFERTILITY** ☐ Primary ☐ Secondary ☐ Treated ☐ Untreated
13	10	GYN	**UTERINE-CERVICAL ABNORMALITY** ☐ Uterine Anomaly ☐ Corrected ☐ Incomp Cx ☐ Cerclage, Removed ☐ Yes ☐ No
14	5		**PREVIOUS UTERINE SURGERY C-Section:** ☐ Classical ☐ Low Trans ☐ Low Vert ☐ Unknown ☐ Hysterotomy ☐ Myomectomy
15	5	PREG. COM-PLICATIONS	**HEMORRHAGE** ☐ Previa ☐ Abruptio ☐ Other 3rd Trimester ☐ Post Partum ☐ Transfusion
16	5		**PREGNANCY-INDUCED HYPERTENSION** ☐ Required Hosp ☐ Required Early Delivery ☐ Developed Eclampsia
17	10		**CHRONIC HYPERTENSION (BP ≥140/90 non-pregnant)** ☐ On Drug Therapy:
18	10		**HEART DISEASE** ☐ Rheumatic ☐ Congenital ☐ Arteriosclerotic ☐ Other / ☐ Surgical Correction ☐ Hx of CHF or Arrhythmia / ☐ No limitation of physical activity ☐ Slight limitation ☐ Marked limitation ☐ Unable to carry on any physical activ. w/out discomfort
19	5		**PULMONARY DISEASE** ☐ Asthma ☐ Chronic Bronchitis ☐ Tuberculosis ☐ Other
20	5	MEDICAL-SURGICAL	**GENITOURINARY INFECTIONS** ☐ Asymptomatic Bacteriuria ☐ Pyelonephritis ☐ Syphilis ☐ Cystitis ☐ Gonorrhea ☐ Genital Herpes
21	10		**RENAL DISEASE** ☐ Glomerulo ☐ Chronic Pyelo ☐ Diabetic ☐ Collagen-vas ☐ Calculi ☐ Other:
22	10		**DIABETES** ☐ A ☐ B ☐ C ☐ D ☐ F-R ☐ Insulin, Pre-preg Dosage:
23	10		**THYROID DISEASE** ☐ Hypo ☐ Thyroiditis ☐ Hyper: treated with ☐ Drugs ☐ Surgery ☐ I-131
24	10		**OTHER MEDICAL** ☐ Phlebitis ☐ Embolus ☐ Collagen-vas ☐ On Drug Therapy: ☐ Hematologic:
25	10		**EPILEPSY** ☐ On Therapy: ☐ Phenobarb ☐ Dilantin ☐ Mysoline ☐ Other:
26	5		**PSYCHIATRIC** ☐ Hospitalized ☐ On Drug Therapy:
27	5		**PREVIOUS OPERATIONS** ☐ Diag D&C ☐ Laparoscopy ☐ Appendectomy ☐ Cholecystectomy ☐ Other:
28	10	HABITS	**EXCESSIVE USE** ☐ Alcohol ☐ Tobacco ☐ Marijuana ☐ Narcotics:
29	5	FAMILY HISTORY	**MATERNAL ONLY** ☐ Hypertension ☐ Multiple Births ☐ Diabetes ☐ Hemoglobinopathy ☐ Other:
30	5		**MAT. OR PATERNAL** ☐ Mental Retardation ☐ Congen Anom ☐ Congen Hearing Loss ☐ Allergies ☐ Other:

HEALTH STATUS INDICATORS

YEARS OF EDUCATION   Mother _____ Father _____
QIET (Ex, G, P, Undet) Calories _____ Protein _____ Iron _____
INSURANCE   ☐ Public   ☐ Private   ☐ None
Carrier _____ / _____
Carrier _____ / _____

ALLERGIES

COMMENTS

SPECIAL COMMENTS FOR DATA ENTRY:

Patient Address		City		State	Zip	Birth Date
Home Phone	Preferred Language	Marital Status M W D SEP S		Last name _____ First name _____ M.I.		
Contact Phone	Race-Ethnicity W B H I A O	Spouse's Name		Patient hospital # _____		
Referred By		Hospital of Delivery				

1 PRENATAL HISTORY

Clinic/physician _____

Patient clinic# _____

Figure 8-2. Problem-oriented perinatal risk assessment system (POPRAS). There are separate scores for (1) prenatal history, (2) prenatal screening, and (3) prenatal flow. This system is used prenatally, intranatally (not shown), and neonatally (not shown) to screen for the high-risk neonate. The score for each can be determined by adding all of the appropriate factors. A score of 10 or more indicates risk. The higher the score, the greater the risk. (Courtesy of C. Hobel and the South Bay Regional Perinatal Project, Harbor General Hospital, Torrance, Calif.)

DATE:			PHYSICAL EXAM										
Normal	Yes	No	Normal	Yes	No	Normal	Yes	No	Normal	Yes	No		
SKIN			LUNGS			ABDOMEN			VAGINA				
HEENT			BREASTS			EXTREMITIES			CERVIX				
MOUTH			NIPPLES			NEUROLOGIC			UTERUS				
THYROID			HEART			PERINEUM			ADNEXA				
						VULVA			RECTAL				

UTERINE SIZE/DATES: ____/____ ☐Comparable ☐Smaller ☐Larger
PELVIS ☐Adequate ☐Borderline ☐Inadequate ☐Clinical ☐X-ray
ABNORMAL FINDINGS

LAB DATA BASE			
Date	TYPE ☐A ☐B ☐O ☐AB	Date	HCT ____ HGB ____
	Rh ☐Neg ☐Pos ☐Du+		HGB ELECT (circle 2)
	ANTIBODY SCREEN ☐Neg ☐Pos		A₁ A₂ A₃ F
	VDRL ☐Neg ☐Pos		S C
	FTA ☐Neg ☐Pos		PPO ☐Neg ☐Pos:
	RUBELLA ☐Neg Titer:		CHEST X-RAY ☐Neg ☐Pos:
	URINE CULTURE:		PAP ☐Neg ☐Infl ☐Pos
			DYSPLASIA ☐Mild ☐Mod ☐Sev
U R I N E	PROTEIN ☐Neg ☐Tr		G-C CULTURE ☐Neg ☐Pos:
	SUGAR ☐1+ ☐2+ ☐5+		FATHER'S Rh ☐Pos ☐Neg
	MICRO ☐Neg ☐Pos		☐Homozyg ☐Heterozyg
	BLOOD SUGAR	FASTING ☐1 HR PP ☐2 HR PG	

Prob. No.	÷	Date Positive	R	Risk Val.	DEVELOPING PROBLEMS				
31				5		PRE-PREG WEIGHT ☐<100 lb ☐>200 lb			
32				10	ANATOMICAL	SIZE-DATE DISCREPANCY			
33				5		SMALL PELVIS			
34				5		Rh NEG ☐Not Sensitized			
35				10		☐Sensitized			
36				5		G-U TESTS ☐Abn Pap ☐Pos GC			
						☐Asymptomatic Bacteriuria			
37				5	POSITIVE LAB	POSITIVE SEROLOGY			
38				5		ANEMIA ☐Mild <11 gms or 27-33%			
						☐Severe <9 gms or <27%			
39				5		ABNORMAL ☐SS ☐AS ☐Thalassemia			
						HGB ☐Other:			
40				10		THREATENED AB ☐Hosp ☐Drug Therapy:			
41				5	EARLY PREGNANCY	EARLY TERMINATION (< 20 wks) ☐Spontaneous ☐Induced ☐Ectopic			
42				5		HYPEREMESIS GRAVIDARUM ☐Hosp ☐Drug Therapy:			
43				10		INCOMPETENT CERVIX ☐Cerclage, Date: ☐Drug Therapy:			
44				10		TORCH ☐Toxoplasmosis ☐Syphilis ☐Rubella ☐Cytomegaloviris ☐Herpes			
45				5	INFECTION	FLU SYNDROME ☐High Fever ☐Gastroenteritis ☐Hosp			
46				5		GENITAL-URINARY ☐Vaginitis ☐Asymp Bacteriuria ☐Cystitis ☐GC ☐Genital Herpes			
47				10		PYELONEPHRITIS			
48				10		DIABETES (in this pregnancy) ☐A ☐B ☐C ☐D ☐F-R Rx: ☐Diet ☐Insulin			
49				10		THROMBOPHLEBITIS ☐Hosp ☐Anticoagulant ☐Embolus			
50				10	MEDICAL-SURGICAL	CARDIOPULMONARY ☐Asthmatic Attack ☐Bronchitis ☐Pneumonia ☐Active TB			
						☐Tachycardia ☐Arrhythmia ☐CHF			
51				10		OTHER MEDICAL ☐Hepatitis ☐Late Anemia ☐Other:			
52				5		SURGICAL ☐Adnexal ☐Appendectomy ☐Other:			
53				5	PSYCHO-SOCIAL	☐Marital ☐Coping & Support ☐Unresolved Grief ☐Family ☐Sexual			
						☐Financial ☐Relocation ☐Prior OB Experience ☐Other:			
54				5	ANATOMICAL ABNORMAL-ITIES	MATERNAL WEIGHT GAIN ☐< ½ lb/wk ☐> 2 lb/wk			
55				10		UTERINE SIZE ☐Suspected IUGR ☐Polyhydramnios ☐Mult Preg ☐Myomata			
56				5		FETAL POSITION ☐Breech ☐Transverse Lie ☐Oblique			
57				5		BLOOD PRESSURE ☐Preg-Induced Hypertension Mild ☐1=BP ≥ 140/90 or ↑30 mm systolic or ↑15 mm diastolic			
						☐2=Proteinuria 1+ or 2+ ☐5 =Persistent Edema			
58				10	ABNORMAL-ITIES OF FUNCTION	☐Superimposed Severe ☐BP ≥ 160/110 or ☐Proteinuria >2+ both after 26 wks GA			
59				10		BLEEDING > 20 WKS ☐Cervical ☐Previa ☐Low-lying ☐Undetermined			
60				5		LABOR, HOSPITALIZED FOR ☐Suspected Premature Labor ☐False Labor >57 wks			
						☐Pharmacologic Rx:			
61				10		POST-TERM > 42 WKS (over 42 weeks from LMP or estimated from early physical exam)			
62						ANTEPARTUM FETAL DEATH			
63						PROTOCOL ☐☐☐☐			

MEDICATIONS

COMMENTS

SPECIAL COMMENTS FOR DATA ENTRY

First Total ____
36 Wk Total ____

PRENATAL SCORE   Sig/Date: ____
Sig/Date: ____

Last name ____ First name ____ M.I. ____
Patient hospital # ____

2 PRENATAL SCREENING

Clinic/physician ____

Patient clinic# ____

Figure 8-2 (cont'd).

Pre-Pregnancy Weight		Height		Age		Term		Premi		Ab-Ectopic		Living		LMP			Quickening		EDC		Corrected EDC	

DATE	WEIGHT (LBS)	TOTAL GAIN	SUGAR ACETONE	ALBUMIN	180	170	160	150	140	130	120	110	100	90	80	70	60	50	GEST AGE	FUNDAL HEIGHT	FETAL PRESENT	FETAL HEART	EDEMA	RETURN VISIT	PHYSICIAN

DATE	BLOOD SUGARS					DATE	AMNIOCENTESIS					DATE	ULTRASOUND					
	FASTING	1 HR FP	2 HR PG				GENETIC	AFP	☐Normal ☐Abnormal					PLACENTA	THOR	BPD	GA	PRES
								CHROMO	☐Normal ☐Abnormal									
								OTHER:										
							LUNG MATURITY	Value:										
								Value:										
							ΔOD:	Date	ΔOD:	Date	ΔOD:							

DATE	REPEAT LAB STUDIES		DATE				SPECIAL TESTS	☐E3 ☐HPL ☐Nonstress ☐Stress ☐Amnioscopy			
	HCT	HGB			CX CULTURE ☐- ☐+	Date		Date			
	HCT	HGB			TITERS:						
	ANTIBODY SCREEN ☐+☐-				TITERS:						
	URINE CULTURE ☐+☐-				OTHER:						

DATE	PROB NO.	PLAN	DATE	PROB NO.	PLAN

DATE ORDERED	ROUTINE PLANS	DATE COUNSELED
	☐Iron ☐Vitamins	
	Nutritional Counseling	
	☐Vaginal Delivery ☐C-Section	
	Childbirth Education	
	Prepared Childbirth ☐Yes ☐No	
	Anesthesia:	
	Breast Feeding ☐Yes ☐No	
	Family Planning ☐BTL ☐Papers Signed ☐Other:	
	Pediatrician/ Newborn Care:	

Last name _____ First name _____ M.I.
Patient hospital #_____

3 PRENATAL FLOW
COUNTY OF LOS ANGELES DEPARTMENT OF HEALTH SERVICES
H-2189 (10-90) 76P963

Clinic/physician _____

Patient clinic # _____

Figure 8-2 (cont'd).

Base-line data

Age 35+... 1
Age 40+... 2
Para 0.. 2
Para 6+... 2
Interval <2 years..................................... 1
Obesity (200 lbs.+[90 kg.+]).......................... 1
Diabetes B, C, D...................................... 2
         F.. 3
Chronic renal disease................................. 1
  with diminished renal function...................... 3
  with increased BUN.................................. 3

Hypertension (preexisting)
  140+......... 1   160+......... 2
  90+   110+

SCORE (circle one)   0   1   2   3

Obstetric history

Abortion
Stillbirth
Neonatal death
Surviving premature infant
Antepartum hemorrhage
Toxemia
Difficult midforceps delivery
Cesarean section
Major congenital anomaly
Baby 10 lbs.+ (4.5 kg.+)

One instance of above................................. 1
Two or more instances in different pregnancies....... 2

Rh isoimmunized mother
+ Homozygous father................................... 2
+ History of erythroblastosis......................... 3

Present pregnancy

Bleeding, early (<20 wk)
  alone............................... 1
  with pain........................... 2
Bleeding, late (>20 wk)
  ceased.............................. 1
  continues........................... 2
  with pain........................... 3
  with hypotension.................... 3
Spontaneous premature rupture of
  membranes........................... 1
  latent period 24 hr+................ 2
Anemia <10 g.......................... 1
       <8 g........................... 2
No prenatal care...................... 2
  <3 prenatal visits.................. 1

Toxemia I... 1
Toxemia II.. 3
Eclampsia... 3
Hydramnios (single fetus)............................. 3
Multiple pregnancy.................................... 2
Abnormal glucose tolerance............................ 1
Decreasing insulin requirement........................ 3
Maternal acidosis..................................... 3
Maternal pyrexia...................................... 1
Pyrexia + FHR >160.................................... 2
Rh negative:
With rising titre..................................... 2
With amniotic fluid
Liley zone III.. 3

SCORE (circle one)   0   1   2   3

Gestational age

28 wk or under.. 4
32 wk or under.. 3
35 wk or under.. 2

37 wk or under.. 1
42 wk or more... 1
43 wk or more... 2

SCORE (circle one)   0   1   2   3   4

Figure 8-3. Example of an antepartum fetal risk score form. This form is used prenatally and at the onset of labor to predict fetal risk. The score can be determined by adding all of the appropriate factors. A score of 6 or more indicates risk. The higher the score, the greater the risk. *Reprinted with permission from* Goodwin, J., J. Dunne, and B. Thomas. Antepartum identification of the fetus at risk. *Canadian Medical Association Journal* (October 18, 1969). 57-64.

perinatal risk; by initiating and utilizing multiple sources and assessment tools for data collection, such as histories, physical examinations, and appropriate laboratory data; and by interpreting data that leads to nursing diagnoses.
2. Plan of care
   Establishing an appropriate plan of intervention with the high-risk perinatal family based on nursing diagnoses by collaborating with the family and other health care

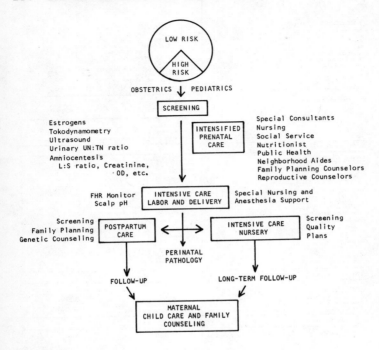

Figure 8-4. The flow of care in the perinatal center. FHR, fetal heart rate; L:S, lecithin:sphingomyelin; OD, optical density; UN:TN, urea nitrogen: total nitrogen. *Reprinted with permission from* Aubry, R. H., and J. C. Pennington. Identification and evaluation of high risk pregnancy: the perinatal concept. *Clinical Obstetrics and Gynecology* (March 1973). 13-27.

providers; by differentiating immediate and long-term health care goals with the family; and by determining and coordinating the plan of action to meet these identified goals.

3. Intervention

   Implementing the interventions with the high-risk perinatal family that are based on the plan of care, including initiating technical procedures and therapeutic regimes; maintaining a therapeutic environment; intervening in life-threatening situations; teaching, counseling, and facilitating family development; preventing further complications; and promoting optimum health development of the high-risk perinatal family.

4. Evaluation

Evaluating the plan of care of the high-risk perinatal family by evaluating the interventions; evaluating the effects of the interventions on the family; evaluating the family's progress toward the identified goals; and initiating changes in the plan of care based on new data and resources and on the environment.

Comprehensive high-risk perinatal nursing care is provided in the interdependent clinical practice areas of maternal-fetal care and maternal-neonatal care.

Nursing practice in the high-risk maternal-fetal area is primarily focused on restorative care for the maternal-fetal unit, with the goal of improving the outcome for the high-risk childbearing family. This care is integrated into the continuum of care needed by the high-risk childbearing family and is extended into the maternal-neonatal areas.

Nursing practice in the high-risk maternal-neonatal area is primarily focused on either restorative care for the mother who becomes or remains at high risk after the birth of the infant, or restorative care for the neonate born with threats to his or her immediate or long-term transition and adaptation to extra-uterine life. Nursing practice within the maternal-neonatal area is a continuation of care initiated during maternal-fetal care and includes supportive care for the family during the fourth trimester, with the goal of facilitating neonatal development and family integration.

The maternal-fetal and maternal-neonatal areas in high-risk perinatal nursing practice are not discrete; they comprise a dynamic system of care throughout the continuum of childbearing events.

Nurses who are interested in maternal and child health as a specialty area of practice are encouraged to pursue further educational endeavors. Numerous workshops, conferences, continuing education, and formal educational programs are available for the advancement of specialized knowledge and skills. The perinatal nursing specialty and nurse-midwifery are two specialized areas of nursing that integrate the normal and high-risk segments of maternal-fetal and neonatal health care. They include the care of all pregnant women, neonates, and their families. These nurses may vary in their area of specialization, but they function within the entire perinatal concept and their goal is the same: to provide optimal health care for the childbearing family.

REFERENCES

1. Babson. 13.
2. American Nurses' Association.

CHAPTER 9

FIRST STAGE OF LABOR

Suzanne M. Smith

The time of labor and birth, though short in comparison with the length of pregnancy, is perhaps the most significant portion of gestation for both the client and her fetus. The physical and psychological changes that occur during labor provide many opportunities for the nurse to use her skills as a caregiver. Although labor and delivery are normal physiological functions, the possibility of variations in, or deviations from, the norm must be recognized and managed as necessary. The physical and emotional well-being of both clients (mother and baby) are ensured by appropriate assessments and intervention.

This chapter discusses the *normal* first stage of labor. Subsequent chapters discuss the second, third, and fourth stages of labor as well as possible deviations from the norm.

PHYSIOLOGY OF ORGAN SYSTEMS IN LABOR

Cardiovascular system

In the normotensive woman, blood pressure, which tends to drop during the midtrimester, will be at or near the prepregnant level as term approaches. Pain, fear, and apprehension may contribute to an increased blood pressure.

The increased metabolism secondary to anxiety and muscle activity during labor results in an increased resting (between contractions) pulse rate.

Changes in both blood pressure and pulse rate while lying in the supine position are caused by compression of the inferior vena cava by the uterus and its contents. This compression results in a decreased venous return from the lower extremities. The decreased return to the right side of the heart leads to decreased filling of the ventricle and a decreased cardiac output.

Significant inferior vena caval compression results in supine hypotension syndrome (in approximately 10 percent of pregnant women at or near term), in which the blood pressure drops precipitously, resulting in a diminished venous return and cardiac output. During labor contractions, however, the blood pressure increases significantly and the pulse rate decreases if the patient is supine. The treatment for supine hypotension syndrome is removal of the cause, i.e., immediate substitution of the lateral position and continued avoidance of the supine position.[1]

Hemopoietic system

During labor, the white blood cell count may become markedly elevated. The cause is unclear, but the elevation may represent a response to the increased muscular activity by the reappearance in the circulation of leukocytes that were previously shunted out of active circulation. The differential count, however, does not normally change from the nonpregnant state. Thus, any shifts should be considered significant.

Fluid and electrolyte balance

There are no characteristic changes in the electrolyte composition of blood or of body fluids during pregnancy and labor. However, urine should be evaluated during labor for the presence of ketones or protein (see below) and for the specific gravity.

Respiratory system

There is a normal state of hyperventilation during pregnancy that is due to an increase in the respiratory minute volume of approximately 26 percent.[2] The hyperventilation results in a blowing off of excessive amounts of carbon dioxide, which decreases the concentration of carbon dioxide in the alveoli and lowers the carbon dioxide tension in the blood, while the oxygen tension in the alveoli remains within normal limits. The plasma bicarbonate levels are also lowered slightly during pregnancy. The result of all these changes is a compensated respiratory alkalosis with a blood pH of approximately 7.42 near term as compared with the average nonpregnant value of 7.35.[3]

The hyperventilation responsible for these changes results from increased central nervous system sensitivity to carbon dioxide tension in the blood, probably because of elevated blood progesterone levels. An additional slight increase in the respiratory rate during labor is normal and reflects the increase in metabolism. Prolonged hyperventilation, however, such as that caused by fear or by improper use of prepared breathing techniques, may result in a noncompensated alkalosis.

Gastrointestinal system

There is a severe reduction in gastric motility, secretion of gastric juices, and absorption of solid foods immediately before and during labor. This results in a virtual cessation of digestion and a prolonged gastric emptying time. Liquids, which are generally not affected by the above changes, leave the stomach in the usual amount of time. In addition, nausea and vomiting are not uncommon during the transition phase or as side effects of some analgesics. Thus, judicious caution is recommended in decision-making regarding oral intake. For these reasons, oral intake during labor is often limited to liquids or easily digestible solids.

Renal system

Polyuria (frequency of urination) is common during labor. It may be the result of increased cardiac output with a corresponding increase in the glomerular filtration rate and renal plasma flow. It is less pronounced in the supine position because of the effect of inferior vena caval compression, which limits cardiac output.

The anatomic relationship of the urinary bladder and the uterus causes various effects. Bladder distention may contribute to a prolongation of labor by obstructing the descent of the presenting part or by impairing effective uterine contractions. Conversely, the pressure of the presenting part may lead to urinary frequency, urinary urgency, and/or stress incontinence. Prolonged pressure, particularly in combination with distention, can result in trauma to the bladder, which leads to subsequent hypotonia, urinary retention, and, eventually, urinary tract infection. These facts point to the importance of continually evaluating the bladder during labor and encouraging the woman to void approximately every 2 hours.

Proteinuria does not usually occur in pregnancy, although slight proteinuria may occur in labor as a result of the increased metabolic activity. One third to one half of women in labor may exhibit proteinuria levels ranging from trace to 1 + . It is more common in primiparas, anemic parturients, or in prolonged labor. A proteinuria level of 2 + and above is abnormal and requires further evaluation, particularly to rule out preeclampsia.

A voided urine specimen may be contaminated by bloody show or amniotic fluid. This may result in a positive test for protein. Although the results cannot be discounted, the coexistence of these other causes must be considered.

Ketonuria in labor is generally caused by maternal exhaustion or distress secondary to dehydration, nutritional deficiency, or other electrolyte imbalances. Attention must be paid to the maintenance of hydration by means of oral or intravenous fluids.

PHYSIOLOGY OF LABOR

Theories regarding the initiation of labor

Although there are many theories that attempt to explain the initiation of labor, the actual cause has never been identified. Most authorities agree that many or all of the proposed theories contain part of the answer.

The theory of uterine stretch (overdistention) proposes that, when the uterus reaches a certain size, labor begins in order to empty the uterus and decrease the size. This theory has been used to explain the premature onset of labor in multiple gestation and in some cases of hydramnios.

Nerve stimulation and pressure on the lower uterine segment, cervix, and vagina by the weight of the presenting part is useful in explaining the onset and progress of labor when the presenting part is engaged and well-applied to the cervix.

Uterine contractility or "working capacity" increases near term. Consequently, contractions may be transmitted from one cell to the next. Thus, contractions can involve the entire myometrium rather than isolated areas — as occurs with Braxton Hicks's contractions (see p. 225).

Changes in the amount of a specific hormone and/or in its proportion with regard to other hormones may influence the onset of labor. Oxytocin has been shown to stimulate uterine contractions, and, thus, is used in the induction or stimulation/augmentation of labor. Progesterone is known to inhibit uterine contractions. Estrogen and prostaglandins produced by the fetus, fetal membranes, and/or uterine *decidua vera* are also implicated in the onset of labor. Certain prostaglandins, which increase before and during labor, have been shown to produce myometrial contractions.

Placental aging may influence the levels of hormone production — particularly of estrogen and progesterone. Changes in the production of cortisol and/or adrenocorticotrophic hormone by the fetus have also been implicated. In addition, there may be an unknown hormone of placental origin that is produced at term.

There is a proposed menstrual cycle association because labor usually begins at the end of 40 weeks or at 10 menstrual cycles after the last normal menstrual period.

Emotional and physical factors may also be implicated in the cause of labor when certain other factors are involved. Many women report a fall or other accident or a severe emotional shock shortly before the onset of labor. In addition, enemas, the use of castor oil, ambulation, sexual stimulation, and other physical activities are effective in some cases.

Uterine physiology

Contractions. The myometrium (uterine muscle) is composed of smooth muscle that possesses the same property as other smooth muscles in the body: the ability to contract and relax in a coordinated manner. Uterine contractions occur when the contraction of one muscle cell stimulates a nearby cell to contract and stimulate another cell. This pattern of contraction and stimulation continues for varying distances over the myometrium. Braxton Hicks's contractions and false labor occur when this mechanism has not become fully developed and coordinated (*see below*).

A specific pacemaker site has not been identified in humans. It is believed that most uterine contractions in labor are initiated near the cornual area of the fundus. Because of the greater concentration of myometrial cells in the fundus, as compared with the lower portion of the uterus, the probability is high that effective contractions are triggered there.

The upper portion of the uterus contains a greater concentration of muscle fibers than do the lower uterine segment and the cervix. When the myometrium contracts, the fibers of both the fundus and corpus of the uterus shorten. However, when the contraction ends and these fibers relax, they do not return to their original size, but maintain a shorter length than before. The property of muscle contraction resulting in a shortened muscle when relaxed is known as brachystasis (or retraction). This continued shortening of the myometrial fibers of the upper portion of the uterus results in a progressive decrease in the size of the uterine cavity and a thickening of the myometrial tissue of the upper portion. These changes supply the force needed to advance the fetus and maintain the advantage gained with each contraction. Brachystasis of the upper segment does not cease until the uterus is empty.

Conversely, the lower portion of the uterus and cervix contain significantly fewer myometrial elements. In addition, these muscle cells are arranged in a more circular pattern, as opposed to the longitudinal pattern of the upper portion. When the uterus contracts, these circular fibers increase in length and are drawn up by the longitudinal fibers, which causes the formation of the lower uterine segment and the effacement of the cervix. The property of muscle contraction resulting in a lengthened muscle cell when relaxed is known as mecystasis. The mecystatic changes of the lower uterine segment are complete when full dilation and retraction of the cervix are achieved.

In normal labor, there is a difference in the pressure produced by each contraction, with the greatest force exerted at the fundus, decreasing throughout the uterus, to the least force exerted at the cervix. In addition to this differentiation in intensity, the duration of contractions also varies. During each contraction, the duration in the middle of the uterus is shorter than in the fundus but longer than in the lower segment and cervix.

The junction of the upper portion of the uterus (in which the muscle fibers have shortened and the uterine wall has thickened) with the lower uterine segment (in which the muscle fibers have lengthened and the wall has thinned) is known as the **physiologic retraction ring**.

If there is an obstruction to the continued dilation of the cervix or to the advancement of the fetus, and uterine contractions continue, the upper portion will continue to thicken with further brachystatic shortening of the muscle fibers and the lower segment will continue to thin. This will result in the formation of a **pathologic retraction ring** (Bandl's ring) as the physiologic ring becomes more pronounced. Rupture of the excessively thinned lower uterine segment is a possibility and results in a life-threatening situation for both the mother and her fetus. Bandl's ring may be visible as an indentation or transverse groove on the abdomen between the symphysis pubis and the umbilicus. It is essential that this situation not be mistaken for a full bladder and that relief of the obstruction or an operative delivery be effected immediately.

Cervical change. The function of the cervix is to retain the products of conception throughout the pregnancy until labor ensues. A clear understanding of uterine contractions (*see above*) will aid in the understanding of cervical physiology.

During pregnancy, the cervical os remains undilated (closed) and the cervical canal remains uneffaced (2 to 3 centimeters long). The consistency of the cervix, however, is slightly softer to the touch than its consistency when the uterus is nonpregnant. Toward the end of pregnancy, effacement begins as the cervix begins to be taken up from above downward and becomes perceptibly softened. Often, slight dilation of the os, particularly in multiparas, also occurs. At the onset of labor, approximately one half of the canal has been taken up (50 percent effaced) and the internal os is dilated to 2 to 3 centimeters.

The mecystatic changes that occur in the lower uterine segment also occur in the cervix. Effacement generally proceeds in conjunction with dilation, becoming complete at 6 to 7 centimeters. When effacement is complete (100 percent), the cervix has been described as "paper-thin." On occasion, 100 percent effacement occurs before significant dilation, and an unskilled examiner may mistake a closed but fully effaced cervix for a fully dilated one.

Cervical dilation is caused by a combination of the mecystatic forces of contractions and the mechanical effects of a wedge: As the uterine contractions exert pressure on the fetal membranes, the hydrostatic action of the amniotic sac dilates the cervical canal. This effect is greatest if the membranes have become loosened from the lower uterine decidua, allowing them to slide through the cervical os during contractions and act as a wedge. In the absence of intact membranes, the presenting part of the fetus functions as the dilating wedge.

The Ferguson reflex is a phenomenon whereby mechanical stretching of the cervix appears to enhance uterine activity. The exact mechanism is not known; however, the risk of inadvertent, iatrogenic cervical trauma or lacerations is significant enough to warrant the avoidance of manual dilation of the cervix in all cases.

The mucous plug. The cervical canal is sealed during pregnancy by a tenacious mucus produced by the endocervical glands. Shortly before or during the early phase of labor, the mucous plug is expelled from the cervix because of initial effacement and/or dilation. If extruded intact, it is generally a thick piece of sticky mucus that may also include some blood. If expulsion of the mucous plug occurs gradually, it may be unnoticed or, perhaps, be mistaken for amniotic fluid.

The amount of blood that accompanies the mucus is highly variable, most frequently only a few drops or streaks. When labor is well established, there is usually some bleeding or bloody show, which is the result of the rupture of capillaries in the cervix, primarily during dilation. Thus, although it is not unusual for labor to be accompanied by significant bloody show, this must be differentiated from frank bleeding, which is an obstetric emergency.

Pain in labor. Uterine contractions in labor are the only physiological contractions of any muscle in the body that may be painful. The experience of pain in labor is dependent on physiological, emotional, and psychological factors. The individual's somatic perception of pain cannot be predicted before labor.

Pain is likely to be most intense during active labor, to be decreased by effective pushing in the second stage, and to be absent, or nearly so, thereafter. In normal labor, most pain is experienced suprapubically. Backache is most frequent in malpositions (especially occiput posterior) and malpresentations (some breeches). Backache is thought to be due to faulty cervical dilation or an improper "fit" of the presenting part within the lower uterine segment or against the cervix.

The following is a list of six mechanisms that have been suggested to describe the cause of pain in labor:

1. Hypoxia of the contracted myometrium, i.e., uterine ischemia (similar to angina pectoris).
2. Stimulation or compression of nerve endings in the lower uterine segment and cervix by the interlocked muscle bundles during dilation.
3. Cervical stretching during dilation.
4. Traction on the peritoneum, adnexa, and supporting ligaments.
5. Pressure on the bladder and urethra.
6. Distention of the maternal soft parts before the advancing fetus.

SIGNS OF IMPENDING LABOR

Physical signs

During the last days or weeks of pregnancy, some women experience one or more of the following signs of approaching labor. None are specific indicators of the onset of labor, nor do they predict the time when labor will begin. However, they do provide evidence that the period of gestation is nearly complete, and this information and reassurance may be used in counseling the client.

Lightening. Lightening is the sensation perceived by the client when the presenting part of the fetus descends into the true pelvis. She may report that "the baby has dropped." In general, with cephalic presentations, the fetal head will be "fixed" on abdominal palpation and engaged, or nearly so, on vaginal examination. This frequently happens approximately 2 weeks before labor in primigravidas. After lightening, the client may find breathing easier as a result of increased space in the upper abdomen, which permits greater room for lung expansion. Conversely, however, she may experience new discomforts that result from the increased pelvic and lower abdominal pressure: urinary frequency, leg cramps, dependent edema, or a sensation of pelvic fullness.

Braxton Hicks's contractions.   These are irregular and generally painless uterine contractions that occur intermittently throughout pregnancy. When perceived by the client, they are often described as a tightening of the uterus or as the "balling up" of the baby. Braxton Hicks's contractions may become increasingly frequent and noticeable as labor approaches, occasionally causing the woman to mistake them for labor. An explanation that the uterine muscle practices for labor, just as other muscles are trained before strenuous exercise, is often beneficial to the client. In addition, she may be advised to use the contractions to practice her breathing, relaxation, or other coping techniques for labor.

Energy spurt.   A "nesting urge" (an energetic feeling or need to accomplish a variety of household tasks) frequently occurs within 24 to 48 hours of the onset of labor. Although it may be permissible for the client to complete one or more of these tasks, she should be forewarned not to overextend herself at this time because she needs to conserve her energy for labor.

Urinary frequency.   The pressure of the presenting part in the pelvis limits the capacity of the bladder and increases the sensation of fullness. In the absence of other signs or symptoms of urinary tract infection, urinary frequency at the end of pregnancy is normal.

Diarrhea.   Diarrhea (or other gastrointestinal symptoms, including indigestion, nausea, and vomiting) may occur within the day preceding labor. Although the cause of these disturbances is unknown, uterine contractions may be stimulated by intestinal irritation. In the absence of other causes of gastrointestinal upset, diarrhea may be viewed as a naturally occurring labor stimulant.

Sleep disturbances.   Sleep disturbances often occur during the third trimester as a result of the "mechanical" adjustments necessitated by the changes in body shape and the increasing weight of the uterus. Many women, however, report additional difficulty or change in their sleeping patterns immediately before labor. As with the energy spurt, the client should be encouraged to conserve her energy and remain resting (even if she is unable to sleep), rather than risk exhaustion before labor.

Loss of the mucous plug.   See page 223.

True vs. false labor

It is necessary to document the onset of true labor as accurately as possible. Incorrect identification of labor may result in unnecessary intervention, which would disrupt normal physiological processes. Conversely, incorrect diagnosis of false labor may result in delivery of the infant without medical attendance. The characteristics of true and false labor are compared in Table 9-1.

INITIAL NURSING ASSESSMENT

Many clients arrive at the hospital in early labor, and it may be necessary to document the existence of labor or complications before continuing with the admission (Table 9-2). When labor or a complication has been demonstrated, a complete data base and assessment is essential to the provision of appropriate nursing care. Therefore, the details of the data base are provided in this section.

Identification

Obtain or confirm previously prepared paperwork, including name, age, parity, etc., according to the record-keeping required by the institution.

History

Labor history. Obtain accurate information concerning the onset, frequency, duration, and intensity of contractions. Determine the presence of bleeding or bloody show and the status of the membranes. If the membranes are ruptured, note the time, color, odor, and amount of leaking fluid. Assess the physical and nutritional status of the client since the onset of labor, including the amount of rest, and the type, amount, and time of last oral intake.

Current pregnancy history. Obtain significant information concerning any antepartum problems or complications, the last normal menstrual period, the estimated date of confinement, weeks of gestation completed, maternal blood type, weight gain, and the results of any special tests, such as ultrasonograms.

Obstetric history (previous pregnancies). Complete the parity statistics. Included should be the number of full-term pregnancies, number of premature pregnancies, number of abortions (whether spontaneous or induced), and number of children currently alive. All information concerning the outcome of each previous pregnancy, type of delivery (spontaneous, instrumental, or operative), length of the pregnancy, infant weight, and condition at birth is also recorded. Special note should be made of any complications of a previous pregnancy, labor, or delivery.

Medical-surgical history. Record allergies to medications in particular, but also to foods or environmental elements. In addition,

TABLE 9-1
Differentiation of True from False Labor

Parameter	True labor	False labor
Contractions Frequency	Increase.	Same or decrease.
	Regular.	Generally irregular, but may be regular for a short period.
Intensity	Progessively stronger.	Same or weaker. (Client may perceive contractions as strong.)
Duration	Progressively longer.	Same or shorter.
Location	Most often felt to begin in the back and to move around to the front (low in the abdomen).	Variable, often felt only at the fundus (high in the abdomen).
Effects of walking, position change, and other activity.	Tend to increase intensity and duration.	Tend to decrease intensity and duration.
Bloody show	May or may not occur.	Does not occur.
Cervix	Change in effacement and dilation.	No change in dilation, possible slight change in effacement.
Diagnosis	True labor is diagnosed by cervical change.	False labor is diagnosed in retrospect.

pay special attention to chronic or recurrent conditions (cardiac, respiratory, renal, anemias, etc.).

Family history. Obtain information concerning the family history of the father of the baby to provide a data base for care of the baby, as well as the client's complete family history.

Psychosocial and emotional history. Assess the emotional status and support systems of the client. The need for, and depth of,

TABLE 9-2
Initial Intrapartum Assessment

Assessment	Nursing diagnosis	Nursing intervention
Rule out complications or significant deviations from the norm.	Normal.	Observe labor or send home, depending on labor status.
	Deviation from the norm.	Consult, admit, or observe, depending on situation and policy.
Note significant risk factors in medical, obstetric, and antepartum history.		
Note absence or presence and extent of vaginal bleeding on history and during examination.		
Confirm or disprove ruptured membranes (*see* Table 9-3).		
Evaluate maternal and fetal vital signs.		
Evaluate emotional and psychological status and coping mechanisms.		
Determine labor status by the following procedure.	Labor established.	Admit and provide care as detailed in Table 9-8.
Elicit labor history.	Uncertain labor status.	Observe for a reasonable time span (generally 1 to 3 hours, depending on policy, etc.) and reassess.
Antecedent phenomena (lightening, energy spurt, bloody show, etc.).		

Assessment	Status	Nursing Interventions

Contraction pattern.
  Onset.
  Frequency.
  Duration.
  Perception of strength.
Rupture of membranes.
Maternal status.
  Nutrition/hydration.
  Rest.
  Excretion.
Perform abdominal examination.
  Leopold's maneuver.
  Contraction status.
Perform pelvic examination.
  Membrane status.
  Labor status.
  Dilation.
  Effacement.
  Presenting part.
  Position.
  Station.
	Not in labor, or prodromal (very early) labor.	Send home. Encourage ambulation (to aid in labor progress, coping ability, or relief of false labor) as appropriate. Encourage rest to conserve energy and prevent maternal exhaustion. Administer sedative if ordered. Encourage light nourishment and intake of fluids. Teach comfort measures as appropriate. Provide appropriate instructions regarding return to hospital or clinic.

Reassess labor status after observation period, if necessary.	Labor established. Uncertain labor status. Not in labor, or prodromal (very early) labor.	See nursing interventions above.

information concerning these topics will vary according to the needs of the individual.

Chart review. Confirm all history-taking information with prenatal care records. In addition, obtain results of all laboratory work during the pregnancy: Papanicolaou (Pap) smear, culture for gonococcus, hematocrit/hemoglobin or complete blood count (initial and subsequent), serology, blood group and Rh factor, indirect Coombs's, rubella titer, sickle cell screening, urinalysis, tuberculosis screening or chest x-ray, and any special tests, such as fasting blood sugar, 2-hour postprandial or glucose tolerance tests, thyroid studies, or other cultures.

Physical evaluation

Perform a physical examination appropriate to the specific needs of the client. The essential elements pertinent to labor management will be included here.

Vital signs. Obtain and record base-line data of temperature, pulse, respirations, blood pressure, and fetal heart tones.

Abdominal examination. Perform a complete abdominal examination:

1. Assess the contraction pattern by resting the palpating hand lightly at the fundus of the uterus. Note the frequency (the time from the start of one contraction to the start of the next), duration (the length of time a contraction is palpable), and intensity. (The intensity is a subjective assessment based on the tenseness of the maternal abdomen or its ability to be indented by the examiner's fingertips at the height of the contraction. If the uterine muscle can be easily indented during the contraction, the contraction is said to be mild. If the muscle is relatively firm during the contraction and cannot be indented at the peak, the contraction is said to be moderate. If the uterus is hard and cannot be indented during much of the contraction, it would be recorded as a strong contraction.)

2. Determine the fundal height by measurement of centimeters or fingerbreadths below the xiphoid process, as appropriate to the institution (*see* Chapter 1).

3. Determine the presentation and position of the fetus (*see* Chapter 1).

4. Estimate the fetal weight while performing Leopold's maneuvers. At best, the estimation of fetal weight by abdominal palpation is an educated guess based on repetitive experience. There is often a range of estimates between practi-

tioners. The accuracy of a given practitioner's estimations is often variable, ranging from very accurate to an error of 1 pound or more in either direction. Many practitioners use the terms "small," "average," and "large" as their estimates, instead of attempting to assign a specific weight. It is important to make an estimation of fetal weight based on the palpation findings (in combination with the fundal height and growth pattern, weight gain in pregnancy, and weights of previous infants) in order to have another parameter available with which to assess the normalness of the situation.

5. Obtain an explanation for all scars that are noted, particularly if no mention of surgery or trauma was elicited in the history. Ascertain the history of any previous uterine surgery.

Speculum examination. *(Never perform a speculum or manual pelvic examination in the presence of frank vaginal bleeding.)* Whether a speculum examination is routinely performed depends on institutional policy and procedure. The purposes for a speculum examination on admission include obtaining a cervical mucus/discharge specimen for culture to rule out infections (including gonorrhea or beta-hemolytic streptococcus), assessing the labor status by visual inspection of the cervix, and determining the status of the membranes and/or evaluating the color of the amniotic fluid (Table 9-3). The use of test paper (Nitrazine or litmus paper) is based on the difference between the normally acidic vaginal secretion pH of 4.5 to 5.5 and the alkaline pH of amniotic fluid of 7.0 to 7.5. The microscopic evaluation for ferning is based on the physical property of air-dried sodium chloride crystals in the amniotic fluid, which assume a fernlike pattern.

Pelvic examination. *(Never perform a pelvic examination in the presence of frank vaginal bleeding.)* The performance of a pelvic examination in the presence of ruptured membranes without labor depends on the institutional and practitioner's policy or directive. Parameters for evaluation during the examination include cervical changes (location, effacement, and dilation), identification of the presenting part, the position and station, and the status of the membranes (*see* Chapter 1 for the procedure and common findings).

Other physical examination elements. Perform other aspects of the physical examination. Other areas of particular concern in pregnancy and labor include the presence and/or extent of edema of the ankles, lower legs, hands, and face; the existence of varicosities, particularly of the legs or vulva; and the assessment of Homans's sign, deep tendon reflexes, and costovertebral angle tenderness.

TABLE 9-3
Assessment of Fetal Membrane Status

Method	Finding	Assessment
Visualization of membranes on speculum examination.	Membranes visible.	Membranes in advance of fetal presenting part are intact (does not rule out possibility of high leak).
	Fluid appears clear, bluish, or milky.	Normal amniotic fluid.
	Fluid appears dark green.	Meconium staining of variable degree. Requires further assessment.
	Scalp and/or hair visible.	Membranes ruptured.
	Fetal buttocks visible.	Membranes ruptured.
Nitrazine paper.*	Yellow (pH 5.0). Olive-yellow (pH 5.5). Olive-green (pH 6.0).	Intact membranes likely, except in presence of minimal fluid or prolonged rupture of membranes.
	Blue-green (pH 6.5). Blue-gray (pH 7.0). Blue (pH 7.5).	Probable ruptured membranes. However, bloody show will also cause an alkaline reaction.
Litmus paper.*	Red (acidic). Blue (alkaline).	Intact membranes. Ruptured membranes.

Ferning‡	Pattern of crystalline ferns.	Ruptured membranes. The presence of vaginal discharge or bloody show can disrupt the pattern.
	No ferning. Only streaks of dry fluid.	Intact membranes. The presence of vaginal discharge or bloody show can disrupt the pattern.

---

*Obtain a specimen of the fluid or discharge from vaginal pool on a sterile swab and touch it to the test paper.

‡Obtain a specimen as above, roll the swab onto a glass slide, and allow it to air dry. Then visualize specimen under the microscope.

DESCRIPTION

The first stage of labor is the period during which the actual work of labor (dilation and effacement of the cervix) is accomplished. (Many clients do not recognize or understand the four stages of labor as constituting a continuum that begins with the onset of effective contractions and ends 1 hour postpartum. In general, to clients, "labor" refers to the first stage and "delivery" refers to the second and third stages.)

The first stage is further divided into three phases: early (or latent), active, and transition (Table 9-4). According to Friedman, an alter-

TABLE 9-4
Phases of the First Stage of Labor

Factor	Latent	Active	Transition
Dilation, *cm*	0-3	4-8	8-10
Effacement, %	Often 100	100	100
Descent of presenting part	Minimal, if at all	Progressive, at moderate rate with beginning flexion of head	Progressive, at maximum rate
Bloody show	May be present; minimal	Probably present; increased quantity	Probably present; heavy
Contractions Frequency	Every 5-20 min, regular, becoming progressively closer	Every 3-5 min	Every 1½-3 min
Duration, *sec* Intensity	15-45 Mild to moderate	40-60 + Moderate to strong	60 + Strong
Duration of phase			
Average, *hr*	4-12	2-5	½-2
Nullipara, *hr*	8-12	2-4	1-2
Multipara, *hr*	4-8	1-3	½-1

native means of identifying these phases includes the latent phase and the active phase, which is then subdivided into the acceleration phase, the phase of maximum slope, and the deceleration phase (Fig. 9-1).[4]

Early labor (latent phase)

Early labor begins with the onset of uterine contractions, which are effective in causing progressive cervical effacement and dilation. It is the longest phase of the first stage, lasting approximately 10 hours in nulliparas and less in multiparas. Dilation progresses to 3 centimeters, and effacement is complete, or nearly so, by the end of early labor. In the "textbook case," the contractions are of mild to moderate intensity, occurring at regular and progressively shorter intervals (from every 20 minutes to every 5 minutes) and increasing in duration (from 15 to 45 seconds).

Active phase

The active phase is so named because the rate of progress, as measured by cervical dilation and descent of the presenting part,

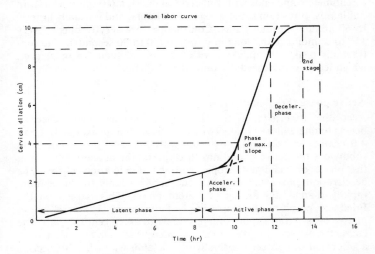

Figure 9-1. The Friedman curve. *Adapted from* Friedman, E. A. Graphic appraisal of labor: a study of 500 primigravidae. *Bulletin of the Sloane Hospital for Women in the Columbia-Presbyterian Medical Center* (June 1955). 43.

becomes more rapid. The active phase begins when the cervix is approximately 4 centimeters dilated and ends at approximately 8 centimeters dilation. The contractions of active labor become more frequent, occurring every 3 to 5 minutes. Contraction strength and frequency cause many women discomfort. Spontaneous rupture of the membranes usually occurs at the end of the first stage of labor, or during the second stage. The normal active phase for nulliparas is 2 to 4 hours, and for multiparas, 1 to 3 hours — although actual labor times vary widely from person to person. Progress in labor is an extremely complex process that depends on the power of uterine contractions, the adequacy of the pelvis, and the weight and presentation of the fetus.

Transition

Although the transition phase is considered a subdivision of the active phase by Friedman (his deceleration phase), the change in the contraction pattern and maternal experience is sufficient to warrant consideration of this phase as a separate entity. It is the shortest phase of the first stage but also the most intense. Transition begins at 8 centimeters and ends with full cervical dilation (10 centimeters). In nulliparas, transition usually lasts 1 to 2 hours, and it usually lasts 30 to 60 minutes in multiparas. Contractions are very frequent (every 1½ to 3 minutes) and long in duration (60 to 90 seconds). The contractions peak very quickly, with little or no time for relaxation, which leads to increased discomfort and difficulty in coping.

Active phase (Friedman)

According to Friedman, the active phase begins when the cervix begins to dilate more rapidly (when the cervix is approximately 2.5 to 4.0 centimeters dilated), and ends with full dilation. Friedman subdivides the active phase into three parts: the acceleration phase, the phase of maximum slope, and the deceleration phase. The acceleration phase begins when the cervix begins to dilate more rapidly than it did during the latent phase. This is seen on the Friedman graph as the "upswing" of the curve. The acceleration phase lasts from approximately 2.5 to 4.0 centimeters. The characteristic upswing of the Friedman curve is usually predictive of a labor that will proceed normally (i.e., a labor with adequate uterine contractions, ample pelvic proportions, and normal fetal weight and presentation). On the other hand, slow dilation during this phase, which is seen as a "flat graph," is a warning sign that labor may be prolonged.

The phase of maximum slope is the time of most rapid cervical dilation. It lasts from approximately 4 to 8 centimeters. Cervical dilation in nulliparas averages 3.0 cm/hr, with a minimum of 1.2 cm/hr. In multiparas, the average is 5.7 cm/hr, and the minimum is 1.5 cm/hr. It takes powerful, coordinated uterine contractions to accomplish this dilation. A normal curve reflects the overall efficiency of these contractions.

The deceleration phase lasts from approximately 8 to 10 centimeters, and is so named because progress may not be as rapid as in the phase of maximum slope. Progress through this phase is reflective of the relationship of the pelvic diameters to the weight and presentation of the fetus.

ADMISSION

Essential admission history

In the event of a rapidly progressing labor or an apparently imminent birth, it is crucial to obtain the most essential information first. The objective is to obtain the *key* material: details can be filled in after the birth or in a few minutes, if the initial expectation of a precipitous delivery is not fulfilled. Table 9-5 provides one set of questions that are listed in order of importance.

This admission history should be obtained by talking with the client while performing a rapid abdominal and pelvic examination. Unless the infant is being born, the nurse must always listen, or have someone else listen, to the fetal heart. The nurse must perform an abdominal palpation quickly so that basic data is available before the pelvic examination is performed. Next, the nurse must perform a rapid but thorough pelvic examination. Of course, if the examination findings do not indicate imminent delivery, there is time to complete the examination and data collection in a more leisurely manner. If at all possible, someone else should prepare the equipment and paper work in this tension-producing situation while the primary nurse and the client build a working rapport. The following is a list of nursing priorities for the initial collection of data:

1. Identification of client and significant other(s), and introduction of personnel.
2. Significant history (*see* Table 9-5).

TABLE 9-5
Essential Admission Questions

Question*	Rationale
1. What is your name?	To rapidly establish rapport and open a direct line of communication.
2. When is the baby due?	To determine the possibility of a pre- or postmature fetus.
3. What number baby is this for you? Any abortions or miscarriages?	To determine parity, which gives a more accurate prognosis regarding the likelihood of a precipitous delivery.
4. Any problems during *this* pregnancy? Were you admitted to the hospital for any reason? Any problems with bleeding, high blood pressure, or sugar? Did you take any medications other than iron and vitamins?	To provide a quick assessment of antepartum risk factors.
5. Did you have any special tests during this pregnancy? Ultrasonogram: a sound picture of the baby? Special blood tests: a long sugar test (glucose-tolerance test or fasting blood sugar and 2-hour postprandial)?	To evaluate antepartum risk factors that the client may not consider to be "problems."
6. Do you have any allergies? Medications (antibiotics, analgesics, or anesthetics)? Food? Environmental factors?	To determine contraindications to analgesia, anesthesia, and other medications.

7. Any problems with other pregnancies?
   Full term?
   Bleeding in pregnancy, labor, or postpartum?
   Babies healthy at birth? Size?
   Type of delivery? Stitches?

   To determine problems with previous pregnancies that may be relevant to this birth.

8. Have you ever been sick? Ever had an operation?
   Tonsils? Appendix?
   Broken bones?
   On any medications?
   See a special doctor?

   To assess maternal health and risk factors.

9. When did your labor start?
   Did your water break? When?
   Any bleeding?

   To obtain a basic labor history.

10. Any problems/illness in your family?
    Diabetes? Hypertension? Heart problems? Twins?

    To identify risk factors for the mother and/or her baby.

*The subquestions should be asked only if additional information about that area is more essential than the remaining areas.

3. Inspection of perineum for signs of imminent delivery, frank bleeding, or spontaneous rupture of membranes.
4. Abdominal examination (simultaneous with history taking). Determination of presentation and position, number of fetuses, estimated fetal weight, and contraction pattern and status.
5. Assessment of vital signs: fetal heart tones, and maternal blood pressure, pulse, respirations, and temperature.
6. Speculum and bimanual examination: collection of specimen(s), assessment of membrane status, assessment of cervical change and status, and station of presenting part.

Nursing interventions after the initial assessment

In a normal situation, the physician is notified of labor status after completion of the data base. In the event of frank vaginal bleeding, the physician must be notified immediately and the nurse must not continue with a vaginal examination of any kind.

If the determination of false labor or very early labor is made, the client may be sent home or admitted for further observation as indicated by institutional or practitioner policy or preference (*see* Table 9-2). The nurse should proceed with the admission of the client to the labor and delivery suite if the decision for further observation was made or as indicated for the following reasons:

1. Medical or obstetric complications.
2. Well-established labor, generally determined by a regular contraction pattern with cervical dilation of at least 3 to 4 centimeters.
3. Emotional and/or social reasons, such as an inability to cope with labor events or extreme hardship or difficulty in traveling between the home and the hospital (e.g., because of weather conditions or great distance).

Admission procedures

The nursing activities and procedures included in the admission process will vary according to institutional and practitioner policy, client preferences, maternal physical well-being, and fetal status. Table 9-6 discusses the specific procedures and variations included in the admission of a client. Table 9-7 discusses the routinely ordered laboratory data, their purposes, and related management.

Not mentioned in the tables are the standard nursing actions for the admission of a client to any unit in the hospital. These include the introduction of staff members responsible for her care and the orientation of the client and significant others to the unit (use of the mechanism to adjust bed position; method to summon assistance; location of bathroom and/or other appropriate facilities such as telephone, kitchen/pantry if permitted to eat or drink, early labor lounge or area permitted for ambulation). Identification bracelet; changing into hospital gown or personal nightgown, if permitted; the location for storage of street clothes, suitcase, etc.; and method to secure valuables are also completed on admission. These nursing actions will be carried out according to specific policies and their appropriateness to each situation.

CONTINUING NURSING ACTIONS DURING LABOR

As labor continues, additional observations, assessments, and nursing actions are essential to confirm the continued well-being of the client and fetus, to document appropriate progress in labor, and to promptly recognize variations of, or deviations from, the norm.

Table 9-8 lists the nursing care activities in labor and their rationales. Table 9-9 lists minimum frequency recommendations for nursing observation in normal labor.

FACTORS INFLUENCING INTRAPARTUM MANAGEMENT DECISIONS

During admission, or shortly thereafter, certain preliminary management decisions are made. These decisions include whether a perineal shave will be performed, and, if so, how much pubic hair will be removed; whether an enema will be administered; and whether an intravenous infusion or oral hydration will be used. In addition to the practitioner's routine and the institution's policy, other specific factors may influence the decisions.

Perineal shave

The possible types of preparation include a full shave, which removes all hair from the mons pubis, labia, and perineum; a mini-prep, which removes hair from the perineum and a portion of the labia; and no preparation at all. The factors to be considered are the amount and distribution of pubic hair, the imminency of delivery, the probability of delivery over an intact perineum versus the need for an episiotomy, and client preference.

Enema

There are several types of enemas that may be administered during labor. These include a soapsuds enema, a tap water enema, and a Fleet or other small-sized, prepared enema. The factors involved in the

TABLE 9-6

Commonly Performed Admission Procedures

Procedure and nursing actions	Rationale	Discussion	Alternative
Perineal shave of the perineum, labia, and mons pubis	To decrease possible contamination of a "sterile" area, thus preventing infection.	Careful attention to aseptic technique during pelvic examination, delivery, and repair of laceration or episiotomy is more important in prevention of infection.	Miniprep of perineum and labia. Miniprep of perineum only. Clipping of long hairs with scissors, but no shave. No prep.
Provide for privacy.	To improve perineal cleanliness.	The nicks that might occur during the prep increase the risk of infection by providing an additional route of entry for pathological organisms.	
Allow the client to assume comfortable position.	To provide easier visibility of the perineum during labor, delivery, and/or postpartum.	Cleanliness is primarily a matter of appropriate instruction and postpartum emphasis on its importance.	
Discontinue shave during contractions.		Perineal visibility is rarely, if ever, impaired by the presence of pubic hair in the normal distribution pattern.	
Leave the client clean and dry afterward.		The procedure itself is often perceived as embarrassing or physically uncomfortable by the client.	
Perform prep as quickly, but as safely and as comfortably, as possible.		Regrowth of pubic hair is generally uncomfortable and irritating.	

Enema

Use water at body temperature for comfort.

Help the client into a comfortable position, preferably the left lateral position, which physiologically enhances bowel function.

Administer fluid slowly and stop flow during contractions if the client complains of cramping.

Provide privacy: the enema will be more effectively expelled, and the client will be more comfortable, if she can use a bathroom rather than a bedpan.

Remain nearby while the enema is being expelled, in case of sudden change in labor contractions, SROM, cord prolapse, or precipitous delivery.

To stimulate uterine contractions.

To reduce the likelihood of contamination of the delivery area by feces.

To improve accuracy of findings and comfort during pelvic examinations.

To provide greater room in the pelvic cavity by emptying the rectum. (Fleet enema or a small tap water enema is sufficient.)

The effectiveness of enemas for stimulation of contractions is controversial and often influenced by outside factors. (Soapsuds enemas appear to be more irritating and thus more effective for this purpose). Diarrhea or previous bowel movements reduce the possibility of contamination. Perineal cleanliness by client or caregivers prevents this as well. Enema is relatively uncomfortable to a client during active labor and may result in her decreased ability to cope with the labor itself. Some clients request an enema for their own comfort if they are constipated. Many clients do not want the enema. If the membranes are ruptured and/or the presenting part is not engaged, an enema may predispose the client to prolapse of the umbilical cord during expulsion of enema fluid. Certain complications contraindicate the use of an enema:

Enema of reduced quantity (e.g., a Fleet or a 250-milliliter soapsuds enema). Delay of enema until specific indication or advantage occurs. No enema.

Procedure and nursing actions	Rationale	Discussion	Alternative
		Premature labor: it is not advisable to risk stimulation of the labor unnecessarily. *Vaginal bleeding (placenta previa or abruption):* stimulation from the enema could increase the severity. *Breech presentation:* risk of cord prolapse is increased.	
Intravenous infusion Use an intracatheter because it provides more freedom of movement of extremity and is more likely to remain properly in place if activity is increased.	To prevent or treat maternal dehydration, as evidenced by ketonuria, vomiting, or physical signs or symptoms (minimal skin turgor, complaints of increased thirst, or concentrated urine). To provide energy for labor.	Some practitioners prohibit all oral intake; others allow clear liquids but prohibit all forms of solid food. Clients receiving oral liquids may not need intravenous fluids to maintain hydration. The nurse must continuously assess the client for indications for intravenous therapy. Restricts maternal use of the extremity and may increase physical discomfort during the insertion procedure and perhaps thereafter.	*Oral fluids:* clear liquids, ice chips, or electrolyte-rich fluids. *Oral nutrition:* fluids with extra glucose or light solids. Intramuscular analgesic if needed. Local or pudendal (rather than regional or general) anesthetic in 2nd stage.
Use sterile technique during insertion.	To have an immediately available route for medication administration for pain relief, induction or stimulation of labor, operative delivery, or obstetric emergencies.		
Use antiseptic or antibiotic ointment or jelly at site of insertion.			
Pay careful attention to anchoring the catheter and the tubing to prevent inadvertent movement.	To be able to replace fluid or blood loss on indication. Predisposing factors for hemorrhage include grand		

multiparity, precipitous labor, prolonged labor, uterine overdistention, oxytocin induction or augmentation of labor, anemia, or blood dyscrasias. If an intravenous line is not in place when hemorrhage occurs, great skill is needed in rapid insertion of the line.

SROM, spontaneous rupture of membranes.

TABLE 9-7
Admission Laboratory Tests *

Type	Purpose	Related management
Hematocrit or complete blood count	Documentation of maternal hemopoietic status.	Considered in management decisions regarding hydration and intravenous therapy.
Blood type and cross-match or hold	Precaution for emergency. Identification of Rh factor, if blood type was not obtained prenatally.	Used for matching blood to be transfused in the event of a hemorrhage. Identifies possibility of Rh incompatibility with fetus.
Blood test for syphilis	Diagnosis of syphilis (often obtained only in nonregistered clients).	Identifies mother and infant in need of treatment in the postpartum period.
Urinalysis	Identification of hydration status, glycosuria, and proteinuria (a sign of preeclampsia and/or infection).	Considered in determining the need for intravenous therapy and/or medications and for identifying complications.

*Normal values for these tests are provided in Appendix B.

decision regarding enema administration include the speed of labor progress or the need for stimulation; the amount of cervical dilation; the status of the lower bowel, such as evidence of a significant amount of feces present as determined during pelvic examination; and client preference. There are certain specific or relative contraindications to the use of an enema that must be ruled out before its administration: the presence of premature labor, unexplained vaginal bleeding, breech presentation, and an unengaged presenting part, particularly in the presence of ruptured membranes.

Nutrition and hydration status

The decision regarding the use of an intravenous infusion versus oral hydration and/or nutrition is also made during labor. Evidence of dehydration or electrolyte imbalance (such as ketonuria, nausea, and/or vomiting), complaints of thirst, and poor skin turgor must be evaluated. The client's ability to tolerate oral fluids or nutrients and her preference regarding eating and/or drinking during labor should be taken into account. As part of the decision to allow oral intake, it is necessary to consider the risk of aspiration of gastric contents, especially under general anesthesia. Certain situations require the intravenous route for medication administration: regional or general anesthesia; operative and, frequently, instrumental delivery; oxytocin induction or augmentation; and, perhaps, the repetitive use of sedation or analgesia. An intravenous line may be needed for blood or fluid replacement in clients at risk for postpartum hemorrhage. Conditions that predispose the client to postpartum hemorrhage include an overdistended uterus as a result of a large fetus, multiple gestation, or hydramnios; precipitous or prolonged labor; oxytocin induction or augmentation; blood dyscrasias; and severe anemia.

ASSESSMENT OF AMNIOTIC FLUID

Spontaneous rupture of membranes

Rupture of the chorionic and amniotic membranes, which surround the fetus, generally occurs during the first stage of labor. During labor, the function of the membranes and amniotic fluid is to act as a cervical dilating wedge during contractions and to protect the presenting part (particularly the fetal skull) from excessive pressure or trauma. Unless there is a specific indication to do so (such as the need for internal fetal monitoring or the need to stimulate labor), it is no longer recommended that the membranes be artificially ruptured. For identification of spontaneous rupture of membranes (SROM) that occurs before the client's arrival at the hospital, *see* p. 231 and Table 9-3.

When SROM occurs after admission, detailed documentation is rarely necessary. The client should be instructed to notify the nurse if she feels a loss of fluid from the vagina. Observation of quantity, color, and odor of fluid as well as an immediate vaginal examination is most often sufficient to confirm or invalidate the diagnosis. A vaginal examination is essential to rule out prolapse of the umbilical cord, particularly if the station of the presenting part had previously been high. The fetal heart tones must also be checked immediately to aid in assessment. Frequently, SROM will occur during a vaginal examination that is being performed for another indication.

Significance of SROM

Once the membranes have ruptured, a primary barrier to intrauterine maternal and fetal infection is removed. Thus, further vaginal examinations must be kept to a minimum and performed under strict aseptic technique. In addition, assessment of maternal temperature should be done more frequently (every 1 to 2 hours).

TABLE 9-8
Nursing Considerations in Labor

Nursing considerations	Rationale	Discussion
Activity Ambulation as desired Bed rest Bed rest with bathroom privileges Allow client out of bed to sit in chair only Allow client out of bed in labor room only	Selected to improve maternal comfort and coping during labor, to encourage the most efficient uterine contraction pattern, and to prevent complications (e.g., cord prolapse or uncontrolled delivery, the latter of which is one of the stated reasons for bed rest).	Factors involved in decision-making include client preference, fetal well-being, effectiveness of uterine contractions, rapidity of labor progress, station of presenting part, and status of membranes.
Labor position Upright, ambulating	Increases maternal sense of normalness and well-being. Increases physiological and effective uterine contractions. Frequently aids in coping techniques or in relief of discomfort. Reinforces the normalness of labor. (Bed rest is generally perceived as required during illness.)	Technically, ambulation increases the difficulty of monitoring fetal-maternal status. Most clients prefer to remain ambulatory, or agree to it when encouraged, and return to bed intermittently for vital signs, fetal heart checks, and indicated examinations. Contraindications to ambulation include ruptured membranes with the presenting part not engaged (increased risk of cord prolapse), sedated or medicated client, frank bleeding (placenta previa or abruptio placentae), moderate or severe preeclampsia, and documented fetal distress.
Supine (most common position in labor, with head of bed elevated)	Facilitates external fetal monitoring to produce valid tracings.	The risk of supine hypotension syndrome and thus of fetal distress is increased. Backache may occur.

Lateral recumbent	Encourages coordination and effectiveness of uterine contractions. May aid in rotation of fetal head to occiput anterior. Reduces supine hypotension syndrome. Increases renal perfusion. May be used as an alternative birthing position in bed.	Contractions are stronger in intensity but less frequent. Rotation results from the forces of gravity. Inferior vena caval compression by the uterus is relieved. Removal of pressure on the vena cava improves blood flow to the kidneys. This position is most useful in occiput posterior and occiput transverse positions, supine hypotension syndrome, and initial intervention with ineffective uterine contractions, variable fetal heart decelerations (resulting from cord compression), and fetal distress.
Knee-chest and all fours	Relieves back discomfort resulting from muscular tension or posterior position of fetus. May help to rotate fetal head. Reduces risk of cord prolapse or of compression, if prolapse has occurred (while preparing for cesarean section).	Some women prefer to deliver in this position.
Fluid administration (by intravenous or oral route)	Maintains hydration. Maintains and replenishes energy supply for the work of labor. Relieves and prevents physical discomfort, e.g., thirst and dryness of mouth and throat.	See Table 9-6. Variables to consider in decision-making regarding route of fluid administration include hospital policy, client preference, and presence of nausea and vomiting.
Administration of antacid	Reduces gastric acidity. Helps to prevent and control nausea during labor. Decreases the likelihood of vomiting in labor or during use of general anesthesia.	Use of antacids is generally based on institutional policy. Frequently used routinely in hospitals that allow oral fluids and/or solids in labor.

Nursing considerations	Rationale	Discussion
Evaluation of vital signs, including blood pressure, temperature, pulse, and respirations	Documents maternal status, and screens for deviations from the norm.	Abnormal blood pressure may help to identify complications such as supine hypotension syndrome and preeclampsia. Abnormal temperature, pulse, and respirations may indicate other deviations, such as infection or dehydration. *See* Table 9-9 for schedule recommendations for obtaining vital signs. Obtain vital signs if changes in maternal status occur (e.g., skin warm to the touch). Obtain vital signs before allowing change in activity or use of analgesia or anesthesia.
Urinalysis (dipstick of each voiding)	Documents maternal status (e.g., hydration and nutritional status and signs of preeclampsia).	*See* Table 9-7.
Observation of contractions and changes in behavior	Indicates labor progress.	Assessment, identification, and documentation of contraction pattern, including frequency, duration, and intensity. The nurse should assess, identify, and document changes in maternal behavior (e.g., ability to cope with contractions, change in desired activity, and change in verbalization or responsiveness to others and environment).
Vaginal examination (Institutional policy determines whether nursing staff may perform vaginal examinations.)	Documents labor progress and identifies deviations from the norm.	Vaginal examinations should be kept to a minimum. They should be performed when the documented findings will be used in making or changing management decisions.

Routine performance of vaginal examinations according to a prescribed frequency (e.g., every 2 hours) should be discouraged because it leads to excessive manipulation, with a potential increase in infections, and it does not provide significant information for management. Behavioral clues and a change in contraction pattern are important parameters of progress in labor. Astute observation may eliminate the need for some vaginal examinations. One essential time for the performance of a vaginal examination is when other criteria indicate full dilation. It is crucial to ensure that the cervix is fully dilated before permitting pushing. This avoids trauma to the maternal cervix and the fetal head. Another important time for performing vaginal examination is immediately after SROM (to check for prolapse of the umbilical cord as well as to document any change in the cervix and in the descent of the fetus).

(*See* Chapter 18 for a full discussion of indications, rationales, techniques, and alternatives to electronic fetal monitoring.)

Fetal monitoring

SROM, spontaneous rupture of membranes.

TABLE 9-9

Recommended Frequency of Nursing Observations
in the First Stage of Labor

Criterion	Latent phase	Active and transition phase
Fetal heart tones	Every ½ hr (more often if variations occur)	Every 15 min (more often if variations occur)
Maternal blood pressure	Every 2 hr Every ½-1 hr if elevated	Every 1 hr Every ½ hr if elevated
Temperature	Every 4 hr Every 1 hr if elevated or if membranes are ruptured	Every 2 hr Every 1 hr if elevated or if membranes are ruptured
Pulse	Every 4 hr	Every 2 hr
Respiration	Every 4 hr	Every 2 hr
Urine dipstick	Every voiding	Every voiding
Contraction pattern	Every 2 hr*	Every 1 hr*
Bloody show and vaginal discharge	Every 2 hr*	Every 1 hr*
Maternal behavior	Every 2 hr*	Every 1 hr*

*Minimum frequency. Assess more often as needed and note time of changes.

Fetal tachycardia is often a sign of fetal infection or of fetal response to maternal infection or elevated temperature. The characteristics of the amniotic fluid should be evaluated (*see below*).

In the event that a vaginal examination after SROM documents prolapse of the umbilical cord, the nurse must *not* remove her examining hand. It is crucial that the presenting part be held up and supported off the cord in order to maintain the integrity of feto-placental circulation. The nurse must, in this instance, call for assistance. An assistant should then notify the physician and prepare for an emergency cesarean section according to hospital policy. This preparation would include notification of the blood bank to cross-match one or two units of whole blood or packed cells; notification of anesthesia personnel as appropriate; preparation of the operating room and equipment or notification of operating room personnel; an abdominal and/or perineal shave; and insertion of a Foley catheter. Continued monitoring of the fetal heart rate is crucial. This can be performed by palpating the pulsation of the cord (being careful not to occlude the vessels).

Amniotic fluid

Normal amniotic fluid.

Appearance/color/odor: The fluid is clear or milky white (caused by fetal epithelial cells or vernix). Amniotic fluid has a characteristic odor that is not foul.

Amount: The amount of fluid seen depends on the amount ahead of the presenting part, particularly when the fetal head is well-applied to the cervix. Approximately 100 to 500 milliliters leaks at the time of rupture. Further leakage generally occurs with contractions because the increased pressure forces fluid from around the fetus. The total normal volume of fluid ranges from 800 to 1,200 milliliters.

Meconium-stained amniotic fluid.

Color: The color depends on the time of passage of meconium relative to the time that amniotic fluid is observed and on the amount of meconium contained in the fluid. Fresh meconium has a green color, which, because of metabolism, becomes brown to yellowish over time.

Significance: In a cephalic presentation, the passage of meconium in utero may signify fetal distress. The existence of old meconium may be significant to current fetal well-being. In the breech presentation, it is often the result of pressure of the cervix on the presenting buttocks.

Intervention: In the presence of known or suspected meconium staining, continuous electronic fetal monitoring is necessary to ensure safety and immediate recognition of fetal distress. At delivery, the baby's nose, mouth, and trachea should be suctioned before the baby's first breath, if possible, to prevent aspiration of meconium.

Bloody amniotic fluid.

Color: Bloody amniotic fluid ranges in color from a bright red to a "port wine" color.

Significance: Bloody amniotic fluid indicates premature separation of the placenta (abruption) or rupture of vasa previa (the presence of the cord vessels within the membranes adjacent to, or crossing, the cervical os).

Intervention: In rare instances, identification or suspicion of vasa previa occurs before rupture of the membranes by visualization or palpation on pelvic examination. In such cases, a cesarean section is indicated. In general, however, the diagnosis is not made until after delivery, when the placenta, cord, and membranes are examined. In the presence of bright red amniotic fluid, rapid preparation for a cesarean section and continuous electronic fetal monitoring are essential. In less critical situations, continuous electronic fetal monitoring and preparation for a possible cesarean section are indicated.

Hydramnios.

Significance: The occurrence of a significant increase in the amount of amniotic fluid above normal levels is called hydramnios. Often, volumes less than three times the normal (approximately 3,000 milliliters) are not clinically apparent as hydramnios. The cause of most cases of hydramnios is not identified. It is generally diagnosed by excessive enlargement of the uterus, often accompanied by difficulty in palpating fetal parts or in auscultating fetal heart tones. Ultrasonography is useful in documenting hydramnios as well as in ruling out fetal anomalies or multiple gestation, both of which often occur concomitantly with this disorder.

Hydramnios is present in association with certain fetal anomalies. These most frequently involve the central nervous system: spina bifida with meningocele or myelomeningocele or anencephaly. Specific medical or obstetric complications of pregnancy may also be associated with hydramnios. These include diabetes mellitus, preeclampsia or eclampsia, and erythroblastosis fetalis with fetal hydrops. Cord prolapse and postpartum hemorrhage are also frequently occurring complications.

Intervention: Nursing intervention in labor includes close monitoring and assessment of both client and fetus.

Oligohydramnios.

Significance: The existence of a severely reduced quantity of amniotic fluid (less than 300 milliliters) is known as oligohydramnios. The cause is unknown, although the most frequently associated condition is malformation of the fetal urinary tract, including obstruction and renal agenesis. Prolongation of the pregnancy beyond term by several weeks may result in relative oligohydramnios.

Intervention: Nursing care during labor is unchanged. However, more frequent evaluation of fetal heart tones or intermittent use of the fetal monitor is indicated.

PAIN DURING LABOR

Pain pathways

Pain during the first stage of labor stems primarily from the uterus. Uterine sensory innervation is derived from the sympathetic nervous system — specifically the tenth, eleventh, and twelfth thoracic nerves.[5] Uterine contractions are thought to stimulate pain receptors by creating an ischemic state during contractions, by stretching the cervix, and by causing traction on the fallopian tubes, ovaries, peritoneum, and supporting ligaments.

During the active phase of the first stage of labor and throughout the second stage, when the presenting part is low enough to distend the lower birth canal and the perineum, additional painful stimuli are transmitted from the lower genital tract through the pudendal nerve via the ventral branches of the second, third, and fourth sacral nerves.[5]

Relief of pain

Any pain relief measures should preserve fetal homeostasis, be simple, and be safe.[6] Obviously, then, the most ideal pain relief is that achieved without the use of narcotics, barbiturates, or other analgesia or anesthesia. The nurse is in the position to provide the most effective pain relief — physical presence, support, and reassurance/teaching. In addition, the nurse may aid the client by teaching or supporting the client's effort to maintain a regimen of breathing, concentration, and comfort techniques according to the type of preparation for childbirth, if any, that is used by the client and her partner. A summary of methods of childbirth preparation is provided in Table 9-10.

Many methods of childbirth preparation use a system of breathing techniques to help the client cope with labor. Deep, slow breathing assists muscular relaxation, and the quiet concentration on the process of breath control gives the client a rhythmic focus of activity. Various schools of childbirth education advocate different methods of respiration. Some encourage diaphragmatic breathing in order to relieve pressure on the uterus, while others teach light, shallow breathing to prevent pressure on the uterus. A suggested sequence of breathing patterns for labor is listed below (Fig. 9-2).

1. In early active labor, when the client is no longer able to talk through her contractions, the nurse should instruct her to take deep abdominal breaths, at a rate of 6/min.
2. In the active phase of labor, a more complex pattern of breathing is begun. The client is instructed to take a deep breath and exhale (a cleansing breath), then to take four very shallow chest breaths followed by a blowing breath, at a rate of about 60/min. At the end of a contraction, the client is instructed to take another deep cleansing breath and relax.
3. During transition, the client may have the urge to push at the peak of a contraction. If so, she may be instructed to take very

TABLE 9-10

Methods of Preparation for Childbirth

Method	Basic principles/beliefs	Coping techniques included
Childbirth without fear: natural childbirth (Grantly Dick-Read)	Fear-tension-pain syndrome. Mystical perception of the childbirth experience (woman's psychological needs emphasized).	First to advocate active role of father of baby. Education to reduce or eliminate fear-tension-pain syndrome. Body-conditioning exercises. Passive relaxation to cope with discomfort. Nonspecific, sleeplike breathing.
Classical conditioning (Russian Pavlovian theory)	Stimulus-response reaction.	Conditioning to interrupt the natural, automatic reflex, which results from the stimulus of contractions (tension/pain perception). Reflex reaction replaced with conscious methods to eliminate or decrease pain or muscular tension.
Psychoprophylaxis (Fernand Lamaze. Marjorie Karmel introduced method to U. S. A. in 1959).	Combination of childbirth without fear and classical conditioning.	Similarities to Dick-Read's method: education to reduce fear of the unknown; active relaxation of muscles not involved in uterine contraction (neuromuscular control); body-building exercises; and emotional support person present during labor. Specific addition of psychoprophylaxis: controlled breathing techniques to deal with different contraction patterns throughout labor.
Variation (Elisabeth Bing)	Utilization of trained montrices and labor-support nurses. Additional variations in breathing techniques. Changes in position for 2nd-stage pushing.	

Psychosexual method (Sheila Kitzinger)	Use of sensory memory as an aid in understanding and working with the body. Recognition of importance of human relationships to the woman during pregnancy.	Husband encouraged to use tactile support in labor. "Hummingbird" breathing (form of mouth-centered breathing). Easy, gentle pushing effort, particularly if client is a multipara. Pushing with relaxed abdominal muscles. Kegel exercise emphasized to help with relaxation during 2nd stage. Pelvic rock performed on all fours (like a cat with arched back).
Husband-coached childbirth (Robert Bradley)	Introduction of the trained, prepared husband to the "birth team."	Emphasis on the primary importance of the husband's presence at labor and delivery. Normal, diaphragmatic breathing — no altered techniques as in other methods. "Gentle pushing" by exhaling throughout 2nd-stage contraction.
Birth without violence (Frederick Leboyer)	Not a childbirth preparation method per se but a method of birth techniques to decrease the stress and trauma of the experience on the newborn.	Gentle pushing. Lighting in birth room kept as low as possible. Speaking in soft, hushed voices or not at all. Avoidance of excessive stimulation of the infant — no slap on buttocks or feet, no holding upside down by the feet. Delayed cord clamping to allow two ways of breathing (i.e., oxygen and carbon dioxide exchange through the placenta and by the infant's lungs). Placement of the infant directly onto mother's abdomen in fetal position. Gentle stroking of the infant's back. Warm, soothing bath (return to the womb) generally administered by the father soon after birth.
Hypnosis	Psychic strength elicited to deal with acquired fears. A form of meditation requiring practice and repeated suggestions throughout pregnancy.	Command of somatic awareness of pain at will by self or hypnotherapist. Directed concentration.

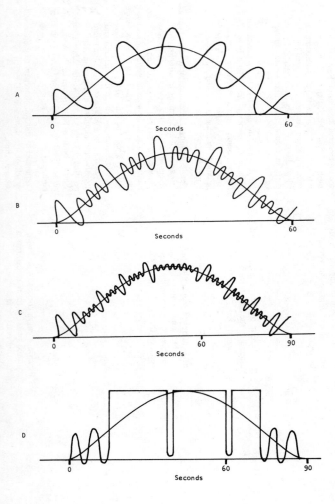

Figure 9-2.   Breathing patterns during labor. The arc represents the contraction. The wavy line indicates breathing rhythm. (A) Early active labor. (B) Active labor. (C) Transition stage. (D) Second stage.

shallow panting or blowing breaths at a rate of about 60/min. After the urge passes, she may switch to another style of breathing. She should be instructed to take a cleansing breath at the end of her contraction.

4. For pushing, the client is instructed to take one or two deep cleansing breaths. Then she is told to take a deep breath, hold it, and push. When she needs to, she should exhale, take another deep breath, and push again. At the end of the contraction, she should take one to two cleansing breaths and relax.

Although the nurse will not be able to achieve expertise in all of the currently available childbirth preparation techniques, he or she should master an effective set of instructions that will assist the majority of clients to achieve a narcotic-free childbirth.

The needs and anticipated emotional responses of the woman in labor and the supportive functions of the significant other and/or the nurse are presented in Table 9-11. In the presence of a well-prepared couple, the nurse may need only to continue the care discussed previously, provide reinforcement of their ability to work with the labor, and suggest possible alternatives or additional comfort and support measures as necessary.

Degree of pain

The degree and severity of pain a woman will experience during labor are influenced by many variables besides the frequency, duration, and intensity of contractions. The client's experiences with the health care system during hospitalizations or injuries, previous labors, or medical illness will alter pain perception. On the other hand, the client who has never dealt with the system or who has never been in a hospital before will be more anxious and, thus, have a heightened sense of discomfort. Cultural norms prescribe the experience of pain in labor. The presence or absence of support systems and the preparation for and knowledge about the childbirth event are important factors in the overall perception of pain. Finally, general health is a variable. Good nutrition, rest, and a positive attitude toward the experience of childbirth produce the optimum background for minimal discomfort. On the other hand, decreased nutritional intake, fatigue, anxiety, fear, or superimposed medical/obstetric illness may increase the labor pain.

Medications

Systemic pain relief. Often, medications may be necessary to help a client to cope with the stress and pain of labor. Specific medi-

TABLE 9-11

Emotional, Informational, and Physical Support

Maternal behavioral changes during labor	Coping techniques and supportive measures
Latent phase Excitement, happy anticipation of the labor and birth. Sense of relief at the end of the pregnancy. Some mild apprehension concerning the unknown experience of labor. Anxiousness to talk.	Encourage normal activity unless contraindicated (ambulation, light nourishment). Provide and participate in distraction techniques (cards, board games, reading). Conserve energy for active labor: encourage rest periods. Foster relaxation during contractions. Do not encourage breathing patterns until above measures are no longer sufficiently distracting. Allow client to ventilate feelings and support their normalness. Provide information concerning the function of labor, realistic expectations concerning labor sensations and hospital and practitioner policies and procedures (especially necessary in the unprepared or unaccompanied client). Encourage frequent urination. Provide appropriate information regarding status of labor, progress, and realistic expectations. Answer questions truthfully (find out any information required and return); do not invent answers. Involve the significant other in all of these activities as appropriate to ability and interest.
Active phase Possible apprehension with ill-defined doubts and fears. Uncertainness of ability to cope with contractions.	Continue activities that are not contraindicated. Encourage frequent position changes if on bed rest. Foster relaxation techniques. Encourage complete relaxation and normal breathing between contractions. Teach and encourage breathing exercises if necessary.

Serious mood: "getting down to work." Desire for companionship and support.

(Specific technique varies according to method of prepared childbirth and perception of each contraction.)
Provide physical comfort measures: ice chips, oral fluids, hard candy, back rub, counterpressure, cool cloths, effleurage, massage of the legs and back.
Encourage voiding.
Administer medications as indicated for relief of pain or to aid relaxation and coping ability.
Praise for a job well done (may need praise after every contraction).
Encourage and support significant other; suggest a break before transition and 2nd stage begin.

Transition
Frequent inability to comprehend or follow directions; need for constant repetition and reinforcement.
Generalized discomfort: leg cramps or shaking, irritable abdomen, nausea with occasional vomiting, hiccuping, burping, perspiration on upper lip and forehead, chattering teeth, severe low backache, flushed face, pain.
Marked restlessness.
Increasing apprehension.
Frustration and bewilderment: ready to give up.
Desire to be left alone or desire for total, close contact (clinging behavior).
Strong urge to push/rectal pressure.
Pulling, splitting, stretching sensations deep in the pelvis.

Encourage relaxation.
Teach and encourage breathing techniques.
Provide comfort measures: counterpressure, back rub, position change for backache; deep breathing or breath holding as needed for nausea; sponge or wet cloth to face; moisten lips.
Administer medication if indicated and desired by client.
Reinforce that labor is nearly over.
Recognize and accept client's irritability.
Reinforce the normalness of labor experiences and sensations.
Do not overload with questions, statements, etc. Avoid interruptions and procedures during contractions.

cations, their indications, contraindications, effects, and adverse reactions on the client and/or her fetus/infant are found in Appendix A. The purpose of specific medications that are administered to promote comfort during labor are listed below:

Analgesics: to relieve or reduce pain caused by uterine contractions, muscle or ligament stretching, pressure on nerves, etc.
Tranquilizers: to decrease anxiety and apprehension, thus increasing the ability to relax and cope with labor.
Sedatives: to allow sleep or greater relaxation during the latent phase when contractions may not be effective but are uncomfortable.
Antiemetics: to control significant nausea and/or vomiting.

The use of medications in labor and the factors to consider in decision-making regarding their use are addressed in Table 9-12.

TABLE 9-12
Medications: Factors to Consider in Decision-Making

General factor	Specific factor
Labor status	Contraction pattern Progress as determined by labor curve Anticipated time to delivery
Maternal status	Vital signs Age/size (height and weight) Medical condition, including complications such as hypertension, diabetes, and history of liver, kidney, or cardiac problems Allergies History of drug use/abuse
Indication for medication	Need for pain relief vs. relaxation Realistic maternal expectation of effect Previous medication: time given, dosage, effect, duration
Fetal status	Gestational age Estimated fetal weight Well-being as determined by fetal heart tones and at-risk factors (e.g., infant of a diabetic mother, pre-eclampsia, postmaturity, and meconium staining)

Regional analgesia/anesthesia. Regional analgesia/anesthesia has the advantage of providing effective pain relief to the specific site of the pain while using a very small amount of medication with minimal effect on the fetus. The physician, nurse anesthetist, or nurse-midwife will administer the regional anesthesia, but the nurse must be able to explain the technique to the client, assist her to cooperate while it is being administered, and monitor both maternal and fetal status after it is administered. The common local anesthetic agents are listed in Appendix A. The types of regional analgesia/anesthesia are illustrated in Figure 9-3.

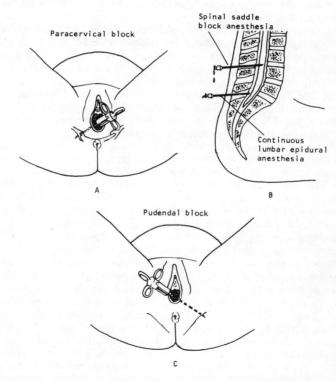

Figure 9-3. Regional anesthesia in obstetrics. (A) Paracervical block; (B) spinal saddle block anesthesia and continuous lumbar epidural anesthesia; (C) pudendal block. *Reprinted with permission from* Ross Laboratories. Clinical Educational Aids. Number 17. Ross Laboratories, Columbus, Ohio.

Paracervical block: The paracervical block is administered during the active phase of labor, when the cervix is dilated between 4 and 8 centimeters. It consists of bilateral injections of local anesthetic into the lateral or posterior lateral fornices of the vagina. An effective block provides excellent pain relief for 1 to 2 hours, depending on the specific anesthetic agent that is used. Occasionally, soon after a paracervical block is administered, fetal bradycardia (lasting up to 10 minutes) occurs. If it does occur, the client should be positioned on her left side, and her fluid intake should be increased. The fetal heart rate will usually return to normal within a few minutes, and, unless there are other insults to the fetus before delivery, the outcome can be expected to be good.

Epidural block: Lumbar epidural blocks may be administered for labor analgesia or for anesthesia for vaginal or cesarean delivery. A continuous epidural block is administered via a catheter that is inserted into the epidural space around the spinal cord. Local anesthetic injected into that space blocks the nerves that enter the spinal cord. The epidural block should not be administered without an intravenous infusion in place. Many physicians prefer to rapidly infuse about 500 milliliters of fluid before administering the block. While the catheter is being inserted, the nurse must help the client sit or lie on her side very still, with her lower back thrust out as far as possible. As soon as the block is administered, the client should be placed on her left side or on her back with the uterus displaced to the left. Her blood pressure, pulse, and respirations should be recorded every 1 to 2 minutes for the first 15 to 20 minutes, and every 15 minutes thereafter because hypotension is a common side effect. Pain relief will last for about 45 minutes to 2 hours, depending on the anesthetic agent that is used. After delivery, the epidural catheter will be removed carefully by the physician or nurse-anesthetist.

Spinal anesthesia: Subarachnoid block (also called spinal anesthesia or saddle block) is administered for delivery of the baby. The dura of the spinal cord is entered, and local anesthetic is injected. The client must sit still, with her head down and her lower back arched out, while the block is being administered. She may need to remain sitting for a few seconds after the medication is injected before assuming the position for delivery so that the local anesthetic can descend to the level of the second, third, and fourth sacral nerves. As with epidural anesthesia, hypotension may result, so it should be administered only after an intravenous infusion has been started, and blood pressure should be recorded afterward every minute for 10 minutes. There is some risk with both epidural and spinal anesthesia of the medication anesthetizing nerves high in the spinal column, thus blocking the nerves involved in respiration. Therefore, emergency equipment and drugs necessary for respiratory resuscitation should be available whenever these forms of anesthesia are used. After delivery, the client should remain flat in bed for 8 to 12 hours to prevent headaches caused by the leakage of cerebrospinal fluid.

Pudendal block: The pudendal block is usually administered immediately before vaginal delivery. It may be administered transvaginally, as shown in Figure 9-3, or through the perineum. It provides anesthesia for the introitus, labia, and perineum. It does not require any specific nursing measures. Depending on the type of medication used, the effects may last from 45 to 90 minutes.

VARIATIONS OF NORMAL LABOR

Premature rupture of membranes if labor ensues

Definition.   SROM before the onset of labor is called premature rupture of the membranes (PROM). The incidence of PROM is approximately 12 percent. Approximately 20 percent of all cases of PROM occur at or before the 36th week of gestation. The cause of most instances of PROM remains unknown. When PROM occurs near or at term, labor will most often (80 to 90 percent) ensue within 24 hours.[7]

Effect on labor.   None.

Nursing interventions.   Because of the increased risk of maternal and/or fetal infection after rupture of membranes, most women will be admitted to the hospital once PROM is documented. Nursing care is essentially the same as for normal labor, with the addition of hourly checks of maternal pulse and temperature and more frequent evaluation of fetal heart tones. An increase in maternal pulse or temperature and/or the development of fetal tachycardia are the most common early signs of developing infection. Foul-smelling amniotic fluid may also herald infection.

Posterior position of the fetus

Definition.   The fetal head, as the presenting part, is positioned such that the occiput (or back) of the head is toward the posterior segment of the maternal pelvis. Approximately 15 to 30 percent of all labors involve occiput posterior positions at some time.[8] The majority of these rotate spontaneously to occiput anterior positions. The remainder are termed persistent occiput posterior. (Delivery mechanisms and techniques are considered in Chapter 10.) Labor with occiput posterior positions is often called "back labor" because the back is where the client perceives the contractions.

Effect on labor. Because of the less than optimal fit of the presenting part against the cervix and within the pelvis, and because of the additional time required for the fetus to rotate spontaneously to the anterior position, the labor tends to be longer. Furthermore, the effectiveness of uterine contractions may be reduced, which also results in a longer labor.

Nursing interventions. Routine nursing care remains the same. The client often requires assistance in determining the most effective relief measures and the most comfortable position for labor. It is believed by some that lying on the same side as the fetal limbs may help in spontaneous rotation. Many women, however, are not comfortable in any one position for long periods, and frequent changes are indicated. Relief measures may include counterpressure at the location of the perceived discomfort, back rubs, ice packs or hot packs applied to the lower back, or pelvic rock exercises.

Supine hypotension syndrome

Definition. Supine hypotension syndrome is a fall in blood pressure that occurs as a result of the pressure of the uterus on the inferior vena cava, which impairs the return of blood to the heart from the lower extremities. The client may complain of feeling faint or dizzy.

Effect on labor. None, unless the condition is allowed to persist, in which case decreased uterine perfusion may lead to episodes of fetal distress.

Nursing interventions. The prevention of supine hypotension syndrome is one goal of nursing care in labor. Encouraging the client to assume a comfortable alternative position will help the nurse to achieve this goal. However, should the syndrome occur, the nurse should immediately turn the client on her left side, thus removing the cause of vena caval compression. Administration of oxygen and/or an increased rate of intravenous infusion, if any, may also be employed until the episode subsides. The nurse should auscultate the fetal heart or obtain a monitor tracing to document fetal well-being.

Hyperventilation

Definition. Hyperventilation is excessive respiration, which leads to the development of alkalosis caused by an imbalance in the oxygen-carbon dioxide relationship during respiration. When conditioned breathing techniques are used in labor, there is a risk that inspiration and expiration will be unequal, thereby resulting in an increase in the amount of carbon dioxide blown off as compared with the amount of oxygen taken in. The client may report a tingling of her hands, fingers, feet, or lips. She may become dizzy or light-headed. In severe cases, she may exhibit air hunger.

Effect on labor.   None. Spontaneous correction would occur in severe cases because the client would faint and resume a normal respiration pattern.

Nursing interventions.   The nurse must help the client avoid hyperventilation by assisting her with breathing techniques. If hyper-ventilation occurs, the client should be instructed to rebreathe carbon dioxide by breathing into and out of a small paper bag that is held over her nose and mouth, or by breathing into her own hands cupped over her mouth. After the contraction is over, the client should hold her breath for several seconds.

REFERENCES

1. Danforth. 329.

2. Danforth. 327.

3. Danforth. 332.

4. Friedman. (1955)

5. Pritchard and MacDonald. 443.

6. Pritchard and MacDonald. 436.

7. Varney. 237.

8. Oxorn. 139.

CHAPTER 10

SECOND STAGE OF LABOR

Suzanne M. Smith

PHYSIOLOGY

The physiology of the organ systems during labor has been described in Chapter 9. Specific changes of the second stage (delivery) are included here.

The **metabolic rate** continues to increase throughout labor, resulting in the greatest elevation of normal temperature at the time of delivery or immediately thereafter. The amount of temperature elevation does not normally exceed 1.8 to 3.6 °C (1 to 2 °F), and any further increase must be evaluated to rule out infection or dehydration.

The **pulse rate** also tends to be somewhat increased during the second stage. As in the first stage, there are variations in the rate during and between contractions, and the effect of maternal position must be considered. As with temperature, the maximum increase in pulse rate is at the time of delivery or immediately thereafter.

The **respiratory rate** is unchanged from the first stage of labor. It is important to remember, however, that voluntary maternal pushing alters the rate during contractions. Therefore, the respiratory rate must be evaluated well after a contraction ends.

Blood pressure changes continue to be mediated by maternal position. (It is important to note that pushing need not be confined to the supine position.) There is a continuation of the blood pressure elevation from the first stage, and there are variations in the blood pressure during and between contractions.

Fetal heart tones must be evaluated more often (preferably after each contraction) during the second stage because the effects of descent and maternal pushing may result in early decelerations of the fetal heart rate. It is crucial to differentiate between early decelerations, which result from head compression, and late decelerations, which result from uteroplacental insufficiency. Refer to Chapter 18 for this differentiation.

DESCRIPTION

The second stage of labor begins when the cervix is fully dilated (10 centimeters) and ends with the delivery of the baby. During this stage, the uterine contractions, enhanced by voluntary and involuntary maternal bearing-down efforts, function to push the fetus through the pelvis and the vagina (the birth canal).

The contraction pattern generally changes noticeably when compared with the transition phase of the first stage. Contractions occur less frequently (often as much as 5 to 7 minutes apart). Their duration is generally similar to that of transition: approximately 60 seconds. Intensity varies from client to client and contraction to contraction. Most often, if the presenting part has engaged or reached the pelvic floor muscles, contractions are expulsive and result in involuntary pushing by the mother.

The second stage of labor is considered to be normal if it results in progressive descent of the fetus and in delivery within 2 hours of full dilation. The average length of the second stage is approximately 30 to 60 minutes, with a normal range of from only one or two contractions to up to 2 hours. In the nullipara, the second stage averages 30 to 60 minutes; in the multipara, it is generally less than 30 minutes. If at any time there is arrest of descent or if the second stage continues beyond 2 hours, evaluation for the specific cause is indicated. Table 10-1 summarizes the characteristics of the second stage.

FORCES OF EXPULSION AND RESISTANCE

The efficiency and effectiveness of the second stage of labor are determined by the interrelationships of a number of factors. They may be grouped into three distinct categories: passageway, passenger (fetus), and powers. The relative importance of any one factor is highly variable and, thus, no attempt is made to identify these elements in order of priority.

TABLE 10-1

Characteristics of the Second Stage of Labor (Delivery)

Aspect	Comments
Dilation	10 cm to birth of infant.
Effacement	Complete (100%).
Descent of presenting part	Progressive.
Bloody show	Often increased (but this varies considerably).
Contractions	
Frequency	May be decreased when compared with transition phase. Every 2-7 min.
Duration	Variable. Generally about 60 sec, but some shorter.
Intensity	Strong and explusive, particularly after presenting part reaches the pelvic floor. Perception of pain may decrease with pushing.
Duration of stage	
Average	Less than 1 hr. Over 2 hr constitutes a prolonged 2nd stage.
Nullipara	30-60 min.
Multipara	Less than 30 min.

Passageway

Passageway refers to the bony pelvis and soft tissue of the pelvis.

Bony pelvis. The pelvic type of the individual as well as its specific diameters and/or abnormalities are important to consider. Refer to Chapter 1 for specific information concerning the anatomy of the bony pelvis.

Pelvic floor musculature. The rigidity and/or elasticity of the muscles themselves as well as the mother's ability to consciously relax them while pushing aid in both descent and internal rotation of the fetal head to the optimal position for delivery.

Perineal structures. The rigidity and/or elasticity of the perineum also affects the length of the second stage. This is more significant, however, in determining the need for an episiotomy or the risk of fetal head compression immediately before delivery.

Passenger

Refer to Chapter 1 for details pertaining to the fetus during labor. Areas of particular concern during delivery include attitude, lie, presentation, position, and molding.

Powers

Powers refers principally to the forces that effect delivery.

Contractions. The quality and efficiency of contractions are of significance in evaluating their effectiveness. Refer to Chapter 9 to review the physiology of contractions. The normal characteristics of frequency, duration, and intensity are summarized in Table 10-1.

Expulsive efforts. Intra-abdominal pressure is increased during contractions of the second stage. A further increase in this pressure occurs with voluntary maternal bearing-down efforts.

MECHANICS OF LABOR

Although they are called the mechanisms of labor, these major steps are primarily related to the movements of the fetus during the second stage.

Descent refers to the progressive movement of the fetus through the birth canal. It occurs throughout labor concurrently with other mechanisms. As discussed in Chapter 1, descent is described by the "station" of the presenting part in the pelvis.

Flexion occurs during the course of labor. When the fetus is fully flexed, the fetal head is forward and touching the chest, and the fetal spine forms a convex curve. Flexion occurs during fetal descent as a result of resistance from the maternal soft tissues. As descent progresses, there is resistance from the cervix, the pelvic sidewalls and their overlying muscles, and the pelvic floor. If it has not already occurred, flexion is completed when the fetus reaches the pelvic floor. If full flexion is not achieved, the progress of labor may be impeded.

Internal rotation brings the anterior-posterior (AP) diameter of the fetal head into alignment with the AP diameter of the pelvis. The most common position at this point is occiput anterior (OA). Internal rotation is essential for vaginal birth, except in the case of a very small fetus. The shoulders (which are entering the pelvis at this time) follow the head only to the oblique angle. Thus, there is a 45-degree lag of the shoulders behind the head, resulting in a twisting of the neck. Internal rotation occurs mainly during the second stage.

Extension of the fetal head is the result of resistance from the pelvic floor, which forces the head upward toward the vaginal opening along the curve of Carus. The nucha (suboccipital region) becomes the pivot point beneath the symphysis pubis, and further uterine contractions and maternal pushing result in the extension of the head, causing the delivery of the occiput and face over the perineum. **Crowning** is the point during extension at which the biparietal diameter is encircled by the vaginal orifice. At the point of crowning, it becomes impossible for the fetal head to regress, and delivery will occur within the next one to two contractions.

Restitution occurs after the head is delivered. It is the untwisting of the neck, which returns the head to correct alignment with the shoulders.

External rotation is the visible manifestation of the internal rotation of the shoulders into the AP diameter. The head rotates to the transverse position at this time.

Lateral flexion along the curve of Carus causes the delivery of the shoulders and body. The anterior shoulder impinges under the symphysis pubis and emerges first, followed by the posterior shoulder and the remainder of the body.

To summarize the mechanisms of labor, the movements of a fetus that enters the pelvis in the left occiput transverse (LOT) position (the most common) are presented below (Fig. 10-1).

Descent and flexion: occur throughout the course of labor.
Internal rotation: LOT to left occiput anterior (LOA) to OA.
Extension: OA and the delivery of the head.
Restitution: OA to LOA.
External rotation: LOA to LOT.
Lateral flexion: causes the shoulders and body to deliver.

In the event that the fetus enters the pelvis in an occiput posterior (OP) position, there are two possibilities for the mechanisms. In the most common, during the mechanism of internal rotation, the fetus will rotate 135 degrees to the OA position. This is called the "long arc rotation," and the remainder of the mechanisms are as described above. To summarize the internal rotation in this instance: left (L) OP to LOT to LOA to OA, or right (R) OP to ROT to ROA to OA. This occurs in approximately 90 to 95 percent of all OP positions during labor (Fig. 10-2).[1]

In approximately 6 to 10 percent of OP positions, however, the internal rotation of 45 degrees results in a persistent OP.[1] This is called the "short arc rotation," and the remainder of the mechanisms are adjusted accordingly (Fig. 10-3). To summarize the internal rotation in this case: LOP to OP, or ROP to OP. In this instance, flexion results in the delivery of the head. The sinciput impinges under the symphysis pubis and becomes the pivot point. The head continues to flex, causing the occiput to deliver (up to the nucha of the neck) over the perineum. The face then delivers from under the symphysis pubis as a result of extension. This has been

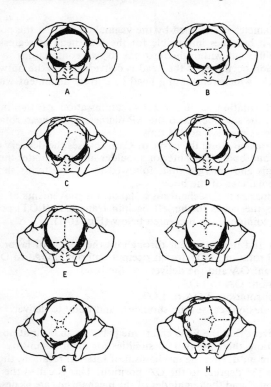

Figure 10-1. The mechanisms of labor. (A) Onset of labor; (B) descent and flexion; (C) internal rotation: left occiput transverse (LOT) to left occiput anterior (LOA); (D) internal rotation: LOA to occiput anterior (OA); (E) beginning of extension; (F) completion of extension; (G) restitution: OA to LOA; and (H) external rotation: LOA to LOT. *Adapted from* Oxorn, H. Oxorn-Foote Human Labor and Birth. Appleton-Century-Crofts, East Norwalk, Conn. 1980. Fourth edition.

called a "sunny-side up" delivery. The changes in the other mechanisms are as follows:

Restitution: OP to LOP, or OP to ROP.
External rotation: LOP to LOT, or ROP to ROT.
Lateral flexion: as above, causes the shoulders and body to deliver.

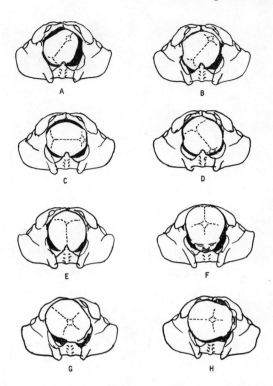

Figure 10-2. Long arc rotation. Most common internal rotation mechanism (135 degrees) if fetus enters the pelvis in an occiput posterior (OP) position. (A) Onset of labor: right occiput posterior (ROP); (B) descent and flexion; (C) internal rotation: ROP to right occiput transverse (ROT); (D) internal rotation: ROT to right occiput anterior (ROA); (E) internal rotation: ROA to occiput anterior (OA); (F) extension; (G) restitution: OA to ROA; and (H) external rotation: ROA to ROT. *Adapted from* Oxorn, H. Oxorn-Foote Human Labor and Birth. Appleton-Century-Crofts, East Norwalk, Conn. 1980. Fourth edition.

EMOTIONAL, INFORMATIONAL, AND PHYSICAL SUPPORT IN DELIVERY

The information presented in Chapter 9 regarding the role of the nurse remains valid in the second stage. Table 9-8 lists the relevant

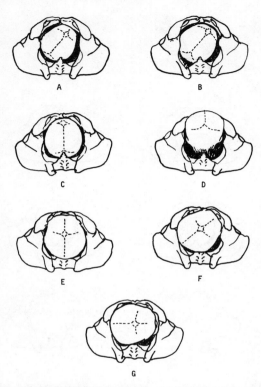

Figure 10-3. Short arc rotation. Internal rotation mechanism that occurs in 6 to 10 percent of all instances when fetus enters the pelvis in an occiput posterior (OP) position. (A) Onset of labor: right occiput posterior (ROP); (B) descent and flexion; (C) internal rotation: ROP to OP; (D) birth by flexion; (E) head falls back during extension; (F) restitution: OP to ROP; and (G) external rotation: ROP to right occiput transverse (ROT). *Adapted from* Oxorn, H. Oxorn-Foote Human Labor and Birth. Appleton-Century-Crofts, East Norwalk, Conn. 1980. Fourth edition.

nursing care activities, with alternatives and rationales, and a discussion of each.

The purposes of nursing observations and assessments are to document continued fetal and maternal well-being, to confirm continued progress in labor (descent of the fetus), and to recognize deviations from, or variations in, the norm during the second stage. Table 10-2

TABLE 10-2

Recommended Minimum Frequency of Nursing Observations in the Second Stage of Labor

Observation	Frequency
Fetal heart tones	After every one or two contractions.
Blood pressure	Every 30 min. Every 15 min if elevated.
Temperature, pulse, and respiration	Every 2 hr. Temperature every hour if elevated, or if membranes are ruptured.
Urine dipstick	Every voiding.
Contraction pattern Bloody show and vaginal discharge Maternal behavior	Continuously: client requires constant nursing presence during second stage.

TABLE 10-3

Emotional, Informational, and Physical Support during the Second Stage of Labor

Maternal behavioral changes	Coping techniques and supportive measures
Strong urge to push, feeling of rectal pressure, need to move bowels. Splitting or burning of vaginal tissues as a result of distention and/or stretching by descending fetus. Increased bloody show. Increasing involvement in birth process. Excitement that birth is imminent. Relief that labor is nearly over. Complete exhaustion after each contraction. Initial difficulty with following directions (e.g., forgetting how to push).	Continue any technique or comfort measure from first stage of labor that was beneficial. Encourage relaxation between contractions to conserve energy. Provide directions for pushing technique. (Technique will vary according to practitioner preference, client's ability, maternal and fetal status, and method of prepared childbirth, if any.) Encourage relaxation of pelvic muscles during contractions and pushing. Provide constant encouragement and reinforcement.

lists the recommended minimum frequency of nursing observations during a normal second stage.

The normal maternal emotions, needs, coping techniques, and supportive measures are presented in Table 10-3.

As stated above, the function of the second stage of labor is the delivery of the fetus. Voluntary and/or involuntary bearing-down efforts (pushing) by the mother accompany uterine contractions to accomplish this function. There are a variety of pushing techniques, and the technique chosen is generally a matter of individual preference. Table 10-4 discusses the various techniques used, and the advantages and disadvantages of each. The positions for labor (lateral, supine, all fours, and knee-chest) that are described in Table 9-8 may also be used for pushing and/or delivery (Fig. 10-4).

The specific maternal and fetal factors that must be considered in determining location for birth are summarized in Table 10-5. The factors to be evaluated in determining the time for transfer to the delivery room are included in Table 10-6.

DELIVERY PROCEDURES

Support person

The nurse generally assumes the responsibility of preparing the support person(s) for the delivery. This preparation begins on admission and continues throughout labor. As delivery approaches, scrub suits, caps, masks, and shoe covers are provided according to institutional policy and the planned birth location. The support person may help in moving the bed to the delivery room, and should then be shown where to stand or sit. The nurse should keep in mind that the support person's function during the birth is to assist and support the client and not simply to be an "interested observer." Both the client and the support person should receive explanations of the equipment available in the delivery room. Any new members of the health care team — e.g., pediatricians or obstetric residents — should be introduced. Needless to say, prior permission should be obtained from the client if nonessential personnel or observers wish to be present at the birth.

Infection

The birth process itself is not sterile. Sterile technique is indicated at the birth to safeguard both the client and her baby from the risks of infection from the hospital environment and the attendants. The client is vulnerable during labor and birth for several reasons. She is in a different environment. Her natural environment would pose little or no threat because she has developed specific antibodies and immune reactions. Her system has not developed these safeguards to the hospital environment and the microorganisms of the staff, other patients, and unfamiliar persons. The newborn possesses most of the immune reactions of the mother, but is even less able to withstand the pathogens in the hospital environment. Furthermore, normal

TABLE 10-4

Pushing Techniques in the Second Stage of Labor

Technique	Advantages	Disadvantages
Involuntary response Bearing-down efforts only in response to natural urge. ("Do what your body tells you.")	Is physiologically normal. Is unlikely to impair placental circulation and, thus, is unlikely to cause fetal hypoxia or acidosis. Allows time for pelvic floor muscles and perineum to distend gradually, decreasing risk of laceration or need for episiotomy. Allows fetal head to accommodate pressure changes slowly.	May cause concern that 2nd stage may be prolonged. May not be appropriate in the event of fetal distress or other need for expeditious delivery. Regional anesthesia may inhibit pushing reflex.
Intermittent pushing Short breath-catching and pushing	Is similar to involuntary response. Can be coordinated and used with regional anesthesia. Can supplement "natural" response in the event of slow progress in descent.	Requires more concentration and coordination than involuntary technique.
Aggressive pushing Lamaze method. Deep cleansing breath, and hold next breath to count of 10 while pushing as hard as possible.	Is useful, in conjunction with episiotomy and/or instruments, to expedite delivery in the event of actual or anticipated complications.	May cause increased fetal head compression or decreased oxygenation of placenta.

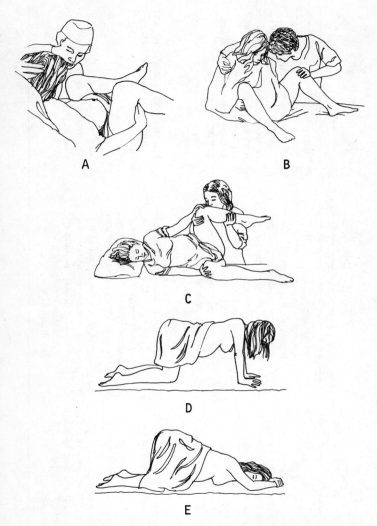

Figure 10-4. Positions for pushing and/or delivery. (A) Dorsal position, (B) lounge-chair position, (C) side-lying position, (D) all fours position, and (E) knee-chest position.

TABLE 10-5

Factors to Consider in Determining Location for Birth

Labor/birthing room in bed	Delivery room in bed	Delivery room on delivery table
Normal fetal heart tones throughout labor. No anticipated problems requiring pediatric assistance or specialized equipment. Progressive labor, with or without oxytocin or regional anesthesia.	Evidence of mild fetal distress. Presence of meconium-stained amniotic fluid. Prematurity. Premature rupture of the membranes.	Significant fetal distress or other indication for instrumental delivery. Multiple gestation. Malposition (face or brow). Malpresentation (breech). Anticipation of significant episiotomy and/or laceration repair. Obesity sufficient to impair attendant's ability to safely conduct the birth. Need for general anesthesia.

TABLE 10-6

Factors to Consider in Timing of Transfer to Delivery Room

Factor	Discussion
Contractions (interval and intensity)	Evaluation aids in estimating expected time of delivery.
Dilation and station versus parity	*Multiparous women* are generally moved to delivery room before full dilation unless other factors indicate a long 2nd stage. *Nulliparous women* are generally not moved until some part of the head is visible between contractions.
Effectiveness of pushing	Speed of progress in descent is important in estimating delivery time.
Fetal well-being or distress	Fetal distress may indicate need to expedite delivery with episiotomy and/or instruments.
Planned procedures	Administration of pudendal or spinal anesthesia, etc., before birth necessitates earlier transfer.
Fetal presentation and position	Some practitioners prefer to delay transfer in breech presentation to reduce the impulse to interfere with normal physiology. In vertex presentation, completion of internal rotation and speed of descent must be evaluated.
Priority	The necessity for delivery room equipment to care for mother and baby must be considered in cases where several women are about to deliver and there are not enough delivery rooms available.

procedures — including venipuncture, vaginal examinations, internal monitoring, artificial rupture of the membranes, etc. — provide potential sites for infection. Once the membranes have ruptured, whether spontaneously or artificially, both the client and her fetus are at greater risk of infection. Lacerations, episiotomy, and the open venous sinuses of the placental site provide portals whereby even normal vaginal inhabitants may become pathogenic.

An understanding of the potential for the development of infection leads to an understanding of the need for aseptic techniques. This does *not* mean, however, that the birth must assume the "aura" of major surgery. Appropriate hand washing, which includes an initial scrub of 5 to 10 minutes and hand washing after caring for each patient or after handling any equipment, is the most important measure for the prevention of infection. The use of full operating room attire is appropriate for births conducted in the delivery room, but is not necessary for birthing room births. In these cases, a simple cover gown or apron for the birth or a change of scrub clothes is sufficient. The birth attendant and any assistants should wear sterile gloves, and hair should be covered or tied back if long. Masks are not necessary unless there is particular risk of respiratory infection. The use of sterile drapes in the delivery room coincides with the use of operating room attire. For deliveries conducted in bed, especially if in the birthing room, a sterile drape under the buttocks to cover the bed sheet is sufficient. Redraping or additional aseptic precautions are indicated in situations that require the repair of an episiotomy or lacerations, third-stage intervention, or control of postpartum hemorrhage. In all cases, the instruments and the sterile field must be handled appropriately. The nurse should not reach across sterile instruments or return used instruments (cord clamp, episiotomy scissors, gauze, etc.) to the sterile field.

Positions

Delivery may be conducted in a variety of positions (Fig. 10-5). Table 10-7 discusses the advantages and disadvantages of each.

Anesthesia

A summary of anesthetic methods used in delivery may be found in Table 10-8. Diagrams of pudendal block and local infiltration are illustrated in Figure 10-6. Specific information regarding anesthetic agents is found in Appendix A.

Episiotomy and laceration

There are two types of episiotomy. A median (or midline) episiotomy extends from the posterior fourchette of the vagina straight through the perineum toward, but not to, the rectal sphincter. A mediolateral episiotomy is cut on an angle beginning at the fourchette toward the ischial tuberosity (Fig. 10-7). Table 10-9 lists the factors to be considered when determining the need for an episiotomy. The advantages and disadvantages of each type are discussed in Table 10-10.

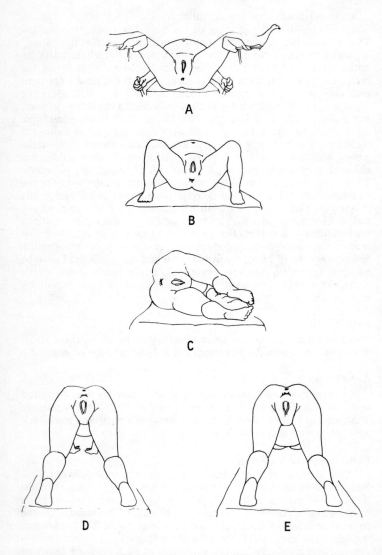

Figure 10-5. Delivery positions. (A) Lithotomy position, (B) dorsal position, (C) left lateral position (D) all fours position, and (E) knee-chest position.

There are four kinds of perineal lacerations. A first-degree laceration involves only superficial tissues: the vaginal mucosa and/or perineal skin, the fourchette, and, perhaps, a small amount of subcutaneous tissue. A second-degree laceration also includes the perineal body and/or perineal muscles: the bulbocavernosus, the superficial and deep transverse perineal, and, perhaps, the levator ani, depending on the depth of the laceration. A third-degree laceration extends through the fascia (capsule) of the anal sphincter and may or may not involve the sphincter itself. A fourth-degree laceration also includes the rectal wall. It is possible, although uncommon, for a fourth-degree laceration to occur without a third-degree laceration occurring first. This is called a "buttonhole fourth." In all other cases, however, the laceration involves all tissues of lacerations of lesser degree.

NORMAL DELIVERY TECHNIQUE

In the event that delivery is imminent and the nurse is either alone or the most qualified individual to conduct the birth, it is worthwhile to have an understanding of the appropriate hand maneuvers. The decision to move to the delivery room or to remain in the labor room will be influenced by several factors: the location of supplies and emergency equipment, and the availability of help from other persons, including family members or support persons. Pediatric attendance should be requested if there is any evidence of fetal distress. Furthermore, if the attendant is not comfortable about delivering a baby, it is wise to have pediatric assistance so that the attendant can be totally devoted to caring for the client.

It is important to maintain a calm appearance and to work *with* the client, her support person(s), and whoever else is present. If the nurse acts in an orderly fashion and provides reassurance that nature is the expert, both the client and the nurse will handle the situation more comfortably.

The most important factor to consider is the safety of the client and her baby. For this reason, an inexperienced attendant is well advised to conduct the delivery in bed rather than on the delivery table. There is then no risk of dropping the baby, and essential equipment can be kept close at hand. When it is evident that the delivery is imminent, the nurse should gather and prepare the necessary equipment (if this has not already been done), scrub as time permits, and put on sterile gloves. The essential equipment consists of two clamps and one pair of scissors for the umbilical cord, a bulb syringe or DeLee mucous trap, several gauze sponges, and a towel or blanket for the baby. A sterile drape should be placed under the client's hips.

TABLE 10-7
Delivery Positions

Position	Advantages	Disadvantages
Lithotomy Can be modified by adjusting the position of the stirrups and/or by providing pillows or a backrest to raise the client's head, shoulders, and back.	Is easiest for the attendant. Provides good visibility of, and access to, the perineum and vagina, particularly for performance and repair of episiotomy. Provides support for the client's legs. Can be used for an uncooperative client: limits mobility and the risk of uncontrolled activity during delivery. Is preferred by some practitioners in case of anticipated shoulder dystocia. Allows mother to view birth by means of a mirror.	Is least physiological: causes compression of the vena cava by the uterus; does not facilitate the forces of gravity. Prevents maternal mobility and position change to aid in mechanisms of delivery for shoulders. Increases the risk of thrombophlebitis, particularly if varicosities are present.
Dorsal Can also be achieved on delivery room table by having the client rest her feet on the lower part of the table, which is lowered (broken) but not fully retracted.	Is similar to lithotomy position in ease for attendant. Avoids the use of stirrups. Allows the client to see the birth by means of a mirror. Is the position of choice in bed for a precipitous delivery or a delivery by an inexperienced person.	Is not physiological: causes compression of the vena cava by the uterus; does not facilitate the forces of gravity. Provides less visibility of, and access to, the perineum than the lithotomy position.
Left lateral	Decreases vena caval compression. Provides good visibility of perineum during birth. Allows mobility of client to aid in delivery of shoulders.	Requires encouragement to assume or remain in this position because many women are unfamiliar with it. Decreases eye contact of attendant with mother.

Position		
	Provides easy access to fetus for suctioning during birth. Is physiological. Is generally more comfortable than the dorsal or lithotomy position.	May require a support person to elevate client's leg during the birth. May cause confusion on the part of the attendant as to the position of the baby and the direction for pressure during birth.
All fours	Does not cause vena caval compression. May be most comfortable for delivery of occiput posterior position. Provides good visibility of perineum during birth.	May require encouragement to assume or maintain this position. May cause confusion on the part of the attendant as to the position of the baby and the direction for pressure during birth. Requires position change after birth for bonding, delivery of placenta, and any repair.
Squatting	Is most physiological for both birth and delivery of the placenta; facilitates forces of gravity.	Provides least visibility of perineum and fetus during birth. Requires position change after birth for bonding and any repair.

TABLE 10-8
Anesthesia

Type	Indications	Nursing care
General (inhalation)	Emergency cesarean section. Need for rapid induction of anesthesia (e.g., difficult instrument delivery or manual removal of the placenta). Need for anesthesia in presence of hypovolemia.	Provide routine postoperative recovery room care, including turning, coughing, and deep breathing. Monitor vital signs closely. Note responsiveness during recovery. Position client so that aspiration is avoided if vomiting should occur during recovery.
Spinal/saddle block	Elective or nonemergency cesarean section. Forceps delivery.	Aid in positioning during procedure. Monitor vital signs closely, especially blood pressure. Blood pressure should be taken every minute for the first 5 min or until stable, and every 5 min for 30 min after it becomes stable. Monitor fetal heart rate: hypotension can lead to bradycardia and/or fetal distress. Note signs of maternal respiratory distress, which might indicate that nerves too high in the spinal column have been anesthetized. Maintain flat bed rest for 8 to 12 hr postpartum to prevent cerebrospinal fluid leakage, which may cause headaches. Note complaints of headaches. Encourage voiding; notify practitioner of bladder distention or failure to void. Encourage oral fluids or maintain intravenous hydration.

Epidural	Elective or nonemergency cesarean section. Forceps delivery. Analgesia for active labor.	Aid in positioning during procedure. Monitor vital signs closely, especially blood pressure because hypotension can result. (*See* Spinal Anesthesia for recommended frequency of measuring and recording blood pressure.) Position client in supine position with bedroll under right side. This prevents compression of the vena cava by the uterus. Monitor fetal heart rate: hypotension can lead to bradycardia and/or fetal distress. Monitor labor and contraction status. Observe for headache, which may result if the dura mater is accidentally punctured.
Pudendal	Spontaneous or low-forceps delivery. Uncomplicated breech delivery. Performance and repair of episiotomy. Repair of significant lacerations, including 3rd and 4th degree.	Explain procedure as necessary (anesthetizes the entire perineum, the vulva, and the clitoris).
Local	Spontaneous vaginal delivery. Performance and repair of episiotomy. Repair of simple lacerations.	Explain procedure as necessary (anesthetizes only the area infiltrated).

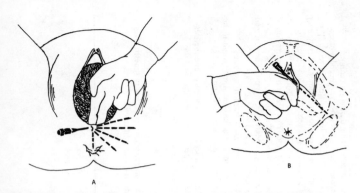

Figure 10-6. (A) Direct infiltration of local anesthesia for mediolateral episiotomy (if there is a midline episiotomy, the procedure is repeated on the opposite side of the perineum), and (B) transvaginal route of administration of anesthesia for pudendal nerve block.

TABLE 10-9

Factors to Consider When Determining Need for an Episiotomy

Indication of need for episiotomy	Contraindications to episiotomy
Android-shaped pelvis	Presence of varicosities of the
Borderline or contracted pelvic	perineum or vulva
outlet	Presence of multiple condylomas
Evidence of inevitable laceration	
Malposition: occiput posterior,	
face, brow, deflexed head	
Malpresentation: breech	
Instrumental delivery	
Prophylactic preservation of	
pelvic muscle integrity	
Short and/or thick perineum	
Prematurity	
Anticipated shoulder dystocia	
Fetal distress	
Large estimated fetal weight	

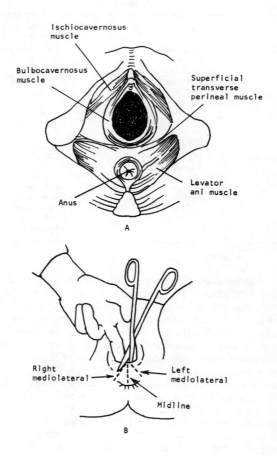

Figure 10-7. Episiotomies. (A) Illustration of the muscles involved in an episiotomy, and (B) episiotomies.

TABLE 10-10

Episiotomy

Type	Advantages	Disadvantages
Median (midline)	Cuts central tendon of the perineum rather than muscle mass. Is technically easy to perform and repair. Associated with less blood loss and pain than mediolateral episiotomy. Heals well with minimal risk of breakdown.	Can result in extension to 3rd- or 4th-degree laceration.
Mediolateral	Provides greater room for manipulations. Has little or no risk of extension involving the rectum.	Cuts through the body of the perineal muscles. Increases technical difficulty of repair. Is more painful. Associated with greater risk of infection or hematoma formation.

The mother should be encouraged to work with her body and her uterine contractions. Long, strong pushing is discouraged because it may increase the difficulty in controlling the speed of the delivery and because it may increase the risk of perineal lacerations. The objective is to allow the advancing head to deliver slowly. To aid in control, it may be necessary to have the client pant but not push during contractions and bear down voluntarily without an accompanying contraction.

As the fetal head distends the perineum, the nurse should apply gentle, steady, and firm pressure on the head in the direction of the perineum in order to maintain flexion. This is accomplished by placing the fingers of one hand together on the top of the baby's head (occiput) near the anterior vaginal opening (Fig. 10-8). The fingers must not slip beneath the labia because they may take up space that is needed by the head for crowning and because they may cause labial lacerations. The speed of advancement is controlled by applying gentle pressure. The objective is to slow the rate of delivery — not to hold or push back the head. The curved fingers and palm are adjusted to the curve of the head as it extends, advances, and emerges from the introitus. It is safe to allow crowning to occur and

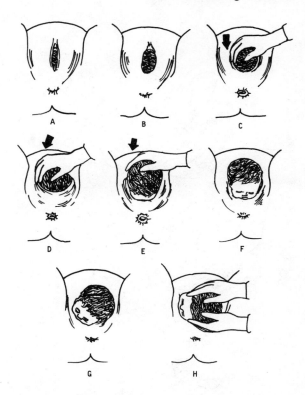

Figure 10-8. Normal birth process with delivery techniques. (A) Anterior-posterior slit; (B) oval opening; (C) circular shape and the beginning of assistance with flexion: the nurse applies cupped fingers to the head and applies light downward pressure; (D) crowning and flexion; (E) extension; (F) birth of the head; (G) restitution; and (H) external rotation.

the head to remain there until the next contraction. However, if the force of the contraction and maternal effort do not extend the head sufficiently to deliver the face, the biparietal diameter or parietal bones should be grasped, and the forehead, face, and chin should be lifted over the perineum. The other hand may be used to gently push back the perineum at the same time, if necessary.

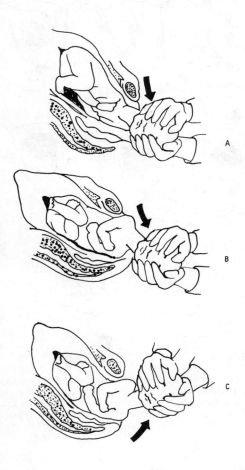

Figure 10-9. Delivery of the shoulders. The pressure direction is indicated by an arrow. (A) Lowering of the baby's head, (B) delivery of the anterior shoulder, and (C) delivery of the posterior shoulder.

After the head is delivered, the mother is instructed to stop pushing until the nurse is ready to proceed. The nurse wipes the baby's face with one or two gauze sponges and suctions the mouth and both nares. The nurse slips his or her fingers along the back of the neck into the vagina and checks the skin folds carefully for the umbilical cord. If present, the nurse gently pulls it forward and over the baby's head (almost all cords are long enough to be slipped over the baby's head). If the cord is too tight and does not slip over the head, it will be necessary to clamp and cut it. In that case, it is necessary to slip two fingers under the cord, apply the two clamps to the cord near each other (making sure they grip tightly), and cut the cord between them. Then the cord is unwrapped from around the neck.

Meanwhile, restitution and external rotation will most likely have occurred. The nurse places her hands along the sides of the baby's face with the thumbs facing toward the top of the head. If there is a delay in external rotation, the head may be turned to the side (the back of the head should be on the same side as the baby's back). The mother is asked to bear down steadily with the next contraction to deliver the shoulders. Firm, steady pressure downward (toward the floor) and outward is applied to deliver the anterior shoulder. Steady upward pressure is then applied to deliver the posterior shoulder and the rest of the body (Fig. 10-9). One hand is slipped along the baby's back to support the baby as he or she is delivered.

After the delivery, the baby may be placed either on the mother's abdomen and chest or on the sterile field. The baby should be removed from the collected amniotic fluid and blood. The mouth and nose are suctioned again as necessary, the cord is clamped and cut, if this has not yet been done, and the baby is dried thoroughly. Unless there is a problem with the baby or the mother, the safest and best place for the baby is in the mother's arms. The pediatrician or others present at the birth can assume responsibility for the newborn, if indicated, so that the nurse can remain with the mother and conduct the third stage of labor (*see* Chapter 11).

It is important to remember that most babies are delivered without problems and that the process of birth is generally simple and straightforward.

REFERENCE

1. Varney. 213.

CHAPTER 11

THIRD STAGE OF LABOR
Suzanne M. Smith

The third stage of labor is a time of rapid physiological and psychological changes for the client. The greatest danger during the third stage is hemorrhage. Careful attention should be paid to ensure the normalcy of the third stage.

The excitement of the birth may cause everyone involved to be less conscientious about monitoring the mother's well-being. This tendency may be magnified if there has been (or is) concern for the well-being of the newborn. The nurse, while sharing in the excitement and/or activity surrounding the birth, must remember to evaluate and care for *both* clients — the mother and her newborn.

This chapter focuses on the care of the mother. Chapter 21 focuses on the care of the newborn.

PHYSIOLOGY

During the third stage of labor, changes in maternal physiology are primarily directed toward the return to homeostasis. Blood pressure, pulse, and respiration all begin to return to normal. As stated previously (*see* p. 269), temperature may remain elevated by 1.8 to 3.6 °C (1 to 2 °F) for 1 to 2 hours postpartum. The decreased gastrointestinal motility and rate of absorption that occur during the first two stages of labor return to normal, unless they are affected by analgesics or anesthetics. The client frequently complains of hunger and/or thirst soon after delivery. Nausea and vomiting are rare. Tremors of the extremities and/or chills are not uncommon, and may be the result of the postpartum release of stress and decrease in metabolism. Finally, particularly after a long labor, the client is often exhausted and needs to sleep.

The third stage of labor consists of two phases: (1) separation of the placenta from the uterine wall, and (2) its expulsion (or delivery). Separation begins immediately after the birth of the baby. The contractions of labor result in a gradual decrease in the size of the uterine cavity (see p. 221). During the second stage, and particularly with the delivery of the baby, uterine size is rapidly reduced, and the uterine cavity is nearly obliterated. The placenta, however, does not decrease in size, and, thus, as the implantation site becomes smaller, the placenta begins to buckle and separate. Cleavage, or placental separation, occurs within the decidua. Part of the decidua is expelled with the placenta, and another part continues to adhere to the myometrium and is expelled in the lochia during involution. Placental separation usually begins toward the center, with the margins remaining attached. The formation of the retroplacental clot is a result of bleeding from the uterine sinuses into the space between the placenta and the uterine wall. Bleeding during the third stage varies greatly, as does the size of the retroplacental clot. It is unlikely that formation of the clot directly causes placental separation, although it may accelerate separation along the margin.

As the placenta becomes separated and the uterus contracts, the placenta is expelled first into the lower uterine segment and then into the vagina. The membranes separate because of a decreased area of attachment and because of the traction caused by the weight of the placenta.

DESCRIPTION

The third stage of labor begins with delivery of the baby and ends with complete delivery of the placenta and membranes. The *average* third stage, without intervention or manual removal of the placenta, lasts about 5 to 10 minutes. However, unless bleeding is excessive, it is not abnormal for it to last 20 or 30 minutes.

Uterine size decreases significantly immediately after delivery of the baby. The location of the fundus is generally slightly below the level of the umbilicus. Uterine contractions resume within 3 to 5 minutes of the birth. Therefore, it is normal for the uterus to feel somewhat soft during the initial part of the third stage. It is important, however, to note uterine consistency in order to recognize the abnormal softness (atony). If the uterus remains soft and also increases in size, bleeding (which is not yet recognized externally) is a possible cause because the placenta prevents its exit from the uterus.

PLACENTAL SEPARATION AND EXPULSION

There are several signs that herald the separation of the placenta: uterine contraction(s), a change in uterine shape from discoid to globular, a rise in the height of the fundus, a visible lengthening of the external portion of the umbilical cord, and a variable amount of bleeding.

In addition, there are other methods that may aid in confirming the diagnosis of placental separation. The empty fundus may become ballottable or freely movable in the abdomen. If the umbilical cord is clamped near the introitus and held while gentle pressure is exerted superiorly on the fundus of the uterus, there should be no retraction of the cord (Brandt-Andrews maneuver). One should, however, try to avoid retracting a contaminated cord into the vagina. Finally, if the cord is followed upward through the vagina, the placenta will be palpable in the upper vagina or cervix. The risk of postpartum infection is increased with both of these methods, and they should be used only when other signs have not confirmed placental separation and when the need to confirm separation outweighs the risks. Furthermore, unnecessary uterine manipulation may increase the risk of uterine inversion or hemorrhage.

Once placental separation has occurred and the uterus has contracted, delivery of the placenta may be facilitated by maternal positions and gentle bearing down efforts, both of which permit gravity and increased intra-abdominal pressure to propel the placenta through the vagina. In the lithotomy and dorsal positions, normal physiology is hindered, particularly if the client is lying relatively flat. In these cases, it may be necessary for the attendant to use gentle cord traction with maternal effort to effect delivery. Care must be taken to "guard" the uterus by applying pressure above the symphysis pubis and to avoid excessive traction in order to prevent uterine inversion.

There are two mechanism of expulsion of the placenta. In most cases, the fetal surface is delivered first and can be recognized by the shiny, smooth appearance of the membranes. This is known as the Schultze mechanism ("shiny Schultze"). Less frequently, the maternal surface appears first at the introitus. The maternal surface can be recognized by its rough, red, and somewhat irregular appearance. Delivery of the maternal surface first is known as the Duncan mechanism ("dirty Duncan").

The risks of the third stage of labor must not be overlooked.

Bleeding during placental separation must be monitored, and appropriate steps should be taken to control hemorrhage, if it occurs. Such a step would involve removal of the placenta. Necessary manipulations and confirmation of placental separation must be performed with close attention to aseptic technique in order to avoid increased risk of infection. Finally, the risk of uterine inversion necessitates that manipulations be kept to a minimum.

OXYTOCIC DRUGS

The use of oxytocic drugs, either routinely or on indication during or following the completion of the third stage, varies greatly among practitioners. There are three principal oxytocic drugs in use: oxytocin (Pitocin or Syntocinon), ergonovine maleate (Ergotrate), and methylergonovine maleate (Methergine). Each of these drugs causes myometrial contractions. Oxytocin is considerably shorter acting than the others. Both ergonovine maleate and methylergonovine maleate are effective for several hours and result in sustained contractions (tetany) (see Appendix A).

The use of any oxytocic drug varies. Prophylactic use is not an uncommon routine in many institutions. The oxytocic drug may be ordered at the delivery of the anterior shoulder or delayed until expulsion of the placenta. Indications for the use of an oxytocic agent may include delayed placental separation, heavy bleeding before or after placental delivery, or the suspicion of retained fragments of placenta or membranes.

The oxytocic drug that is used depends on the speed and duration of action desired and the maternal condition. Both ergonovine maleate and methylergonovine maleate may cause an increase in blood pressure and, thus, are contraindicated in women who have been, or who are, hypertensive or in women who have cardiac disease. Additional specific information concerning those medications is provided in Appendix A.

EXAMINATION OF THE PLACENTA

As soon as possible after delivery of the placenta (i.e., once any bleeding has been controlled and the mother's vital signs are stable), a thorough inspection of the umbilical cord, membranes, and placenta should be performed. The examination should include evaluation for completeness of the placenta and notation of any abnormalities in the placenta, membranes, or cord.

Before inspection of the maternal surface is performed, gauze sponges are used to remove any adherent clots. Both maternal and fetal surfaces are inspected and palpated. The membranes must be held up to determine their completeness or the presence of ragged edges, which are suggestive of retained fragments. The severed end of the cord must be wiped in order to note the number of vessels. Table 11-1 includes the items that are examined, the normal and abnormal findings, and their possible significance.

MATERNAL AND NEWBORN NEEDS

Although the third stage of labor is short in comparison with the first and second stages of labor, the newborn, the mother, and her support person(s) have significant needs. Normally, the family expresses concern for the well-being of the newborn, and a desire to see, touch, and hold the baby. The nurse and/or attendant must remember to keep the family informed. If there is a problem, such as neonatal distress, it is crucial that they be told that the baby is being cared for expertly and that all possible help is being provided. In addition, the nurse should provide the family with as much detail as possible concerning the situation.

A healthy infant's primary needs are a patent airway and a stable body temperature. Basic care includes positioning to aid postural drainage, and further suctioning with the rubber bulb syringe or the DeLee mucous trap. The infant may require stimulation (e.g., massage) to aid in the institution of the respiratory cycle, and he or she will need to be dried off to minimize heat loss. When these immediate steps have been completed, if the mother and her baby are both well, it is ideal to give the baby to the mother for attachment. The nurse can assist the mother and her family to become acquainted with the baby and thus facilitate the attachment experience (*see* Chapter 14).

The mother should at least have the opportunity to see and touch her baby and identify his or her sex. Further information concerning the care of the normal newborn is found in Chapter 21.

In addition to concern for her baby, the mother is also interested in her own condition. She generally wants to know if stitches are necessary and how much bleeding has occurred, or she may ask to see the placenta. In a normal situation, she is relaxed and happy, and may evidence emotional release by laughing and/or crying. Some women become very talkative, whereas others, after obtaining vital information, rest or go to sleep. Chapter 12 discusses the fourth stage of labor, and Chapter 14 discusses the initial attachment and mothering tasks that continue after the last stage of labor.

TABLE 11-1
Placental Examination

Item	Characteristic	Normal finding	Abnormal finding	Significance and possible causes of abnormal finding
Placenta	Size, shape, and weight	15-20 cm diameter. 1.5-3.0 cm thick. Discoid. Approximately one sixth of the infant's weight.	Larger/heavier.	Intrauterine syphilis. Erythroblastosis. Maternal diabetes mellitus. Large-for-gestational-age infant.
			Smaller/lighter.	Maternal diabetes mellitus. Intrauterine growth retardation.
	Color	Dark red; membranes gray.	Pale, lightened color.	Fetal anemia. Erythroblastosis.
			Pale, yellow, or gray.	Intrauterine syphilis.
			Green.	Meconium staining.
	Odor	Characteristic odor; not malodorous.	Malodorous.	Amnionitis.
	Membranes	Two, which are separable.	Not applicable.	Not applicable.
Maternal surface	Appearance	Separate cotyledons, which fit together exactly; margin continuous.	Irregular margin or blank spaces.	Possible retained fragments or cotyledons.

		Normal	Variation	Significance
		Calcifications: variable areas of gritty-feeling white deposits. Infarcts: white, firm, nodular deposits of various sizes.	Extensive calcifications or infarcts.	Postmaturity. Severe maternal hypertension (chronic, preeclampsia, or eclampsia). Intrauterine growth retardation. Intrauterine demise.
	Other	None.	Cysts.	Generally benign.
			Edema.	Severe maternal disease (cardiac, diabetes, or nephritis). Severe erythroblastosis. Intrauterine demise.
Fetal surface	Appearance	Smooth and shiny.	Not applicable.	Not applicable.
	Blood vessels	Intact.	Disappearance at the margin, or broken appearance.	Succenturiate lobe.
	Insertion of cord	Insertion between margin and center. Marginal insertion (Battledore): normal variation.	Velamentous insertion (vessels exit from cord and travel variable distance through membrane to placenta).	Increased risk of vessel rupture, which may lead to fetal hemorrhage and/or exsanguination.
			Vasa previa (presentation of vessels at cervical os or in membranes ahead of fetus).	Same as above.

Item	Characteristic	Normal finding	Abnormal finding	Significance and possible causes of abnormal finding
Cord	Number of vessels	Two arteries, one vein.	Only one artery.	Multiple fetal anomalies.
	Length	50-55 cm (slightly longer than baby).	Short (less than 50 cm).	Fetal distress. Delay or failure of descent. Shoulder dystocia. Abruption.
			Long (longer than 55 cm).	Nuchal, shoulder, or body cord.
	Configuration	Curving of vessels.	True knot.	Fetal anoxia or death from tightened cord.

CHAPTER 12

FOURTH STAGE OF LABOR
Margherita Modica Hawkins and Angela Portale

The fourth stage of labor is defined as the first hour after the expulsion of the placenta. It initiates the puerperium, and it marks the beginning of the major physiological changes from the pregnant to the nonpregnant state. The fourth stage is a physically and psychologically dynamic period for both the client and her infant.[1,2] This chapter will briefly review the maternal physiological and emotional changes that occur during the early postpartum period after vaginal delivery.

MATERNAL PHYSIOLOGICAL CHANGES

Uterine involution

The walls of the uterus shrink, contract, and clamp down over the placental site and its blood vessels. Blood, shreds of placental membrane, decidual tissue, and other debris are shed as lochia rubra. A leukocyte granulation wall builds in the basal layer of the endometrium, which, when combined with the bactericidal potential of blood serum, acts as a defense mechanism against the bacteria. The venous plexus surrounding the vagina begins to refill, which helps to restore the distended vagina and perineum to their original size. Blood and serum from the infiltrated and edematous perineum begin to be absorbed.

Cardiovascular system

Possible vagal nerve counterregulation in response to increased sympathetic activity during labor and delivery may cause a decrease in pulse rate. The circulating blood volume begins to increase as a result of fluid transport from the extracellular space into the systemic circulation. The number of leukocytes, which is elevated during labor and delivery, continues to rise. The erythrocyte sedimentation rate may rise to as high as 50 millimeters within the first hour. Fibrinogen remains elevated with an increase in the number of thrombocytes.

Renal system

Diuresis occurs as a result of the transport of the expanded extracellular fluid. The glomerular filtration rate remains the same as it was during pregnancy.

Endocrine system

The client's breasts begin to produce colostrum as a result of the rapid drop in estrogen and progesterone levels. Luteal and placental hormones recede.

MATERNAL EMOTIONAL CHANGES

The taking-in phase begins

The fourth stage of labor is a time of physical recovery and restoration. The client may be excited, exhibiting varying degrees of exhilaration and, possibly, even euphoria. The emotionally healthy client's physical needs for relaxation, sleep, and nourishment may outweigh the need to form the family unit. The client's immediate responses will vary according to the length and intensity of labor. Perceived positive or negative experiences may also affect passage through this phase.[3]

BASIC NURSING CARE OF THE CLIENT

The immediate postpartum period is well known as a critical time in the mother's recovery. Every mother should be closely observed by a well-trained nurse who is in constant attendance.

It is the responsibility of the nurse during this recovery period to be familiar with the client's medical-obstetric history and her psychosocial status. It is extremely important for the nurse and all others caring for the client to bear in mind the length of labor and delivery and any experiences the client may have had during that time. These factors will have an impact on the client's responses during the fourth stage. These basic techniques must be considered when individualizing care for each family. Table 12-1 provides a sample plan of care for the client at this time.

REFERENCES

1. Rovinsky. 21-23.

2. Vorherr. 1-12.

3. Brown and Hurlock.

TABLE 12-1
Fourth Stage Nursing Care Plan

Parameter	Nursing intervention	Outcome
Immediate postpartum maternal care.	Perform overall, quick, general physical assessment of mother. Check IV site, if present, for integrity. Measure and record blood pressure, pulse, and respirations every 15 min during 1st hr. Explain to the client what will occur during this stage. Identify teaching needs. Record all assessments and interventions. In presence of stable condition, provide liquids and diet as tolerated.	Client is relaxed with procedures and nurse's activities, asks questions, etc. *Minor* fluctuations of vital signs can be expected during 1st hr.
Uterine fundus is firm to palpation.	Check fundal height, consistency, and location every 15 min during 1st hr. Assess lochia with the client supine and in lateral position. Administer standard oxytocic drugs as ordered (*see* Appendix A). Record all assessments and interventions.	Uterus remains firm and at the midline, passing only enough lochia to saturate one pad in the hour. *Uterus becomes boggy (soft and spongy) and/or there is more than one lochia-saturated pad in the hour.
*Uterus is soft and spongy with heavy lochia.	Massage uterus and check at more frequent intervals as needed according to client response. Express clots from uterus. Check bladder for distention (*see below*). Record all assessments, interventions, and results. Maintain IV therapy until client is stable.	Uterus attains firmness, and bleeding abates. *Heavy bleeding continues and uterus remains boggy.

*Uterus fails to attain firmness, and heavy bleeding continues even after nursing interventions.	Notify physician and record. Prepare the client for return to the surgical area for inspection. Maintain or restart IV therapy. Have blood volume expanders on hand. Perform blood type and cross-match, with blood on hand to administer, if needed. Evaluate vital signs frequently.	Client stabilized, hemorrhage ceases.
Urinary bladder palpated but undistended.	Check for distention every 15 min. Encourage the client to void if bladder is filling. Record all assessments, interventions, and results.	Bladder may not be full at this time. *Bladder becomes distended and is easily palpated, with the uterus deviated to the left or right.
*Urinary bladder distended.	Encourage spontaneous voiding: provide privacy, produce sound of running water, assist the client to assume normal position for voiding, pour warm water over perineum, encourage the client to increase her intra-abdominal pressure by blowing up a balloon or blowing through a straw, and/or give oil of peppermint to inhale. (If the client has had spinal or epidural anesthesia, she may not feel the urge to void.) Record interventions and results.	The client voids ≥100 ml and empties her bladder. *The client is unable to void, or voids <100 ml with the bladder remaining distended.

Parameter	Nursing intervention	Outcome
*Bladder remains distended.	Notify physician or nurse-midwife. Catheterize gently and slowly, using scrupulous sterile technique. Record time and results of catheterization. Be sure floor nurse has been notified that patient has had early catheterization. Send urine for culture and sensitivity.	Bladder is no longer distended, and uterus returns to the midline.
Discomfort of perineum because of birth trauma and/or episiotomy.	Check perineum for integrity. Place sterile ice pack at perineum for comfort and to decrease swelling. Instruct the client in cleansing of perineal area and use of sterile sanitary pad. Encourage the client to sit with legs together to promote healing. Instruct the client to start Kegel exercises when ready. Medicate with analgesics, when necessary, as ordered. Record all assessments, interventions, and results.	There is no redness, edema, or discharge, and the suture line is approximated well. *Hematoma, if present, is identified. *Suture line is not approximated, or there is oozing from the episiotomy site.
*Hematoma (vaginal or perineal).	Note any increase in size since last postpartum check. Apply ice pack. Notify physician or nurse-midwife who may want to perform thorough examination of vaginal walls. Record all assessments, interventions, and results.	No increase in size is noted.
*Episiotomy is oozing or suture line is not approximated.	Notify physician or nurse-midwife. For oozing, apply gentle, steady pressure with a sterile dressing to the site, or reapply ice pack. If site is not approximated, prepare the client for return to the surgical area.	The wound is closed and hemostasis is achieved.

Client is initiating breast-feeding.	Provide warm, open, loving, and private atmosphere for new family unit. Assist mother in finding comfortable position for feeding. Encourage interaction with father or significant other by explanation and demonstration of ways he or she may participate. Allow baby to suck each breast for 5-10 min (depending on nipple toughness). The baby should be allowed to nuzzle breasts for as long as mother and baby desire.	The family is interacting and talking. The baby, who is adapting to the breast, may not grasp nipple but just lick and nuzzle at this time. The atmosphere is relaxed and comfortable.
Maternal-infant (family-infant) attachment process is beginning (see Chapter 14).	Provide safe, quiet, open atmosphere; carry out all comfort measures as necessary. Maintain maternal-child contact as much as possible. Include father or significant other. Encourage the client to explore her infant. Encourage skin-to-skin contact between mother and infant, and father and infant. Follow family's desires as much as possible. See Chapter 21.	The client shows signs of interest in baby. Father or significant other participates or interacts. *The client evinces disinterest or hostility.
*Outward disinterest or hostility.	Check physiological status of the client, and attend to all of her physical needs as soon as possible. Remember that the client's need for rest during this time may prevent outward acts of maternal-infant attachment. Provide information on the baby as indicated. Alert postpartum nursing staff to observe whether this behavior continues. Begin to establish professional psychosocial support system.	Maternal-infant attachment is facilitated by the health care team.

IV, intravenous.
*An asterisk is an indication of an unwanted, distressing, or untoward condition or outcome. The nurse should assess for possible presence and intervene as described.

CHAPTER 13

THE ROLE OF THE NURSE IN ALTERNATIVE BIRTH SETTINGS

Judith Melson

The most common setting for women giving birth in America is in an acute care hospital. In this setting, nurses, residents, interns, and medical students provide day-to-day care under the direction of an obstetrician who may perform only the actual delivery. Many of the protocols for patient care in the obstetric setting, where the majority of women are healthy, are similar to those in other areas of the hospital, where illness predominates.

Alternative birth settings, designed with the idea of emphasizing the naturalness or "wellness" of childbirth, include hospital birthing rooms, birth centers, and home birth services. In these settings, a nurse-midwife frequently assumes overall management of the birth as well as the prenatal and postpartum care in collaboration with an obstetrician who provides medical consultation and coverage for the service. In alternative birth settings, nurses take on a variety of responsibilities, including childbirth education, assisting at birth, community nursing, and administration.

The advantage of the alternative birth setting to the client is more control of the events surrounding birth, such as her activity, her eating and drinking patterns, positions for comfort during labor and birth, the presence of the companions of her choice during the labor and birth, and minimal fear of separation from her baby after birth. In addition, practices in alternative settings generally discourage such interventions as early rupture of the membranes, intravenous feedings, induction and/or stimulation of labor, shaving of pubic hair, administration of drugs, and use of enemas.

The advantage for the family is that they are allowed to be present and are supported by a staff that treats the birth process as a normal physiological event. In addition, family members who are not present for the birth are allowed to join the parents and new infant shortly after birth. An atmosphere is thus created that reinforces the normalness of birth.

The advantage for the health care providers is the opportunity to work with parents in a situation that provides for continuity of care, thereby allowing for maximum teaching, support, and enhancement of the strengths and well-being of the woman and her family.

HISTORICAL OVERVIEW OF ALTERNATIVE BIRTH

Although the term "alternative birth setting" was coined in the 1970s, many examples existed in the United States before that time. The most famous of these examples is the Frontier Nursing Service started in Hyden, Kentucky, in 1925, by Mary Breckenridge. Breckenridge introduced the British system of nurse-midwifery to America and was able to provide service for some of the most economically disadvantaged women and families in the nation. A Metropolitan Life Insurance Co. study showed that, in spite of the socioeconomic risk involved with these women, their maternal mortality rate for the years 1925 to 1951 was 9.1/10,000 live births, as compared with 34/10,000 for the rest of Kentucky and the United States.[1]

In New York City from 1931 to 1951, the Lobenstine Midwifery Clinic, in association with Maternity Center Association, established a home delivery service to meet the needs of low-income women in the upper Manhattan community. Many of these women had anemia and poor nutrition and would be considered high-risk clients today. Because they had no money for hospital care, the alternative service was desparately needed. As in Kentucky, the maternal mortality rate was lower than the national average.[2]

Trends in hospitals

The trends in hospital births (generally involving more affluent women) consisted of more and more control of the birth process being assumed by the physician. Some common practices included twilight sleep, general anesthesia, denial to fathers of the option to share in the birth process, separation of mothers and infants, induction of labor, and early rupture of the membranes.

In the late 1940s, women began to express their unhappiness with the philosophy that was changing birth into a cold and unconscious surgical procedure.

Beginning of the consumer movement

Grantly Dick-Read, the father of natural childbirth, was invited to Yale University in 1947, where his visit resulted in the establishment of one of the first rooming-in units. This began the consumer movement in the area of childbirth. The next 10 years witnessed the founding of the International Childbirth Education Association (ICEA) and the American Society for Psychoprophylaxis in Obstetrics (ASPO). Both of these organizations quickly established branches in many cities across the country, providing education for prospective parents, with an emphasis on childbearing as a natural process. In many cities, parents elected to be together during birth, and they were instrumental in getting hospital practices changed. In Washington, D. C., in 1965, only 1 of 16 hospitals allowed fathers to be present at birth. By 1970, as a result of consumer pressure, all but the city hospital had opened the delivery room door to fathers. As parents experienced normal births, they began to question the idea that women in normal health should deliver in an acute care hospital, with its emphasis on sickness and disease. Thus, the movement toward alternative settings for birth was initiated.

The movement in the 1960s and 1970s

In the 1960s, self-educated and apprentice-trained lay midwives began providing home birth services in California, New Mexico, Tennessee, Texas, and Massachusetts. The hospital birthing room concept, started in Connecticut in the 1960s, caught on quickly. Fathers were even allowed to be present at cesarean sections. In 1975, nurse-midwives set up the first contemporary nurse-midwifery home birth service in collaboration with two physicians. The Maternity Center Association in New York opened one of the first independent birth centers in 1975. All of these changes occurred in the face of opposition and resistance from factions of the medical establishment. As more and more alternative birth settings develop, the controversies still continue.

ETHICAL AND LEGAL CONSIDERATIONS

Ethical considerations

Some physicians have called home birth "child abuse." Others have said that home is the safest place to give birth. Physicians, midwives, nurses, and parents can be found to represent both points of view. Although birth at home is the most controversial issue, there are some people who are also opposed to the concept of birth centers. Although some physicians do believe that birth outside of the hospital is truly unsafe, one of the factors behind some of the opposition is the potential economic impact of alternative birth settings on hospital utilization and physicians' practices.

It is important for the nurse to be aware of the community's sentiments regarding alternative birth settings. Before deciding to become involved in alternative birth settings, nurses will want to know the preparation, background, and competence of the health team members they will be working with; the safety record, risk factors, and emergency provisions of the services; and general information about the families to be served.

Legal basis for practice

The legal basis for practice should be known by everyone involved in alternative birth settings. For instance, in New Mexico, nurse-midwives, state-licensed midwives, and physicians may deliver babies at home; in Massachusetts, it is illegal for anyone but a physician to perform a home birth. In some states, birth centers need to be approved by the Board of Health. Nurses will find that in many states they can be reimbursed by insurance companies for their role in a home birth.

Malpractice insurance

Each nurse will want to carry malpractice insurance, unless it is clear that the nurse is covered by the institutional policy. Most carriers of malpractice insurance for nurses cover the nurse's practice in hospitals, community health services, hospices, offices, birth centers, and home births. If there is any doubt, it is best to directly question the insurance company.

Contracts with clients

When employed in a hospital that provides a birthing room for patients, the nurse need not have a special contract with the client. However, when a family directly hires a nurse to assist them at birth wherever it will occur, the nurse is wise to establish a clearly written contract that includes the family's expectations of the nurse and the nurse's expectations of the family. A specific payment plan should be included in the contract.

THE ROLE OF THE NURSE

The nurse who works in an alternative birth setting may be required to act more independently than if he or she were employed in a maternity unit with a large nursing staff. Therefore, previous experience in nursing practice is highly recommended. Good intrapartum experience, involvement in prenatal education, and postpartum and breast-feeding counseling are especially useful. If this experience in not available, the nurse can become an apprentice to an experienced nurse working in the alternative birth setting.

Working closely with families, extended families, friends, and children, rather than with one "patient," requires a high level of communication skills. In addition, the nurse will be an educator, counselor, supporter, and physical caretaker when indicated. Frequently, and particularly when hospitalization is required, the role of the nurse will include being a patient advocate within the health care delivery system. The specific knowledge, skills, and equipment that the nurse should have for working in alternative settings are listed below.

Knowledge required
1. A thorough understanding of the mechanisms and the process of labor and birth.
2. Labor coaching and support principles.
3. Normal physical and emotional changes that occur as labor progresses.
4. Assessment of fetal status, including interpretation of fetal heart rate patterns.
5. Assessment of maternal status and interpretation of data, including blood pressure, reflexes, contraction pattern, affect, ability to cope, dilation, effacement, station, and fetal position.
6. Knowledge of emergency care.
7. Postpartum evaluation and anticipatory guidance.
8. Physiology and technique of breast-feeding.
9. Principles of communication.

Skills required
1. Pelvic examination: effacement, dilation, station, and position.
2. Abdominal examination: Leopold's maneuvers, status of contractions, and fetal heart tones.
3. Use of a Doppler device and a variety of fetoscopes.
4. Initiation of intravenous therapy.
5. Cardiopulmonary resuscitation for adults and infants.

6. Intramuscular and intravenous administration of medications.
7. Emergency birth techniques.
8. Fundal massage for postpartum bleeding.
9. Suprapubic pressure in case of shoulder dystocia.
10. Labor support techniques.
11. Postpartum physical assessment of the mother.
12. Newborn assessment.
13. Breast-feeding counseling.
14. Communication skills.

Other requirements
1. Nursing license in state(s) where practicing.
2. Positive and realistic attitude about the birth process.
3. Personal support systems that assist the nurse in working irregular hours.
4. Telephone, paging system, and well-functioning automobile.

Because both birthing room and birth center births are designed to create a "homelike" birth situation, home birth will be discussed in detail first.

HOME BIRTH

In the United States, the majority of home births are attended by midwives and nurse-midwives, and a small number are attended by physicians. In the rest of the world, the midwife is the primary on-site provider in a home birth, with the physician or consultant available by telephone.

The nurse-client relationship

Nurses who work with home birth families are usually contacted by the couple, who have obtained the nurse's name from a midwife or physician. The nurse may act in either one or several of the following roles: childbirth educator, teacher of special home birth preparation classes, or birth assistant. The nurse who will be a birth assistant may be hired directly by the couple for a fee. The birth assistant's responsibilities should include visiting the home during the client's 37th week, being available and on call for her from her 37th to 42nd week, attending the labor and birth, and visiting a minimum of two times during the postpartum period.

In some situations, two or three nurses share being on call for a group of women and families in their community so that each nurse is not constantly on call. This arrangement works well for nurses who, in addition to assisting at home births, hold other jobs or have small children.

The primary provider and the nurse

The primary provider is the person who will sign the birth certificate, and is usually a certified nurse-midwife or a physician. It is important that the nurse have confidence in, and be comfortable with, this person. The nurse and the provider need to discuss the conduct of the labor and birth so that there will be harmony during the birth. Arrangements for postpartum visits should also be discussed. In general, this responsibility is divided between the nurse and the provider.

Advantages of home birth

In addition to the above-mentioned advantages for all alternative settings, couples who wish to have home births are able to be in a familiar, comfortable setting without institutional policies or constraints. Most couples who have decided on home birth have considered the risk-benefit factors and have decided that home is at least *as* safe as the hospital setting. Home birth can be less expensive, if hospitalization is not required. However, the family should have the means to pay the midwife or physician, the nurse, and, if necessary, the hospital.

Disadvantages of home birth

The main disadvantages involved in home birth are listed below:

1. Distance from the hospital (in many cases).
2. Potential emotional trauma and upset if hospitalization is needed at the last minute.
3. Potential opposition of the medical community. (This may result in emergency treatment being denied or delivered antagonistically.)
4. Client's inability to evaluate and select the provider at the hospital.
5. Lack of equipment and personnel to handle unanticipated emergencies.

Sometimes the total burden of postpartum care is exhausting for the husband if there are no other friends or relatives in the area. For the provider, one of the main drawbacks of home birth is that it entails the complete service and attention of a physician or nurse-midwife and a nurse for the entire course of labor; however, those practitioners involved in home birth feel that their rewards are significant enough to outweigh this drawback.

Requirements and contraindications

To be eligible for a home birth, a woman must be in excellent health and free from major risk factors. In addition, she needs a suitable home with a telephone and such basic necessities as running water, a sewer, heat, and cooking facilities. She needs to have a support system that will provide postpartum care for at least the first 3 days. She must make adequate preparation for the birth, keep her prenatal appointments, and be compliant and openly communicative with the provider.

Contraindications to home birth include medical problems such as high blood pressure, diabetes, heart conditions, and anemia; social problems such as a poor support system, lack of resources for adequate hospital backup, inadequate housing, and irresponsibility; and logistical problems such as living too far from providers, no emergency transport available, living too far from hospital backup, etc. Home birth is also contraindicated when the client is having a home birth to please someone else, lacks a realistic appreciation of the potential risks, or is ambivalent.

Preparation

Preparation is of the utmost importance in achieving a happy and satisfying home birth experience. Both the parents and their children should be advised to prepare by reading, by attending childbirth preparation classes, and by going to prenatal visits together when possible. The entire prenatal period becomes a course on staying healthy during pregnancy and learning about birth.

Prenatal data. Each woman should know her blood type, blood pressure pattern, fetal growth pattern, and hematocrit and other test results. In essence, she should be informed of her normalcy each time it is verified. In addition, she should be told whenever something is amiss and what corrections are needed. This reassurance and guidance build essential confidence and trust that grow throughout the pregnancy.

Education. Regular prenatal classes and prenatal classes aimed at home birth couples are essential. There are several national organizations that offer these classes, including Home Oriented Maternity Experience (HOME) and the Childbirth Education Association (CEA). Many of the nurses who act as birth assistants for home birth couples also teach classes for them.

Supplies. Parents should be provided with a list of supplies and resources that they will need to purchase or have on hand. This list includes the following items:

For the delivery

A firm bed. (Use plywood under the mattress, if necessary.) An easily removable plastic mattress cover or inexpensive shower curtain to protect the mattress.

Plastic pillow covers (optional).

A small pile of newspapers. (Used to cover the carpet and/or floor.)

A large trash receptacle with plastic bags to fit.

A medium-sized round bowl for the placenta.

A new roll of paper towels for hand washing and cleaning up.

Two dozen sterile 4'' × 4'' gauze pads.

Two dozen disposable underpads (available from drug stores or through mail-order catalogs).

One bottle of benzalkonium chloride (Zephiran) 1:750, for pelvic examinations.

A Fleet enema.

A 2- or 3-ounce rubber bulb syringe to suction the baby.

Clean towels and washcloths.

A flashlight with new batteries.

Two telephone books or large catalogs wrapped in a plastic bag to place under the client's buttocks, if necessary.

A heating pad or hot-water bottle.

Extra ice, broth, juices, and/or teas of the client's choice.

Honey.

A telephone.

Copies of a detailed map to help the provider locate their home at night. It should include landmarks, address, and telephone number.

A place for the midwife, physician, or nurse to lie down for rest.

Food and snacks for the midwife or physician, nurse, and family.

For the baby

Four to six receiving blankets (which need not be new).

Disposable diapers for the first stools.

A shirt, kimono, or gown (washed, if new) to dress the baby.

Soft towels and washcloths.

A thermometer (for axillary temperature).

Alcohol and cotton balls.

A tape measure.

For breast care

Hydrous lanolin or vitamin E (plain capsules) or vitamin A and D ointment.

Two nursing bras with cup fasteners that can be opened with one hand.

Clean white cotton handkerchiefs for nursing pads. (These can be easily washed and reused.)

The prenatal home visit

Prenatal visits, an extremely valuable part of any obstetric service, are essential for a successful home birth program. The visit provides the nurse with the opportunity to observe the interaction of family members in their own environment, to assess the family's well-being, and to recognize the special needs that they may have, which the nurse may then communicate to the entire team that is working with the family.

Ideally, the home visit should occur in the client's 36th or 37th week. When the home visit is scheduled, it is helpful to have everyone present who is planning to be present at the birth. The nurse may then review the birth process with everyone and answer any additional questions. Grandparents who are coming from out of town at the time of birth to help the parents should be encouraged to read the *HOME Manual*[3] and/or some other popular book on home birth (*see* Bibliography).

At this visit, the nurse should check the client's blood pressure, check her urine for sugar and acetone, observe for swelling of the extremities or face, question the client as to her general health, listen to the baby's heartbeat, and ascertain the position of the baby abdominally (to rule out transverse lie). All this data should be recorded on the client's chart, including any special needs determined by the nurse.

The home visit provides the nurse with the opportunity to establish a special relationship with the family, to build trust, to enhance the family's knowledge base, and to fill in any gaps in their preparation. Anyone who has not had an opportunity to listen to the baby's heartbeat should do so at this time because this experience seems to initiate or enhance the prenatal attachment process as well as to "create reality" for relatives or friends.

The last item to be reviewed with the client and her family is how to reach the nurse and the midwife or physician when she thinks she is in labor. The client is instructed to call very early when she first thinks she is in labor and to stay in touch until it is time for the nurse and the midwife or physician to come to her home. This allows for planning for weather conditions, rush-hour traffic, baby-sitters, office hours, etc.

The nurse should check the entire list of supplies to be certain that the family has obtained everything it will need. This also provides the opportunity to review the function of each item and to review the emergency birth procedures with the father or significant other. In addition, the nurse should know where the mother keeps her supplies in case of very rapid labor.

In the last week of pregnancy, parents are instructed to make up their bed for the birth. The procedure involves covering the bed with a shower curtain or plastic sheet that can be easily removed, and an old sheet. Many people prefer to make up a clean bed and cover it with the shower curtain and the old sheet so that, after the birth, the shower curtain and old sheet can be removed, leaving a clean bed underneath. It is a good idea to advise parents to plan to use a plastic sheet for the first few days postpartum to prevent any soiling of the mattress. At the beginning of labor, the bed should be ready, all the equipment should be in one place, and extra ice should be in the freezer.

The nurse should ask the client about any special requests or plans that she wishes the nurse or the midwife to implement at the time of birth. These requests should be noted on the chart by the nurse so that they will be apparent to everyone giving care at the birth. These requests may include who she wants to cut the cord, in which position she wishes to give birth, her desires regarding picture-taking, lighting, a Leboyer bath for the baby, etc.

Prenatal reading, education, and preparation are essential to prepare a woman for successful breast-feeding. The prenatal home visit is a good time to review the breast-feeding process and to offer suggestions for reading.

Other details. The parents should keep one car full of gas at all times, in case hospitalization becomes necessary. The nurse should make sure that the telephone numbers of the rescue squad, consultant, and backup hospital are readily available. If the parents wish to take pictures, advise them to keep the camera loaded, because family and friends may not know how to load it. Some women like to have favorite things on hand, such as flowers or special music. Some may also wish to have a special toy, food, or gift for the other children. Complete and thorough preparation contributes to a peaceful, calm, and unhurried atmosphere.

First stage of labor

Latent phase. In general, the client has been instructed to notify the nurse and the midwife or physician as soon as she is aware of any contractions. Close contact is maintained during the latent or early phase of labor. The nurse will visit the client and her family as soon as there is a regular labor pattern in order to assess progress of labor.

On entering the client's home, it is important for the nurse to be with her and observe her behavior for 10 to 20 minutes before proceeding with the obstetric examination, unless, of course, the nurse ascertains that the labor is progressing very rapidly.

The obstetric examination.   The obstetric examination includes three parts: (1) general physical status, including blood pressure determination and assessment for the presence of edema; (2) an abdominal examination, including palpation of contractions, assessment of fetal heart rate, and Leopold's maneuvers; and (3) a pelvic examination, including assessment of dilation, station, etc.

When observing the client's general well-being, the nurse needs to use his or her knowledge of the normal behavioral responses to the phases of labor. For instance, extreme pain in early labor is not normal and could indicate an exhausted, poorly nourished woman, a potential cephalopelvic disproportion, or an abnormal fetal position (*see* Chapter 16). If there is blood pressure elevation or edema, the nurse should check reflexes and ask about headaches and blurred vision (*see* Chapter 17).

When performing an abdominal examination on a woman in early labor, the nurse should assess the strength, frequency, and duration of contractions. Each nurse needs to develop manual skill to assess contraction strength. If the palpating hand is placed just above the client's navel, contractions can be felt with ease because of the lack of adipose tissue close to, and around, the navel in most women. Leaving two fingers near the client's umbilicus, and keeping them still, provides the most information for the nurse and the most comfort for the mother (*see* Chapter 9).

The abdominal examination also includes an assessment of fetal well-being. The nurse can make this assessment by listening to fetal heart tones with a fetoscope throughout the course of several contractions in early labor. This technique provides a valid indication of fetal well-being (*see* Chapter 18). If one hears decelerations in early labor, hospitalization will most likely be indicated, and the midwife or physician should be notified immediately.

The pelvic examination provides the nurse with much information about the condition of the cervix and the position of the baby (*see* Chapter 1). In the home setting, sterile gloves, Zephiran, and lubricating jelly are used. As soon as the obstetric examination is complete, the nurse alerts the midwife or physician as to the progress of the client. It is advisable for the nurse to share all information with the client while the examination is progressing.

Active phase.   As soon as the active phase of labor begins, the midwife or physician, in addition to the nurse, should be present. Some couples like to be by themselves in their room during labor.

The nurse and the midwife come in only as necessary to evaluate the status of the client, the fetus, and the progress of labor. Other families prefer to have the nurse or midwife assist with labor support. Many women have to be encouraged to verbalize their needs and wishes. In most situations, it is advisable for the nurse and the midwife or physician to take turns resting, in case the labor is long or another case follows immediately.

Assessment of the fetal heart rate should be performed approximately every 15 minutes in the active phase of labor (more frequently if there is any doubt about fetal status). Once again, listening throughout the course of several contractions provides the nurse with the most information about the fetus and its adaptation to labor. Most home birth services own a small Doppler device. With this instrument, it is possible to monitor the fetus with the mother in any position. It is important for the nurse to be familiar with the significance of various fetal heart rate patterns and to report any irregularities.

Frequently, the client who is in labor at home experiences a shorter and more comfortable active phase. Consequently, the nurse has to be even more alert for signs of transition.

In preparation for the baby's birth, the nurse must be mindful of the environment. The ideal room temperature is at least 23.9°C (75°F), which may mean turning off the air conditioning in summer or turning up the heat in winter. Baby blankets may be carefully warmed in the oven. Everything in the room should be prepared for the birth at this point.

The nurse should be thoroughly familiar with all of the equipment in the midwife's or physician's home birth bag (Table 13-1). Sterile packages are set out at this point and left unopened. If there are small children and/or many people around, equipment may be set out later, during the second stage.

Second stage

During the second stage, the fetal heart should be auscultated approximately every 5 minutes. Once again, the use of a Doppler device allows the client to push in almost any position she chooses without having to lie back so that fetal heart tones can be heard. If the client is on her side during the second stage, blood flow to the uterus is increased and the contractions are usually strong and effective. Long periods of breath holding and very hard pushing are to be avoided if at all possible because of the fetal decelerations that frequently accompany this kind of pushing. Sitting up and squatting are other positions that women choose for effective and comfortable pushing (*see* Chapter 10).

TABLE 13-1
Home Birth Bag Equipment

Type	Equipment
Medications	Oxytocic drugs to contract the uterus after birth (e.g., oxytocin [Pitocin], methylergonovine maleate [Methergine], ergonovine maleate [Ergotrate]). Local anesthetic (e.g., lidocaine [Xylocaine 1%] for repair of episiotomy or lacerations). Silver nitrate for the baby's eyes. Injectable vitamin K. 1,000 ml of 5 percent dextrose in ½ normal saline or in lactated Ringer's.
Instruments	Delivery set (sterile wrapper that can serve as sterile field when opened, two kelly clamps, scissors, ample number of 4" × 4" gauze sponges, and a rubber bulb syringe for suction). Suture set (needle holder, scissors, ample number of 4" × 4" gauze sponges, with appropriate wrapper to make a sterile field). Optional: ring forceps. Sterile DeLee mucous trap with catheter. Urinary catheter, size 14 French. Cord clamps and cord clamp cutter. Sterile 2-cc and 5-cc disposable syringes. Size 25 and 21 needles, intravenous catheters (Medicuts, Angiocaths), extension tubing, etc., for starting intravenous infusion, if indicated. Cord blood tubes (plain and with anticoagulant). Vacutainer or other equipment to draw blood from client. Doppler device. Blood pressure apparatus and stethoscope. Fetoscope. Mirror. Flashlight. Sterile gloves.
Other	Lubricating jelly. Uristix for glucose and protein determinations. Extra packages of sterile 4" × 4" gauze sponges. 2-0, 3-0, 4-0 chromic catgut suture for repairs. Measuring tapes. Baby scale. Ambu bag (infant size), laryngoscope, and endotracheal tubes.

Type	Equipment
The nurse's bag	Fetoscope.
	Blood pressure apparatus.
	Stethoscope.
	Two cord clamps.
	Scissors.
	Rubber bulb syringe.
	Sterile gloves.
	Flashlight.
	Tubes for cord bloods (plain and with anticoagulant).

Many women like to have hot compresses applied to the perineal area for comfort and to aid in relaxation. Tap water and washcloths work very well because the thick washcloths retain the water's warmth for a long time. Many midwives and physicians participating in home births use warm oil to lubricate the perineum and the vulva. A heavy oil, such as olive oil, works very well and can be warmed on the stove. The nurse may be asked to pour the warm oil over the perineum, the crowing head, and the midwife's sterile gloves.

The nurse should be mindful of all people in the room throughout the labor and continue to teach them and reassure them about the normalcy of the process that they are observing. Pushing noises are often distressing to those people unacquainted with normal labor. Comparing labor to a strenuous athletic event is often helpful. Making noise during labor often provides energy release, and it is preferable not to direct the client to be quiet during labor.

Birth

In preparation for the birth, a small sterile field is set up that contains two clamps, scissors, 4'' × 4'' sterile gauze, and a rubber bulb syringe or DeLee mucous trap. Occasionally, lidocaine hydrochloride (Xylocaine) may be indicated. Clean underpads are placed under the client's buttocks. Newspapers are placed around the side and foot of the bed to prevent amniotic fluid from dripping onto the rugs or floor. The warmed baby blankets should be within easy reach and can be kept warm by a hot-water bottle. More warm oil may be indicated. The nurse who assists at home births should become familiar with the preferences of the midwives and/or physicians he or she assists, as well as with the wishes of each client.

The birth should be slow and unhurried, with gentle pushes as the head is crowning. The nurse should listen to the fetal heart frequently during this period, and may hold a mirror for the client who wishes to see the birth. The midwife or physician may ask the nurse to suction the baby. Suctioning may be delayed until the shoulders and body of the baby are born. As soon as the infant breathes, the midwife or physician places the baby on the mother's abdomen. It is the nurse's primary concern at this time to keep the baby warm. The warmed blankets are used to pat the baby dry and to wrap the baby. The mother and father are encouraged to put their hands under the blanket and gently massage the baby's skin. They are also encouraged to speak to the baby, who knows their voices and is stimulated by them.[4] Occasionally, parents are shy about talking to the baby, and the nurse can assist them by setting an example.

At this point, the cord should be cut. The nurse and the midwife or physician do nothing but support the attachment process with gentle encouragement over the next few minutes while watching for signs of neonatal distress, placental separation, or complications.

Some babies will breast-feed at this time and, if there are any signs of readiness, it is advisable to begin. Breast-feeding will aid in contraction of the uterus, consequent expulsion of the placenta, and prevention of bleeding. Signs of readiness for breast-feeding in the first hour of life are tongueing (a motion that is similar to licking one's lips) and the more obvious "fist in mouth." Tongueing and lip motion appear to increase when the mother speaks to the baby.

Family members and friends at birth

Each woman and her family determine who will be present at birth. As long as everything is normal, the nurse and the provider usually do not alter her plans.

Most parents have strong feelings about having their children present at birth. It is generally advisable to support their choice instead of trying to change their minds. There are several books available for educating the children (see Resources list at the end of this chapter). The nurse will be able to help the family prepare the children for whatever their participation will be. The one essential factor is that there be another adult present in the house who is responsible for the children and who can handle them. It is advisable to make minimal proscriptions about what the children's participation will be. If the client decides she does not want them present, they must leave the room. (All children must be allowed to leave at any point during the process. In addition, they must understand that they may be asked to leave at any time.) The children's caretaker must be prepared by the mother before the birth in order to be familiar with the children's likes and dislikes. The children's caretaker is usually a relative or friend with whom they are very comfortable. Table 13-2 summarizes the behaviors of children during births.

Third stage

Attachment and family gathering take place during the third stage. The mother may now invite persons to be with her who were waiting outside the room. They should know that they will be asked to leave the room if any complications arise at any time. Families usually

TABLE 13-2

Behavior Characteristics of Children during Home Births

Age group	Characteristics
yr 2-3	Have very short attention span. Will wander in and out of the room. Can be very demanding on their mothers. Are often happiest staying with a neighbor and seeing the baby right after birth. Are usually not very interested in the experience and prefer to play with the new toy grandmother brings.
4-8	Like to have the door to the birthing room open so they can come and go. Will be quiet when asked. Have a beginning sense that their mothers need some cooperation from them, which they can give. Love to get things for parents and the midwife and nurse or to show where things were kept. Are occasionally tearful if their mother exhibits much pain. Need to be prepared for pushing noises, or will be frightened. Need to be reassured and told that what is happening is normal.
8-12	Will come and go throughout labor. Can be very helpful for fetching things. Are more concerned with pain at this age and are bothered by suturing, blood, etc. Need reassurance about what is normal. Think the cord is "yukky" and generally would not like to cut it. Like to have a small job, e.g., writing down time, etc. Often have a hard time being still and quiet.
13 and over	Depending on the child, can be very supportive of the parents at this age. Some sons uncomfortable with their mother's body.

have many questions about vernix, the umbilical cord, milia, and normal newborn responses. The nurse and the midwife have the important role of teaching about normal newborns at this time.

It is necessary to frequently observe the perineum for blood loss and to feel the fundus for firmness. Both of these procedures can be handled discretely so as not to disturb the attachment process. In addition to the classic signs of placental separation (*see* Chapter 11), uterine cramping and discomfort indicate that the uterus is attempting to expel the placenta. Often, more time is allowed in the home setting for the delivery of the placenta so as to not interfere with maternal-infant attachment. Some mothers will want to hold their babies through the delivery of the placenta and any suturing that may be necessary. Other mothers will want the father to hold the baby until they are finished with any potentially painful experiences.

Fourth stage

Although oxytocic drugs are used less frequently in the home setting than in hospitals, the nurse must be prepared to administer them quickly, if so requested. In addition, the nurse will assist with any necessary surgical repair. Because lighting is often inadequate for suturing at home, the nurse may need to hold a flashlight aimed at the perineum and/or to support one of the mother's legs while the repair is completed. Repairs in bed are not easy, and the nurse must become innovative at discovering ways of making the procedure more comfortable for all who are involved. Placing two telephone books or catalogs in a large plastic bag under the mother's buttocks will often improve exposure. Or the mother may move her buttocks to the edge of the bed, where the nurse and another person can support her legs during suturing.

Many women want to take a shower as soon as the placenta is delivered, the uterus is well contracted, any suturing is completed, and the baby has nursed on both sides. Women who do not feel like showering should be given a bed bath at this time. A clean bed is prepared. The infant is given a thorough examination by the midwife or physician, usually with the family looking on. Food is prepared for the new mother and, after she has eaten, more nursing is indicated before the baby enters his sleepy period (*see* Chapter 21). Barring complications, the nurse and the midwife usually stay about 2 or 3 hours after the birth. The mother is checked frequently for bleeding, a firm fundus, and the status of her pulse and blood pressure.

The birth certificate and careful charting of the events of the labor and birth should be completed and then reviewed by the nurse and the provider. Application of silver nitrate to the infant's eyes is delayed until the family has had ample opportunity to attach with the baby. In a few states, parents can waive the requirement for silver nitrate by signing a release form. However, in most states it is mandatory, and the midwife or physician may be censored for not administering it. The injection of vitamin K for the newborn has become an American routine. Parents should be invited to discuss the pros and cons of this routine with their pediatrician before the birth.

First day instructions

The family should be instructed to make sure that the baby breast-feeds about every 2 to 3 hours during the first 24 hours. This will ensure an ample and early milk supply to the baby, early passage of meconium, and the maximum benefit from colostrum. Breast-feeding also ensures a well-contracted uterus, minimal bleeding for the mother, increased parent-infant attachment, and a reduction in the incidence of sore, cracked, or bleeding nipples. The mother should note how frequently the baby voids and when he passes meconium.

Neonatal complications such as jaundice should be discussed, and parents should be instructed to call the nurse or the midwife if any questions arise.

The mother does not need to stay in bed all day, but she must rest frequently. It is highly recommended that she breast-feed lying down because this will ensure frequent rests. She should be told to do no heavy cooking or cleaning in the first week. Extra bleeding is often the first sign of overexertion. At the first sign of any extra bleeding, the mother is instructed to save all her perineal pads in a plastic bag, go to bed, and call the nurse or the midwife/physician.

Because of their healing property and the comfort they provide, sitz baths are recommended twice a day regardless of whether or not there was suturing. Sitz baths are also recommended more frequently if the mother's perineum is painful. Sitz baths may be started within 12 hours after birth and will often help with any stiffness that may result from pushing.

Extra fluids, frequent voiding, good food, and rest are the order of the day.

Postpartum home visits

The first postpartum home visit should occur between 18 and 36 hours after the birth, and it may be made by the nurse or the mid-wife. Within 12 hours after the birth, most services check in by phone with mothers who have recently delivered. When the visit is made, a brief history is taken of the baby's and mother's activities since the nurse left. Special attention should be given to the frequency of breast-feeding, stooling of the baby, voiding of the mother and her baby (Do both have adequate fluid intake?), amount of bleeding the mother has been experiencing, whether she has passed clots, and her general well-being.

The nurse then performs an examination of the mother (*see* Chapter 19) and the infant (*see* Chapter 21), especially noting the baby's color to rule out jaundice. From this point on, the management of mother and baby in the home is very similar to the nursing management in the hospital. Most home birth services require that a pediatrician see the baby within the first 24 to 48 hours. Some pediatricians or family practice physicians will make home visits, which relieve the mother of having to take the baby out during the first few days. In other cases, grandmother or father may take the baby to the pediatrician's office.

At this time, it is very important to provide the opportunity for the mother (and family) to ask questions about events that occurred during the birth and to express their feelings. The mother's impressions of what occurred, after a day's reflection, may be very different from those of the nurse or the provider. Frequently, a woman sets very high standards for herself, and any crying out, complaining, laceration/episiotomy, or complication is seen as a "failure" instead of the "perfect" birth she had envisioned. The nurse is often able to counsel the mother and to assist her to resolve negative feelings that she may experience about the birth.

Complications

In spite of frequent reports to the contrary, life-threatening emergencies rarely occur *without previous warning* during the childbearing process. All women need to have an experienced and observant nurse and midwife or physician with them throughout labor. Without constant surveillance by experienced personnel, warning signs of complications may not be noticed. This lack of constant observation leads to the belief that many labor complications occur without warning.

The nurse planning to attend home births should be familiar with the signs, symptoms, and treatment of obstetric emergencies (*see* Chapter 17) and discuss them with the attending midwife or physician. In addition, the nurse will want to be sure that the telephone numbers of the rescue squad, consultant, and backup hospital phone numbers are near the client's telephone and on the client's chart. The nurse will also want to review the skills in the skills list (*see* p. 317) that he or she has not performed frequently.

Each family is encouraged to attend classes that prepare them for home birth. These classes should include a session in which the incidence and handling of complications is discussed in detail. In areas where special classes are not available, the home birth service should provide this instruction. The *HOME Manual* covers the risk-benefit controversy in detail and is highly recommended reading for parents, relatives, nurses, midwives, and physicians involved with home births.

All potential home birth clients are carefully screened on their initial entry into the service and throughout their prenatal care to rule out complications and to transfer them to the appropriate service as indicated. In healthy women, the probability of complications occurring during labor is about 10 to 15 percent.

In a midwifery home birth service near Washington, D. C., statistics indicate that 26 percent of the women had to be transferred out of the home birth service. In the antepartum period, 11 percent of the women "risked out" for such reasons as preeclampsia (3 women out of 532), hypertension (5), placenta previa (1), herpes (2), multiple gestation (2), breech presentation (5), postmaturity (6), and various other causes. During the intrapartum period, 13 percent (71 women out of 532) were transferred to the hospital (Table 13-3). Most of the women were able to be transported to the hospital by car, and the local ambulance service was used in approximately 10 percent of the cases. All of the above births resulted in live, normal newborns. The overall cesarean section rate for all women accepted into this service was 6.5 percent.

In making the decision to be involved in alternative birth settings, the nurse should be fully informed of the statistical record of the service with whom he or she will be working, and should discuss the management of emergencies or complications.

In educating parents for any alternative birth setting, the ethical issues surrounding the death of the newborn should be discussed. Parents need to be aware of the fact that if their baby should die in the hospital for any reason, the sympathy of society will be with them. Everyone will feel that the parents had done everything they could for the infant even if the baby dies from iatrogenic causes. If their infant should die in an alternative birth setting, even if the cause of death should be a congenital anomaly incompatible with life, there will be those friends and relatives who will say, "If only you had had the baby in the hospital, maybe something could have been done."

> A couple who lose their baby at home will experience deep guilt and regret for their decision unless they have fully accepted the particular set of risks involved in the choice for home birth. Life is fraught with risk. At best we choose one set of risks against another. . . .[5]

TABLE 13-3

Sample Statistics of Intrapartum Women Transferred from Home Birth Services*

Reason for transfer	Number of women transferred
Failure to progress, first stage	21
Failure to progress, second stage	15
Breech presentation	10
Prolonged rupture of membranes	7
Fetal distress	7
Premature labor	5
Meconium staining	1
Mentum posterior position	1
Elevated blood pressure	1
Bleeding	1
Cord prolapse	1
Pain	1

*Statistics are drawn from a home birth clinic near Washington, D. C. During the intrapartum period, 13 percent (71 women out of 532) were transferred to the hospital. (*See* text for discussion.)

OUT-OF-HOSPITAL BIRTH CENTERS

Although home birth is a safe alternative for many families, some families do not feel safe with it. Of these families, many have chosen the out-of-hospital birth center, which has been defined as "an adaptation of a home environment to a short-stay, ambulatory, health care facility with access to in-hospital obstetrical and newborn services; designed to safely accommodate participating family members and support people of the woman's choice; and, providing professional preventive health care to women and the fetus/newborn during pregnancy, birth, and the puerperium."[6]

In 1971, Booth Maternity Center in Philadelphia opened its doors as a maternity hospital, using physicians and nurse-midwives as providers and offering comprehensive family-centered care. At a time when maternity units were beginning to notice a decline in numbers, Booth Maternity Center reached its capacity by 1975. Parents drove from New Jersey, Delaware, and other cities in Pennsylvania to use this innovative facility that encouraged the presence of support people, allowed ambulation and food and drink during labor, and encouraged rooming-in and breast-feeding. Although Booth is actually a hospital (it has the capacity to perform cesarean sections), it did provide a stepping-stone toward the birth center concept.

In 1975, the Maternity Center Association in New York City opened a model out-of-hospital birth center. Its programs include comprehensive prenatal care offered by nurse-midwives with consultation from the center's attending obstetricians and pediatricians, 12-week childbirth classes, home visits, labor and birth at the center in a homelike atmosphere, postpartum recovery for 4 to 12 hours, postpartum home visits by the visiting nurse service, and close follow-up during the first 6 weeks postpartum. This innovative program for maternity health care has served as a model for the nation.

In Reading, Pennsylvania, Dr. Robert McTammany and Sandra Perkins head a team of physicians and midwives who utilize a "continuum concept."[7] Their prospective clients have three options for place of birth: home, birth center, and hospital birthing room. They may use the prenatal services of the physicians or midwives in the hospital, and the midwives attend the births at the clients' homes. If complications arise at home or in the birth center, the same team of providers cares for the client after her transfer to the hospital. Table 13-4 lists the 1979 clients' choices for their delivery site.

Throughout the United States, nurses are functioning in a myriad of roles in birth centers. Many nurses have been instrumental in initiating birth centers and other options in their communities. Some are owners or co-owners and serve as both administrators and staff. Other nurses are hired by the centers, and some are directly employed by the families they serve.

Anticipatory guidance and education about normal birth processes and preventive health measures are priorities for nurses working with maternity clients in any setting. This role is essential in alternative settings. Providing all maternity care in one setting generally allows for a continuity of nursing care that may not be available to nurses

TABLE 13-4
Sample Distribution of Client Choices for Delivery*

Site	Number of women	Percentage
Hospital	159	58
Birth center	68	25
Client's home	48	17

*Statistics are drawn from the McTammany Nurse-Midwife Clinic, Inc., Reading, Penn. Total number of clients was 275. All babies were delivered by nurse-midwives.

working in hospitals. For many nurses, job satisfaction is very high when there is an opportunity to build an ongoing relationship with their clients.

Families choose birth centers because they offer a homelike childbirth experience. Consequently, the role of the nurse throughout the childbearing experience is similar to that described under the section on home birth.

The birth center provides a central point around which all staff and client activities revolve. This system is more cost-effective than the home birth service in terms of the nurse's travel time and energy. It also necessitates the nurse's involvement in institutional matters such as developing and revising policies; procuring appropriate equipment; managing supplies; and participating in the center's programs, including parent education and family orientation. In brief, the nurse makes a commitment to the smooth functioning of the center so that parents and staff are satisfied. Most birth centers provide a unique opportunity for the nurse to have a positive impact on families in the prenatal, intrapartum, and postpartum periods.

IN-HOSPITAL BIRTHING ROOM

A birthing room is an adaptation of a room or suite of rooms in a hospital obstetric unit that is intended to provide a homelike setting that is conducive to family-centered labor and birth experiences.

In response to the national increase in home births and to pressure from consumers, many American hospitals have introduced "birthing rooms." A 1981 survey of the state of Washington revealed that 31 percent of the state's 82 hospitals with maternity services had birthing rooms available and another 32 percent had plans for a birthing room. Of the 30 hospitals that did not plan a birthing room, 24 had fewer than 500 deliveries per year.[8]

Whether birthing rooms are a success depends more on the philosophy of the staff than it does on the physical aspects of the room. In some hospitals where there is little commitment to homelike births, the birthing rooms go unused. Even if the nursing staff is very supportive, the parents usually will have made plans with their physician before they enter the hospital. If the physician is comfortable with the use of the room, it will be used regularly. If not, it will be empty much of the time. A home-style birth can occur in any surroundings. However, the attitude of the staff is what creates the ambiance. In some institutions, changing the physical surroundings helped the staff to relax some protocols and increase sensitivity regarding parents' wishes to be involved in decision-making regarding their care.

SUMMARY

In all settings, nurses are called upon to give safe, individualized, family-centered care to their clients. Nurses who work in alternative birth settings must assume even more responsibility for providing a wide range of expert nursing care: from teaching preventive care to performing technical skills during an emergency. Because of the close contact with the client and her family, nursing in alternative settings provides a great deal of satisfaction for both the client and the nurse. Because of the demand by consumers for this type of care, it seems probable that more and more nurses will provide care in alternative birth settings in the future.

RESOURCES

Books for children

The Flight of the Stork. Bernstein, A. Delacorte Press, New York.

Inside Mom. Coveney, S. St. Martin's Press, Inc., New York. 1977.

Children at Birth. Hathaway, M., and J. Hathaway. Academy Publications, Sherman Oaks, Calif. 1978.

A Baby Is Born. Levine, M., and J. Seligmann. Western Publishing, Racine, Wis. 1978.

Where Did I Come From? Mayle, P. Lyle Stuart, Inc., Secaucus, N. J. 1973.

Where Do Babies Come From? Sheffield, M., and S. Bewley. Alfred A. Knopf, Inc., New York. 1973.

Making Babies. Stein, S. Walker & Co., New York. 1974.

Organizations and resources

Alliance for Perinatal Research and Services (APRS), 321 South Pitt St., Alexandria, Va. 22314.

American College of Home Obstetrics (ACHO), Suite 600, 664 North Michigan Ave., Chicago, Ill. 60611.

American College of Nurse Midwives (ACNM), 1522 K St., Suite 1120, Washington, D. C. 20005.

American College of Obstetricians and Gynecologists, Washington, D. C.

American Foundation for Maternal and Child Health, Inc., 30 Beekman Pl., New York 10022.

American Society for Psychoprophylaxis in Obstetrics (ASPO), 1411 K St., N. W., Washington, D. C. 20005.

Association for Childbirth at Home, International, 16705 Monte Cristo, Cerritos, Calif. 90701.

Home Oriented Maternity Experience (HOME), 511 New York
Ave., Takoma Park, Washington, D. C. 20012.
International Childbirth Education Association (ICEA), P. O. Box
20048, Minneapolis, Minn. 55420.
La Leche League International, 9616 Minneapolis Ave., Franklin
Park, Ill. 60131.
Maternity Center Association, 48 East 92nd St., New York 10028.
National Association of Parents and Professionals for Safe Alterna-
tives in Childbirth (NAPSAC), P. O. Box 267, Marble Hill, Mo.
63764.

REFERENCES

1. Ernst.

2. Varney. 58.

3. Ventre et al. 12.

4. Klaus and Kennell. 63.

5. Ventre et al. 62-63.

6. Cooperative Birth Center Network.

7. Ernst et al. 569-587.

8. Dobbs and Kirkwood.

CHAPTER 14

PARENT-INFANT ATTACHMENT

Elizabeth Luginbuhl

In the last 60 years, birth and death events have been removed from the home and brought into the hospital. Until 10 or 15 years ago, little attention was paid to the effect of separating infants and mothers in the early postpartum period. However, clinical researchers began to consider the significance of separating newborns and mothers during the birth experience. The research results and the recommendations made by clinical experts have greatly changed contemporary obstetric/neonatal practices. As a result, the current trend is to allow the mother and her infant to be together as much as possible immediately after birth. It is believed that early contact between the mother and her infant enhances attachment (bonding) between the two. It is the responsibility of clinical practitioners to provide a birthing milieu that supports and nurtures the family during this important time.

ATTACHMENT

Attachment may be defined as a unique relationship between two people that is specific and endures through time.[1] It is characteristic of all large, ground-living primates (including humans) to live in social groups that are made up of both sexes and all ages.[2] There is reason to believe that an interrelationship between members of a given group of living entities must be perpetuated for survival and protection.[2]

In terms of birth, attachment is a reciprocal interaction mediated by infant and maternal behaviors. Primary infant attachment behaviors include sucking, clinging, following, crying, and smiling.[3] Primary maternal attachment behavior is directed toward reducing the physical distance between the infant and herself.[4] With every experience of interaction between mother and child, the response is intensified.[5] Mother-to-infant and infant-to-mother interactions that can occur simultaneously in the first days of life are described in Table 14-1.[6] These interactions begin the acquaintance process as the parent and her child slowly begin to develop a secure, predictable future. Parent-infant attachment is more than a relationship that is held together by some force or influence; it is a commitment made by parents to care for and love their offspring, and, in so doing, to safeguard future generations.

TABLE 14-1

Maternal-Infant Interactions That Occur Simultaneously in the First Days of Life

Mother to infant	Infant to mother
Touch	
Mothers approach their nude infant with fingertip touching of extremities, then proceed to massaging, stroking, and encompassing the trunk with the palm of their hand.	Newborns become quiet when exposed to the natural beating of the human heart (tentative finding).
Eye to eye	
Mothers of full-term infants seem interested in their babies' eyes and hold the infant in the en face position. Mothers first feel love, and the baby "becomes a person," when the infant begins to look at the environment.	Infants can see and follow movements at birth.
High-pitched voice	
Mothers speak to infants in a high-pitched voice.	Infants are attracted to speech in the high-frequency range.

Mother to infant	Infant to mother
Crying	
	Infant's crying causes increased blood flow to mother's breasts, which promotes lactation.
Entrainment	
Infant's movement may stimulate and reward mother to continue speaking.	Over time, the infant moves in rhythm to adult speech.
Time giver	
Mother helps infant reestablish wake-sleep patterns. Mother tends to hold infant more when he is in alert state.	When infant is in alert state, he is ready to respond to the parent.
Breast-feeding	
T and B lymphocytes and macrophages found in breast milk protect the infant against potentially dangerous enteric pathogens.	Breast-feeding and/or licking mother's nipple leads to release of oxytocin in the mother and increases uterine contraction. Serum prolactin (which induces milk secretion) increases in the postpartum period when licking, sucking, or tactile contact occurs.
Bacterial flora	
In the first minutes of life, mother transfers to infant her mixture of respiratory organisms and protects the infant from hospital-acquired strains.	
Odor	
Mothers report that each of their infants has his own scent.	Breast-feeding infants can identify their mother's breast pad by the 5th day of life.
Heat	
Mother provides enough body heat to maintain infant's temperature when wrapped infant is placed on mother's chest.	Infant is unable to protect himself from heat loss at birth.

Adapted from Klaus, M. H., and J. H. Kennell. Maternal-Infant Bonding: The Impact of Early Separation or Loss on Family Development. C. V. Mosby Co., St. Louis. 1976. p. 67-82.

FACTORS THAT INFLUENCE ATTACHMENT

Parental factors

It is important to note that although early contact between the parent and infant influences attachment, there are other factors that contribute to the development and quality of attachment. Each parent's potential for attachment will be determined by a long history of interpersonal relationships, past experiences with this or previous pregnancies, and absorption of cultural values and practices. Figure 14-1 illustrates the major influences on parenting behavior and some possible disturbances that may result.

Infant factors

Obviously, one of the most important influences on attachment is the infant. Although infants initiate most of the interaction with caregivers, they differ significantly in individual behaviors (e.g., how much they cry, how consolable they are, and how much stimulation they can process).[7] The Neonatal Behavioral Assessment Scale (NBAS) by T. Berry Brazelton provides a tool for assessing neonatal characteristics and individuality. The NBAS is a 27-item scale that provides a means of assessing the state and the interactive behavior of the newborn. (The term "state" refers to characteristics that regularly occur together: body activity, eye and facial movements, breathing, and the level of response to external stimuli [e.g., handling] and internal stimuli [e.g., hunger].)[8] Many of the items on the NBAS are summarized in Blackburn's Infant State and Infant State-Related Behavior Charts, which provide succinct descriptions (and their implications) of newborn state, behavior, interactive potential, and individuality (Tables 14-2 and 14-3). By demonstrating the NBAS to the parents, the nurse can provide visible evidence of the newborn's unique characteristics, strengths, and abilities, thereby enhancing the acquaintance process and facilitating attachment.

Hospital and staff practices

Administrators, physicians, midwives, and nurses should do their utmost to assist the new or expanding family. Facilities and practices should provide an environment for homelike births. Parents should participate in decisions relating to labor, birth, and postpartum care. They should be able to choose the birth experience that satisfies their needs.[9]

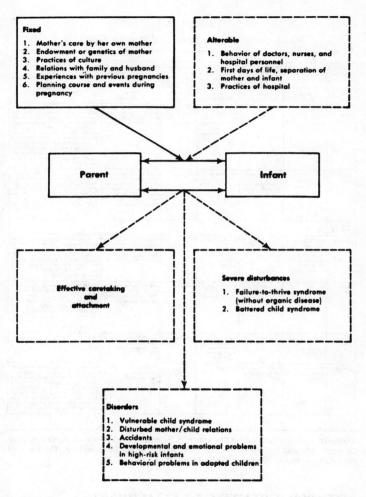

Figure 14-1. Schematic diagram of the major influences on maternal behavior and the possible resultant disturbances. Solid lines represent unchangeable determinants; dotted lines represent alterable determinants. *Reprinted with permission from* Klaus, M. H., and J. H. Kennell. Maternal-Infant Bonding: The Impact of Early Separation or Loss on Family Development. C. V. Mosby Co., St. Louis. 1976. p. 13.

TABLE 14-2
Infant State Chart (Sleep and Awake States)

STATE is a group of characteristics that regularly occur together: body activity, eye movements, facial movements, breathing pattern, and level of response to external stimuli (e.g., handling) and internal stimuli (e.g., hunger).					
SLEEP STATES	CHARACTERISTICS OF STATE				IMPLICATIONS FOR CAREGIVING
	Body Activity	Eye Movements	Facial Movements	Breathing Pattern	Level of Response	
Deep Sleep	Nearly still, except for occasional startle or twitch.	None.	Without facial movements, except for occasional sucking movement at regular intervals.	Smooth and regular.	Threshold to stimuli is very high so that only very intense and disturbing stimuli will arouse infants.	Caregivers trying to feed infants in deep sleep will probably find the experience frustrating. Infants will be unresponsive, even if caregivers use disturbing stimuli (flicking feet) to arouse infants. Infants may only arouse briefly and then become unresponsive as they return to deep sleep. If caregivers wait until infants move to a higher, more responsive state, feeding or caregiving will be much pleasanter.
Light Sleep	Some body movements.	Rapid eye movements. (REM), fluttering of eyes beneath closed eyelids.	May smile and make brief fussy or crying sounds.	Irregular.	More responsive to internal and external stimuli. When these stimuli occur, infants may remain in light sleep, return to deep sleep, or arouse to drowsy.	Light sleep makes up the highest proportion of newborn sleep and usually precedes wakening. Due to brief fussy or crying sounds made during this state, caregivers who are not aware that these sounds occur normally may think it is time for feeding and may try to feed infants before they are ready to eat.
AWAKE STATES						
Drowsy	Activity level variable, with mild startles interspersed from time to time. Movements usually smooth.	Eyes open and close occasionally, are heavy-lidded with dull, glazed appearance.	May have some facial movements. Often there are none, and the face appears still.	Irregular.	Infants react to sensory stimuli although responses are delayed. State change after stimulation frequently noted.	From the drowsy state, infants may return to sleep or awaken further. In order to awaken, caregivers can provide something for infants to see, hear, or suck, as this may arouse them to a quiet alert state, a more responsive state. Infants left alone without stimuli may return to a sleep state.
Quiet Alert	Minimal.	Brightening and widening of eyes.	Faces have bright, shining, sparkling looks.	Regular.	Infants attend most to environment, focusing attention on any stimuli that are present.	Infants in this state provide much pleasure and positive feedback for caregivers. Providing something for infants to see, hear, or suck will often maintain a quiet alert state. In the first few hours after birth, most newborns commonly experience a period of intense alertness before going into a long sleeping period.
Active Alert	Much body activity. May have periods of fussiness.	Eyes open with less brightening.	Much facial movement. Faces not as bright as quiet alert state.	Irregular.	Increasingly sensitive to disturbing stimuli (hunger, fatigue, noise, excessive handling).	Caregivers may intervene at this stage to console and to bring infants to a lower state.
Crying	Increased motor activity, with color changes.	Eyes may be tightly closed or open.	Grimaces.	More Irregular.	Extremely responsive to unpleasant external or internal stimuli.	Crying is the infant's communication signal. It is a response to unpleasant stimuli from the environment or from within infants (fatigue, hunger, discomfort). Crying tells us infants' limits have been reached. Sometimes infants can console themselves and return to lower states. At other times, they need help from caregivers.

Reprinted with permission from Blackburn, S. Sleep and awake states of the newborn. *In* Duxbury, M., and P. Carroll, editors. Early Parent-Infant Relationships, The National Foundation—March of Dimes, White Plains, N.Y. 1978. p. 21.

RESEARCH PERTAINING TO ATTACHMENT

Recent clinical research in the field has shown that early and extended contact between parents and infants fosters an increase in desirable parental caretaking behaviors, such as fondling and caressing. This supports the hypothesis of a "sensitive period" in the first minutes and hours of the baby's life.[10] Predictable patterns of maternal behavior (e.g., touching and holding) have been described,[11,12] and recent research has shown that the newborn is capable of responding to more environmental cues than was supposed, e.g., infants turn their eyes and heads to follow a moving stimulus, and they move their eyes in the direction of a complex auditory stimulus such as speech.[13,14]

MATERNAL TASKS AND NURSING INTERVENTION DURING THE PERINATAL PERIOD

Prenatal tasks

It has been suggested that there are three areas that the nurse can assess during pregnancy to predict how the mother will react to the infant immediately after birth. First, and least important, what attitude does the woman have toward the pregnancy? Did it interfere with career plans? Does she feel comfortable? (It should be noted that women who initially regret their pregnancy have just as good a chance as anyone else of having a healthy relationship with their babies. They may, however, need more adjustment time.) Second, how does the woman refer to the fetus? Does she intellectualize the growth of the fetus as if it were a lump? Or does she think of it as a human being endowed with certain characteristics and movements? The more she identifies with infant characteristics in utero, the shorter will be the time lapse from when the baby is born to when the mother begins to have maternal feelings. Third, what does the woman predict her baby will be like? Will she play a nurturing role to feed it, bathe it, etc.? Or will she be afraid of it and think of the baby more as an older child and in terms of the dreams she has for it? A data base, which includes this information, may be extremely helpful in planning postpartum care.[15]

Because physical changes are more evident during pregnancy, psychological and emotional preparation may be overlooked. It has been suggested that if a woman has difficulty accepting passivity, contemplation, and being waited on — all of which are characteristics of the second and third trimesters — she may have difficulty with giving and receiving from her infant. Also, if in the past her relationship with her own mother lacked nurturing, this factor is likely to surface and affect her ability to prepare for her new role.[16]

Binding-in has been described in terms of a child's being incorporated into the mother's entire self-system during pregnancy. A woman who does not successfully bind to the idea of her child during pregnancy may not be ready to take in the infant immediately after delivery.[17] Furthermore, the assumption that all women automatically feel motherly after birth may cause a mother to become frightened that something is wrong with her and may even hinder the mother-child relationship.[18] The nurse should be receptive to those mothers who need more time adjusting to the birth of their infant.

TABLE 14-3
Infant State-Related Behavior Chart

BEHAVIOR	DESCRIPTION OF BEHAVIOR	INFANT STATE CONSIDERATION	IMPLICATIONS FOR CAREGIVING
ALERTING	Widening and brightening of the eyes. Infants focus attention on stimuli, whether visual, auditory, or objects to be sucked.	From drowsy or active alert to quiet alert.	Infant state and timing are important. When trying to alert infants, one may try to: 1. unwrap infants (arms out at least) 2. place infants in upright position 3. talk to infants, putting variation in your pitch and tempo 4. show your face to infants 5. elicit the rooting, sucking, or grasp reflexes. Being able to alert infants is important for caregivers, as alert infants offer increased feedback to adults.
VISUAL RESPONSE	Newborns have pupillary responses to differences in brightness. Infants can focus on objects or faces about 7-8 inches away. Newborns have preferences for more complex patterns, human faces, and moving objects.	Quiet alert.	Newborns' visual alertness provides opportunities for eye-to-eye contact with caregivers, an important source of beginning caregiver-infant interaction.
AUDITORY RESPONSE	Reaction to a variety of sounds, especially in the human voice range. Infants can hear sounds and locate the general direction of the sound, if the source is constant and remains coming from the same direction.	Drowsy, quiet alert, active alert.	Enhances communication between infants and caregivers. The fact that crying infants can often be consoled by voice demonstrates the value this stimulus has to infants.
HABITUATION	The ability to lessen one's response to repeated stimuli. For instance, this is seen when the Moro response is repeatedly elicited. If a noise is continually repeated, infants will no longer respond to it in most cases.	Deep sleep, light sleep, also seen in drowsy.	Because of this ability families can carry out their normal activities without disturbing infants. Infants are not victims of their environments. Infants can shut out most stimuli, similar to adults not hearing a dripping faucet after a period of time. Infants who have more difficulty with this will probably not sleep well in active environments.
CUDDLINESS	Infant's response to being held. Infants nestle and work themselves into the contours of caregivers' bodies versus resist being held.	Primarily in awake states.	Cuddliness is usually rewarding behavior for the caregivers. It seems to convey a message of affection. If infants do not nestle and mold, it would be wise to discuss this tendency and show the caregivers how to position infants to maximize this response.
CONSOL-ABILITY	Measured when infants have been crying for at least 15 seconds. The ability of infants to bring themselves or to be brought by others to a lower state.	From crying to active alert, quiet alert, drowsy, or sleep states.	Crying is the infant behavior that presents the greatest challenge to caregivers. Parents' success or failure in consoling their infants has a significant impact on their feelings of competence as parents.
Self-Consoling	Maneuvers used by infants to console themselves and move to a lower state: 1. hand-to-mouth movement 2. sucking on fingers, fist, or tongue 3. paying attention to voices or faces around them 4. changes in position.	From crying to active alert, quiet alert, drowsy, or sleep states.	If caregivers are aware of these behaviors, they may allow infants the opportunity to gain control of themselves instead of immediately responding to their cues. This does not imply that newborns should be left to cry. Once newborns are crying and do not initiate self-consoling activities, they may need attention from caregivers.
Consoling by Caregivers	After crying for longer than 15 seconds, the caregivers may try to: 1. show face to infant 2. talk to infant in a steady, soft voice 3. hold both infant's arms close to body 4. swaddle infant 5. pick up infant 6. rock infant 7. give a pacifier or feed.	From crying to active alert, quiet alert, drowsy, or sleep states.	Often parental initial reaction is to pick up infants or feed them when they cry. Parents could be taught to try other soothing maneuvers.

Chart continues on next page

BEHAVIOR	DESCRIPTION OF BEHAVIOR	INFANT STATE CONSIDERATION	IMPLICATIONS FOR CAREGIVING
MOTOR BEHAVIOR AND ACTIVITY	Spontaneous movements of extremities and body when stimulated versus when left alone. Smooth, rhythmical movements versus jerky ones.	Quiet alert, active alert.	Smooth, nonjerky movements with periods of inactivity seem most natural. Some parents see jerky movements and startles as responses to their caregiving and are frightened.
IRRITABILITY	How easily infants are upset by loud noises, handling by caregivers, temperature changes, removal of blankets or clothes, etc.	From deep sleep, light sleep, drowsy, quiet alert, or active alert to fussing or crying.	Irritable infants need more frequent consoling and more subdued external environments. Parents can be helped to cope with more irritable infants through the items listed under "Consoling by Caregivers."
READABILITY	The cues infants give through motor behavior and activity, looking, listening, and behavior patterns.	All states.	Parents need to learn that newborns' behaviors are part of their individual temperaments and not reflections on their parenting abilities or because their infants do not like them. By observing and understanding an infant's characteristic pattern, parents can respond more appropriately to their infant as an individual.
SMILE	Ranging from a faint grimace to a full-fledged smile. Reflexive.	Drowsy, active alert, quiet alert, light sleep.	Initial smile in the neonatal period is the forerunner of the social smile at 3-4 weeks of age. Important for caregivers to respond to it.

Reprinted with permission from Blackburn, S. State-related behaviors and individual differences. *In* Duxbury, M., and P. Carroll, editors. Early Parent-Infant Relationships, The National Foundation—March of Dimes, White Plains, N.Y. 1978. p. 29-30.

Delivery tasks

Work done by Klaus et al. on extended maternal-infant contact in the first 3 days after birth showed a significant increase in en face and fondling behavior at a 1-month filmed feeding analysis of the extended contact group.[19] Research of this kind has changed delivery room practices. Extended contact between parent and infant should be offered whenever possible, and parental reaction to the infant and to each other should be noted.

During the dynamic physical and emotional events of labor and delivery, the observations made by labor and delivery room staff — which focus on: How does the mother look? What does the mother say? What does the mother do? — have been shown to be good predictors of families with the potential for parenting success or failure.[20]

Postpartum tasks

During the postpartum period, the mother may be tired and worried about bodily changes, a painful episiotomy, or engorged breasts.[21] The nurse should provide comfort measures and assist the mother at this time to replenish the energy she will need to meet her infant's needs.

It is believed by some researchers that humans model themselves after significant others and that mothers will look to the nurse, who is usually female, more than to other medical professionals.[22] The nurse, then, is in a unique position to work with the mother, evaluate her needs, teach infant care and behavior, and coordinate follow-up care as needed.

Attachment assessment

The assessment of attachment during the phases of the pregnancy cycle should be included in the obstetric data base. Continuity of assessment from the prenatal to the postnatal period helps with setting priorities and planning care. Coordination of resources in the community and hospital (e.g., social services and nursing) provides for better assessment and implementation of supportive services when indicated. A sample guide for the assessment of attachment during the perinatal period is illustrated in Figure 14-2.

Mothers who consistently manifest low-level attachment behaviors — such as an absence of en face, holding the baby away from the chest and abdomen, a lack of eagerness for feeding time, allowing the baby to ingest air from the nipple, a lack of desire to burp the baby, and an appearance of tension or depression — require additional support and intervention.[23,24] Personification of the infant and strengthening the maternal image will foster the acquaintance process.

Support system care planning

So that each family can reach its potential of parent-infant health, coordination and communication between health care services are essential. Building support systems and maximizing resources early in the pregnancy contribute to effective care planning. The following is a list of suggestions to consider when planning supportive care for the childbearing family:

Assignment of primary care nurse for prenatal, labor and delivery, and postpartum care.

Social service caseworker evaluation and support during prenatal, labor and delivery, and postpartum care.

Preparation for childbirth classes with significant other.

Tour of labor and delivery and postpartum units.

Identification and introduction to community health care worker in the prenatal period.

Prenatal home assessment by community health care worker, if indicated.

Facilitation of a period of extended contact in the immediate postpartum period.[25]

If the infant was born by cesarean section, immediate initiation of contact with the father.[26]

Delay of eye medication (such as silver nitrate) for the infant until parents have had early contact.[27]

Encouragement of rooming-in with readily available staff for teaching and consultation.[25]

Postpartum parent education class on infant care, behavior, and development, with flexibility for educational level and ethnic content.[25]

Acknowledgment of the mother's ability or sincere efforts to comfort, feed, soothe, and sense her baby's needs.[28]

Discharge planning to include the need for support measures:[25]

    Visiting nurse services.

    Close well-child care follow-up.

    Supportive others.

    Homemaker.

    Mental health and family service agency.

    Family planning.

    Sibling day-care.

PARENT-TO-INFANT ATTACHMENT IN SPECIAL CIRCUMSTANCES

High-risk newborn

The birth of a premature, sick, or malformed baby can have a significant effect on parent-to-infant attachment. Long-term separation and hospitalization, in addition to an uncertain outcome, can interrupt and delay the attachment process.[29] Observations have been made throughout the world on the incidence of infant battering and failure to thrive and on their relationships to early separation at birth.[1] Budin, author of the first text in neonatology, found that some mothers abandoned babies whose needs they did not have to meet. He designed glass-walled incubators so that the mothers could see their infants and participate in their care. With these changes, mothers remained attentive to their infants' needs.[30]

Health care practitioners can offer much support and guidance to the families of high-risk newborns. Negative parental reactions to sick, premature, and malformed infants can range from disbelief to resentment. The nursing staff should be well prepared to assist the family in both expert technical care and in a counselor role. The following is a list of recommendations for working with the families of high-risk newborns:[31]

Evaluate and reevaluate the stages of grief reactions (i.e., shock; denial; anger, sadness, and anxiety; equilibrium; and reorganization).

If possible, provide the parents with an opportunity to see and touch their infant, if the baby has to be quickly moved to a neonatal intensive care unit or to another hospital.

Encourage the father to accompany the infant to the intensive care unit or to follow the transport team to the different hospital.

Provide detailed explanations of equipment and procedures to both parents as soon as possible. A booklet describing care and equipment should be given to the parents. (Protect the parents from seeing frightening and painful procedures.)

Provide daily information regarding the infant's condition, strengths, and individual characteristics. (This can be accomplished by telephone 24 hours a day or by a visit to the mother's hospital room, if possible. A photograph provides some contact for the mother while she is physically separated from her child.)

Encourage grandparents, brothers, sisters, and/or significant others to visit and share in the birth of the infant.

Arrange for scheduled meetings with the parents, depending on the critical nature of the infant's condition.

Allow the parents to adjust to the sick newborn at their own pace.

Inform the parents of the benefits of touching and stroking their sick newborn (e.g., decreased apnea).

Encourage and support the mother who wishes to express breast milk for the infant during the period of separation.

If the infant progresses, be optimistic in discussions with the family; however, avoid giving false hope. (Never say "brain damage" unless 100 percent certain that the baby is damaged or retarded.)

Facilitate ways in which the parents will experience positive feedback from their baby, such as noting when the baby quiets down when spoken to, focuses, or cuddles.

Record parental phone calls and visits. Fewer than three visits in 2 weeks should alert the staff to the possibility that the parents may need additional help in adjusting to the health of their infant.

Be a patient listener.

Collaborate with other disciplines as necessary (e.g., social services, chaplain, and physician).

Encourage the parents to "nest" (spend one or two nights at the hospital with their infant) before discharge.

Multiple births

Attachment to multiple-birth infants requires special consideration. It may be difficult for a mother to form a close attachment to more than one infant at a time. Monotrophy, as described by Bowlby in discussing the child's tie to his or her mother, is the tendency to respond instinctively to a particular individual or group of individuals rather than indiscriminately to many.[32] Often, mothers feel that they first attach to their twins as a "unit." Once the mother is attached to the unit, individual personalities emerge and individualization takes place.[33]

The following list of major points should be considered when caring for parents of multiple births:[33]

Allow the parents to express any ambivalent feelings regarding multiple births.

If twins are discovered or suspected during labor and delivery, tell the parents immediately. This facilitates attachment to the second baby.

Encourage the mother to hold her babies immediately after delivery, if possible, first together, then separately.

Keep the babies side by side in the nursery. This reinforces the reality of having twins.

Bring both babies to their mother at the same time for feeding.

Help the parents to treat each baby as an individual.

Observe for disparate behavior, such as holding one twin close while the other is held at a distance. (Encourage verbalization of any favoring of one twin over the other, and gently draw the parents' attention toward the infant receiving less attention.)

Allow more time for attachment to multiple births than to a single birth.

If possible, both babies should be discharged from the hospital at the same time. (If one infant remains in an intensive care area, make arrangements for frequent visits or telephone calls.)

(If one infant dies, it is difficult to attach to the surviving infant while grieving occurs.)

Maternal sensory impairment

Many interactions that occur in the attachment process involve the senses (e.g., eye-to-eye contact, hearing, and entrainment).[34] A deaf or blind mother will need more time and assistance in getting acquainted with her infant. Alternative senses compensate when sensory deprivation exists.[34] Supportive care for the sensory-impaired mother includes the following actions:[34]

Use therapeutic touch in nursing care activities to relate a feeling of warmth and understanding.

Encourage the mother to have close physical contact with the infant (e.g., cuddling and rocking).

Encourage rooming-in.

Assist the mother with identifying cues that will help her sense her infant's needs.

Encourage the mother by acknowledging success in her caretaking abilities.

ATTACHMENT ASSESSMENT FORM*

NAME_____ AGE_____ MARITAL STATUS: Single___ Married___ Separated___

GRAVIDA_____ PARA_____ AB_____ DELIVERY DATE_____

EXPECTED DATE OF CONFINEMENT_____ METHOD OF FEEDING_____

SUMMARY OF LABOR AND DELIVERY (anesthesia, complications, presence of a supportive person):

_____

_____

_____

_____

DIRECTIONS: This form is provided to systematically assess and record the components of the attachment process based on information obtained from available records, observations, and interviews with the parent(s) and other health care providers.

PRENATAL

	YES	NO	COMMENTS
Planned the pregnancy	___	___	_____
Confirmed the pregnancy	___	___	_____
Accepted the pregnancy	___	___	_____
Received early prenatal care	___	___	_____
Described fetal movement	___	___	_____
Personalized the fetus	___	___	_____
Asked what the fetus was like in utero	___	___	_____
Attended prenatal classes	___	___	_____
Planned for infant's needs	___	___	_____

*This form (pages 74-77) may be reproduced

Figure 14-2. Sample attachment assessment form. *Reprinted with permission from* Kang, R. Parent-infant attachment. *In* Duxbury, M., and P. Carroll, editors. Early Parent-Infant Relationships. The National Foundation—March of Dimes, White Plains, N. Y. 1978. p. 74-77.

PRENATAL

	YES	NO	COMMENTS
Thought of possible names	___	___	_____
Client in good health	___	___	_____
Father of infant involved	___	___	_____

AREAS OF CONCERN: _____

DELIVERY PERIOD (Birth through 4 hours)

	YES	NO	COMMENTS
Accepts sex of infant	___	___	_____
Calls infant by name	___	___	_____
Calls infant by affectionate terms	___	___	_____
Comments on beauty of infant	___	___	_____
Realistically appraises the physical appearance of the infant	___	___	_____
Looks and reaches out to infant	___	___	_____
Touches infant	___	___	_____
Smiles at infant	___	___	_____

AREAS OF CONCERN: _____

Figure 14-2 (cont'd).

FIRST POSTPARTUM DAY *(From birth through first day)*

	YES	NO	COMMENTS
Calls infant by name	___	___	
Describes infant in affectionate terms	___	___	
Offers positive comments about infant's physical appearance	___	___	
Finds family resemblances	___	___	
Looks and reaches out to infant	___	___	
Hugs and touches infant	___	___	
Kisses infant	___	___	
Smiles at infant	___	___	
Expresses positive emotional feelings to infant's father or significant other	___	___	
Experiences average discomfort	___	___	
Welcomes visitors	___	___	

AREAS OF CONCERN: _____

POSTPARTUM PERIOD *(From second day to 6 weeks)*

	YES	NO	COMMENTS
Wants to be near infant	___	___	

Figure 14-2 (cont'd).

POSTPARTUM PERIOD (From second day to 6 weeks)

	YES	NO	COMMENTS
Enjoys caring for infant	___	___	_____
			_____
Holds infant close	___	___	_____
			_____
Feels infant belongs to her	___	___	_____
Feels infant notices her	___	___	_____
			_____
When away, thinks about infant	___	___	_____
Verbalizes warm comments about infant	___	___	_____
Recuperates with little difficulty	___	___	_____
Responds sensitively and appropriately to infant	___	___	_____

AREAS OF CONCERN: _____

_____

_____

_____

_____

Figure 14-2 (cont'd).

Infant death

If the infant is born dead or dies in the postpartum period, the parents should be permitted to see and hold their dead infant, if they so desire.[35] This facilitates the mourning process and confirms reality. Although it is never a pleasant assignment, the nurse who assists the family at this time should offer support in the following ways:[36]

Provide the parents with a photograph of the infant, before or after death, if possible.

Remain with the parents, unless they prefer otherwise.

Provide a comfortable and quiet area where the family can have privacy.

Prepare the infant appropriately (e.g., bathe and dress, if necessary, and swaddle in an infant blanket).

Discuss funeral arrangements openly and honestly.

SUMMARY

Assessment and facilitation of parent-infant attachment in the early postpartum period are nursing challenges. Each family has its own unique set of strengths and liabilities as it approaches this important step in life. Helping the childbearing family get the best possible start has lasting effects. A caring attitude, practiced in a professional and competent manner, represents the highest level of nursing intervention. Parent-infant attachment is basic to the survival of future generations. As such, it must be handled by sensitive, gentle facilitators.

REFERENCES

1. Klaus and Kennell. (1976) 2.
2. Bowlby. 62-63.
3. Bowlby. 180.
4. Bowlby. 239-241.
5. Bowlby. 272.
6. Klaus and Kennell. (1976) 67-82.
7. Korner.
8. Blackburn. 21.
9. Young.
10. Klaus and Kennell. (1976) 50-59.

11. Klaus et al. (1970)
12. Salk.
13. Goren et al.
14. Turkewitz et al.
15. Caplan. 86-93.
16. Caplan. 65-95.
17. Rubin. (1975)
18. Neikirk. 69.
19. Klaus et al. (1972)
20. Gray et al.
21. Kang. 71.
22. Rubin. (1967)
23. Klaus and Kennell. (1970)
24. Lamper. 72-83.
25. Kerns et al.
26. Young.
27. Klaus and Kennell. (1976) 95.
28. Jenkins and Westhus.
29. Young.
30. Klaus and Kennell. (1976) 3.
31. Klaus and Kennell. (1976) 151-179.
32. Klaus and Kennell. (1976) 83.
33. Gromada.
34. Mcrae.
35. Klaus and Kennell. (1976) 235.
36. Wooten.

CHAPTER 15

ANTEPARTUM DEVIATIONS

Kathleen Buckley

This chapter focuses on some of the more common deviations that arise during pregnancy which may threaten the health of the client or fetus. It includes the medical management and nursing actions involved with each deviation. One of the most challenging nursing goals is to help the client with health deviations to appreciate the normal psychophysiological changes that occur with pregnancy and to help her understand and cope with the manifestations of illness. Deviations from health during pregnancy place added stress not only on the client but also on the entire family structure. The nurse must be the active leader in coordinating the health care team's efforts to bring about the best possible outcome for the client, her baby, and her support systems (family).

ANEMIA

Definition

Hematocrit is the volume percentage of red blood cells in whole blood. Hemoglobin is the oxygen-carrying pigment in red blood cells. Any condition that lowers the level of hematocrit or hemoglobin in the blood will result in less red blood cells and, therefore, less oxygen and nutrients being transported throughout the body.

Anemia may be defined as a condition in which the hemoglobin level is below 10 grams or the hematocrit level is below 30 percent.

In pregnancy, the blood plasma volume may expand by as much as 50 percent. This physiological dilution begins in the first trimester, peaks in the second, and stabilizes thereafter. A corresponding two- to four-point drop in hematocrit during the second trimester is a normal result of this process.

Types of anemia

Iron deficiency anemia.   A pregnant woman who has insufficient stores of iron and an inadequate dietary iron intake is prone to developing iron deficiency anemia. The iron demands of a fetus are at least 800 milligrams, and a twin gestation may exceed a 1,000-milligram requirement. Without adequate stores of iron, the body produces fewer, pale (hypochromic), and small (microcytic) red blood cells.

Folic acid deficiency anemia.   A pregnant woman who does not have an adequate dietary intake of high-quality animal protein or uncooked, green leafy vegetables is prone to developing folic acid deficiency. This deficiency results in fewer and larger (macrocytic) red blood cells. The fetus has large metabolic requirements for folic acid and its derivatives. Frequently, clients also develop nausea, vomiting, and/or anorexia, any of which further aggravates the nutritionally deficient state.

Glucose-6-phosphate dehydrogenase anemia.   Deficiency of the enzyme glucose-6-phosphate dehydrogenase (G6PD) is an inherited defect that occurs in approximately 15 percent of black women. Certain foods and drugs may produce destruction of red blood cells in these women (Table 15-1). Hemolysis may also occur with infection or acidosis.

Beta-thalassemia minor.   This hereditary disorder occurs when an abnormal autosomal gene from one parent combines with a normal gene from another, resulting in reduced or absent production of the globin chains of hemoglobin. The levels of hemoglobin A_2 are elevated, and target cells are usually seen in the complete blood count. This disorder is often misinterpreted as iron deficiency because it produces a hypochromic microcytic anemia.

Although beta-thalassemia minor produces anemia, it also confers increased resistance to malaria. It is most often seen in persons of Mediterranean, Central African, and Asian descent.

Fetal outcome will vary: if both parents have beta-thalassemia minor (a heterozygous condition), their baby has a 25 percent chance of developing thalassemia major (homozygous), which is also known

TABLE 15-1

Drugs Causing Hemolytic Reaction in Clients with Glucose-6-Phosphate Dehydrogenase Deficiency

Nitrofurans	Antimalarials	Antipyretics and analgesics	Sulfonamides	Others
furaltadone (Altafur) furazolidone (Furoxone) nitrofurantoin (Furadantin) nitrofurazone (Furacin)	Pamaquine Pentaquine primaquine phosphate quinacrine hydrochloride (Atabrine hydrochloride) quinidine quinine quinocide	acetanilide acetophenetidin (Phenacetin Empirin) acetylsalicylic acid Aminopyrine Antipyrine Para-aminosalicylic acid	n-2-acetylsulfa-nilamide Salicylsulfapyridine (Azulfidine) sulfacetamide sodium (Sulamyd) sulfamethoxyprid-azine (Kynex, Midicel) Sulfanilimide sulfapyridine sulfisoxazole (Gantrisin)	acetyl phenyl-hydrazine chloramphenicol chloroquine hydro-chloride dimercaprol (Bal) fava beans methylene blue nalidixic acid (Negram) naphthalene (moth balls, moth spray) phenylhydrazine Probenecid Tolbutamide (Orinase) vitamin K (water soluble)

as Cooley's anemia. These offspring usually do not live past young adulthood. It is possible to diagnose this problem at the 18th to 20th week of gestation through analysis of a fetal blood sample.

Sickle cell trait.   Sickle cell trait is an inherited defect in approximately 8 percent of American blacks.

Sickle cell trait is associated with iron and folic acid deficiencies. It is also associated with an increased incidence of bacilluria. An unusual reduction of oxygen tension (e.g., sudden depressurization in an airplane or inadequate oxygenation during inhalation of anesthesia) may trigger a sickle cell crisis.

If both parents have the sickle cell trait, they may have a baby with sickle cell disease.

Other types.   Chronic blood loss and chronic infection may also produce a hypochromic microcytic anemia. Bleeding gums, frequent nosebleeds, or intestinal parasites may deplete iron stores to such a degree to decrease the hematocrit level.

A client with a history of repeated infection (e.g., urinary tract or upper respiratory tract) may also develop an anemia as a result of decreased production and increased destruction of red blood cells. Hypochromic microcytic anemias that do not respond to iron or folic acid therapy may represent anemias that result from an unrecognized infection.

Medical management

A battery of diagnostic studies (Table 15-2) will determine the specific etiology of the anemia. Treatment depends on the causative factor(s).

Iron deficiency anemia.   An iron supplement (200 mg/day) should be prescribed.

Folic acid deficiency.   A folic acid supplement (1 mg/day) should be taken, and dietary intake of folic acid should be increased (*see* Table 5-4).

G6PD.   Iron and folic acid supplements are prescribed. The client must be taught to avoid drugs and foods that may produce a hemolytic reaction (*see* Table 15-1).

Beta-thalassemia minor.   Iron therapy is *not* recommended. The father of the baby should be screened for the trait. If he has the trait, further diagnostic studies are in order.

Sickle cell trait.   Iron and folic acid supplementation should be prescribed, and the sources of both should be increased in the diet (*see* Table 5-4).

Other types.   Hypochromic microcytic anemias respond when the blood loss is decreased or the infection is identified and treated.

TABLE 15-2

Diagnostic Studies Used to Evaluate Anemia *

1. Complete blood count with indices and reticulocyte count.
2. Serum iron.
3. Total iron binding capacity.
4. Hemoglobin electrophoresis.
5. Glucose-6-phosphate dehydrogenase.
6. Stool culture for ova and parasites.

*See Appendix B.

Nursing actions

1. Explain the appropriate causative factors of anemia and the purpose of diagnostic studies.
2. Review the importance of taking iron and/or vitamin supplements.
3. Counsel the client to take iron with a glass of orange juice (vitamin C enhances iron absorption). Iron should also be taken between meals in order to aid absorption.
4. Teach the client about food sources of iron and folic acid:
   a. Iron: liver, iron-fortified cereal, lima beans, baked beans with molasses, spinach, liverwurst, and egg yolks.
   b. Folic acid: liver, eggs, milk, green leafy vegetables (uncooked).
5. Clients with G6PD deficiency should know that there are certain foods and drugs that they may not use. Make sure that they are provided with a list of contraindicated medications to carry with them at all times (*see* Table 15-1).
6. Refer couples with beta-thalassemia minor trait or sickle cell trait for genetic counseling and evaluation early in pregnancy, if appropriate.

DIABETES MELLITUS

Definition

Diabetes mellitus (DM) is a metabolic disease in which the islands of Langerhans in the pancreas fail to produce sufficient insulin. Because insulin transforms glucose into glycogen, converts glucose into fat (lipogenesis), affects transfer of amino acids into cells, and affects the rate of protein synthesis, any actual or relative deficiency produces a starvation-type syndrome that is characterized by hyperglycemia, ketonuria, and dehydration.

The client usually exhibits the classic signs of polyuria, polydipsia, and polyphagia. Other signs and symptoms include weight loss, weakness, fatigue, pruritus, delayed wound healing, and/or pain in the fingers and toes.

Although DM is an inherited disorder, other factors (e.g., environment, hormone levels, and immunologic variables) can effect the onset.[1] It is a recessive trait, with 20 percent of the population not diabetic but able to pass on the gene, and 5 percent diabetic.[1]

Pregnancy and DM

Before the discovery of insulin in 1921, DM and pregnancy were a life-threatening combination for both the mother and the fetus. The maternal mortality rate was 25 percent, and fetal death was 60 percent.[2]

Pregnancy changes many normal relationships in body fuel metabolism. Circulating levels of glucose and amino acids are decreased, and free fatty acids, ketones, and insulin secretion are increased. The fetus draws glucose and amino acids continuously from the maternal circulation. These tremendous alterations in metabolism are normal. Pregnancy is termed a diabetogenic state because of the decreased reactivity to insulin that begins in the third trimester.

Medical management

A superimposed deficiency of insulin on the normal, but profound, fuel metabolism alterations poses multiple risks for the mother and baby. Careful management depends on prompt diagnosis. Any woman who presents with a suspicious history or symptoms should be screened for DM with a fasting and 2-hour postprandial blood sugar test (Table 15-3). If one of these values is elevated, further testing with a 3-hour glucose tolerance test is indicated. An oral glucose tolerance test is considered abnormal or diagnostic for DM if two or more values are abnormal (*see* Appendix B). Because reactivity to insulin is altered in the third trimester, it is important to screen clients well before that time. (The 28th week of gestation is recommended.) A thorough history and physical examination are then necessary to classify the severity of the disease (Table 15-4). Class A DM is usually managed by diet alone. Class B and greater DM require both dietary and insulin management (Table 15-5).

Close collaboration of the entire health care team is vital in order to ensure a successful outcome. The primary goals include the prevention of ketoacidosis, toxemia, infections, hyperemesis gravidarum, and intrauterine death. The client should be seen weekly or biweekly until the 28th week of gestation, and then weekly thereafter. Careful evaluation of maternal cardiovascular and renal func-

TABLE 15-3
Screening for Diabetes Mellitus

Family history of diabetes in siblings, parents, or grandparents.
History of large babies (>4,000 g).
History of poor fetal outcome: term stillborn, term infant with respiratory distress syndrome, congenital anomalies, repeated miscarriage, or prematurity.
Maternal obesity (20% above standard weight for height).
Maternal age (≥35 yr).
Hydramnios.
Glycosuria (≥2 episodes).
Repeated monilial vaginal infections.
Grand multiparity.
Hypertension.

TABLE 15-4
White's Classification of Diabetes

Class	Characteristics
A	Gestational diabetic; no symptoms.
B	Onset after 20 yr of age; duration of 0-9 yr, no vascular disease.
C	Onset before 10 yr of age; duration of >20 yr; vascular disease; retinitis; calcification in lower extremities.
E	Calcified pelvic vessels.
F	Nephropathy.
R	Malignant retinitis.

Adapted from Nelson, B., L. Gillespie, and P. White. Pregnancy complicated by diabetes mellitus. *Obstetrics and Gynecology* (January 1953). 219.

tioning are required. The frequency of laboratory testing of blood sugars, urine, and blood urea nitrogen levels depends on the severity of the disease. Prolonged hospitalization may be necessary to control the disease.

Placental functioning and fetal growth and well-being are monitored frequently by ultrasonography, urinary or plasma estriols, lecithin:sphingomyelin ratios, and non-stress testing. DM (other than class A) is associated with fetal demise after the 36th week of gestation. The etiology is thought to be premature placental aging or maternal acidosis. Therefore, delivery of class B or greater diabetics

TABLE 15-5

Insulin: Types and Action Curves*

Action	Insulin	Duration of action	Peak effect
		hr	*hr*
Fast	Regular Zinc	6	2-3
	Semilente	12	3-6
Intermediate	Globin Zinc	18	6-8
	NPH	24	8-12
	Lente	24	8-12
Long	Ultralente	36	10-30
	Protamine Zinc	36	16-24

*Note: All types of insulin are available in three different strengths: 40, 80, and 100 U/ml. A unit of insulin (25 mg/ml) has the same potency regardless of its strength. In order to avoid medication error, insulin should always be measured in a syringe that is calibrated for that strength *only.*
Adapted from Thorn, G. W., R. D. Adams, E. Braunwald, K. J. Isselbacher, and R. G. Petersdorf, editors. Harrison's Principles of Internal Medicine. McGraw-Hill Book Co., New York. 1977. Eighth edition. p. 575.

is usually indicated before the 37th week. Class A diabetics are not allowed to carry the fetus past the 40th week of gestation. Because a diabetic fetus tends to be large and the placenta ages more rapidly, cephalopelvic disproportion and/or fetal distress have pushed the rate of cesarean section to 70 percent. Fetal respiratory distress syndrome and prematurity are responsible for the majority of neonatal deaths. Fetal malformations account for approximately 20 percent of these deaths.[3]

Nursing actions

1. Explain the physiological basis of the disease to the client. Specifically, she should understand the following points:
   a. Basic carbohydrate metabolism and the role of insulin.
   b. Definition of DM.
   c. Effect of DM on metabolism.
   d. Effect of DM on the fetus.
2. Coordinate efforts of health care team — obstetrician, internist, social worker, nutritionist, public health nurse — to maximize effectiveness of care.
3. Urge client to keep all clinic appointments.
4. Review role of good nutrition in normal pregnancy.

5. Emphasize nutrition as a means to control diabetes. (Check with physician and nutritionist for exact details of prescribed diet.)

6. Counsel avoidance of the following high-sugar foods in the diet to prevent marked swings in blood sugar levels: candy, chewing gum, honey, syrup, molasses, fruit (canned with sugar), dried fruit, pastries and cakes, soft drinks sweetened with sugar, jellies, jams, preserves, ice cream, and table sugar.

7. Stress the importance of developing a consistent pattern of food intake (no skipping meals) and a similar total calorie intake from day to day to prevent a severe insulin reaction.

8. Review activities of daily living, rest needs, and exercise patterns. The client should avoid fatigue and/or overexertion because they may decrease carbohydrate tolerance.

9. Emphasize the importance of reporting any localized skin infection or any systemic illness to the physician immediately.

10. Teach the client to recognize the signs and symptoms of diabetic coma and insulin shock (Table 15-6).

11. Review personal hygiene and care of teeth, skin, and feet.

12. Review special precautions for cutting fingernails and toenails. (Note: in class B or greater diabetes, the physician may want to do this.)

13. Teach the client to test urine for sugar and acetone (as necessary).

14. If insulin is required, teach the client the technique of parenteral administration.

15. Instruct the client in the purpose and technique for collection of any specific tests: 24-hour urine for estriol determination; fasting and 2-hour postprandial sugar; and glucose tolerance.

16. Suggest that the client wear a special bracelet or necklace in order to alert the medical team to her condition (in case of diabetic coma or insulin shock).

17. Discuss appropriate medical management with the client: the possibility of hospitalization, early delivery, and/or cesarean section.

18. Refer all clients on insulin to a visiting nurse association for home follow-up of all treatments, medications, and dietary regimens.

DRUG DEPENDENCE

Definition

"The female drug addict who appears in the clinic because of pregnancy is perhaps the most pathetic of all drug addicts. Our treatment

TABLE 15-6

Signs and Symptoms of Diabetic Coma and Insulin Shock

		Diabetic coma (hyperglycemia)	Insulin shock (hypoglycemia)
Signs			
	Onset	Slow	Rapid
	Skin	Dry	Sweating
	Reflexes	Normal or absent	Positive Babinski's sign
	Eyeballs	Soft	Normal
	Color	Florid	Pallor
	Urine	Sugar	Negative for sugar
	Breath	Acetone odor	Normal
	Breathing	Slow, labored (Kussmaul's)	Shallow
	Pulse	Rapid	Normal
Symptoms		Thirst	Nervousness
		Nausea/vomiting	Hunger
		Headache	Weakness
		Abdominal pain	Paresthesia
		Dim vision	Blurred vision
		Dyspnea	Stupor, convulsion
		Constipation	Psychopathic behavior

Reprinted with permission from Dickason, J., and M. Schultz. Maternal and Infant Care: A Text for Nurses. McGraw-Hill Book Co., New York. 1975. p. 453.

of her surely tests our humanity, our degree of civilization and our medical knowledge.... Pregnancy and the birth of the baby represent to her the last claim to a worthwhile purpose for her entire being."[4]

Indeed, for clients who are chronic users of heroin or methadone this may be so, but chemical dependence in our society is much more pervasive and a much more subtle problem. Alcohol, nicotine, caffeine, barbiturates, marijuana, amphetamines, and vitamins have all been used to excess.

Definitions of drug abuse vary, ranging from "feeling normal on drugs" to "compulsive use of drugs."[5] Some say that during pregnancy the use of any drug is an abuse because it may be harmful to the fetus. It is probably safe to say that the use of any drug (or anything, for that matter) *to excess* is not healthy for either the mother or the fetus. Specific drugs that may harm the mother or baby are listed in Table 15-7.

Medical management

Heroin and methadone users need to be enrolled in a maintenance program as soon as possible. The fetus will have a much better chance for a healthy outcome if the client is maintained on a consistent dose of methadone. Any attempt to decrease or terminate methadone use also produces fetal withdrawal, and may actually cause fetal demise. Fetal and maternal withdrawal are most safely managed after delivery.

Most heroin users and some methadone maintenance clients will use a variety of other drugs. It is important to elicit this information.

Chronic drug abusers have been described as depressed, paranoid, manipulative, and passive-aggressive. The first clue to drug abuse may be the presence of this psychological presentation. The intensive efforts of the entire health care team — obstetrician, public health nurse, nutritionist, social worker, and psychiatrist — are required to work effectively with chronic drug abusers.

During labor and delivery, it is important to continue methadone dosage on a regular time schedule and to assure the client that this will be the management. This prevents clients from taking "street drugs" just before admission to labor and delivery. It also protects the fetus from severe withdrawal symptoms immediately after birth. The client may also need analgesia. As a general rule, methadone maintenance clients have a low tolerance to pain and a high tolerance to the effects of narcotics. They may safely be medicated with narcotics. Other types of drugs, such as barbiturates or sedatives, are usually avoided because their effects are not reversible in the infant.

After delivery, the infant may show signs of withdrawal. The longer the drug abuse habit and the higher the dosage of the drug, the more likely will the baby show signs of withdrawal (Table 15-8).

Heroin withdrawal usually occurs within the first 4 days after birth. Methadone withdrawal may occur after the baby is discharged from the hospital, and it may be more severe than heroin withdrawal. Treatment includes sedation with paregoric, chlorpromazine, or diazepam, and maintenance of nutrition and hydration status.

The abuse of other substances is harder to elicit and to quantify. Many clients will not think of coffee, cigarettes, or an occasional cocktail as drug abuse. History taking and counseling must be geared to increased maternal awareness of the risks to fetal outcome.

TABLE 15-7
Drugs Abused During Pregnancy

Drug	Maternal complications	Newborn complications
Amphetamines	Agitation Malnutrition Vasculitis Psychological dependence	Congenital heart defects (suspected)
Barbiturates	Malnutrition Central nervous system depression Hypertension Anxiety	Low birth weight Withdrawal syndrome (large doses) Vitamin K deficiency Neonatal jaundice
Cannabis	None known	Bradycardia Electroencephalogram changes

Alcohol	Malnutrition
	Liver disease
	Bone marrow suppression
	Pneumonia
	Delirium tremens
	Brain damage
		Low birth weight
		Fetal alcohol syndrome:
		  Mental retardation
		  Microcephaly
		  Withdrawal

Hallucinogens	Agitation Psychosis	LSD: fetal chromosome damage (suspected)
Cocaine	Excitation Euphoria Decreased sensation of fatigue	Prenatal effects unknown Studies suggest cardiac anomalies Respiratory distress and cardiac insufficiency before birth
Heroin	Toxemia Premature rupture of membranes Breech Abruptio placentae Postpartum hemorrhage Malnutrition Endocarditis Hepatitis Abscess Pulmonary infection Anemia Venereal disease	Low birth weight Withdrawal syndrome
Methadone	Depends on use of other drugs	Withdrawal
Cigarette smoking	Spontaneous abortion Placenta previa Abruptio placentae Lung cancer Cardiovascular disease	Low birth weight Prematurity
Caffeine	Nervousness Diuresis	Fetal limb malformation Hyperirritability

TABLE 15-8
Symptoms of Neonatal Withdrawal

Hyperirritability
Tremors
Shrill, high-pitched cry
Ravenous appetite, but poor sucking ability
Sweating
Sneezing and yawning
Vomiting/diarrhea
Weight loss

Adapted from Scipien, G. M., M. Barnard, M. Chard, J. Howe, and P. Phillips. Comprehensive Pediatric Nursing. McGraw-Hill Book Co., New York. 1975. p. 298.

Nursing actions

1. Explain to the client the maternal and fetal risks of drug abuse.
2. Emphasize the role of good nutrition in pregnancy.
3. Coordinate the efforts of the health care team through the antepartum, the intrapartum, and, *especially,* the postpartum period.
4. Because the client may develop many obstetric complications (e.g., toxemia, placental abruption, and premature rupture of membranes), teach her the signs and symptoms of these complications. Instruct her to seek medical attention immediately, if the signs occur.
5. Assure the client that methadone will be available while she is in the hospital.
6. Coordinate visiting nurse follow-up in the postpartum period.
7. Work with the local social services and the Bureau of Child Welfare to ensure an appropriate home environment for the newborn.

HEART DISEASE

Definition

Certain normal cardiovascular changes occur during pregnancy:

1. Increased maternal blood volume, which increases 40 to 50 percent, is responsible for hemodilution and will result in a drop in hematocrit levels in approximately 50 percent of all clients.
2. Maternal heart rate increases by approximately 10 beats/min.

3. Maternal cardiac output reaches 40 percent above nonpregnant levels. The cardiac output peaks at 28 weeks, coinciding with a decrease in blood pressure in the second trimester. Maternal cardiac output decreases in the third trimester, and it should be normal at birth.

The two most common causes of heart disease seen in pregnancy are rheumatic heart disease (RHD) and congenital anomalies.

RHD accounts for 60 to 80 percent of cardiac disease during pregnancy. Scarring of the mitral valve from rheumatic endocarditis produces mitral stenosis — the most common valvular lesion of RHD. The scarred rigid mitral valve obstructs the flow of blood into the left ventricle. In order to maintain adequate cardiac output, the left atrial pressure increases. Pulmonary and venous capillary pressure increase, resulting in exertional dyspnea — the cardinal symptom of RHD. If the pulmonary capillary pressure becomes too great, fluid is forced from the capillaries into the alveoli, thereby producing pulmonary edema.

In pregnancy, the risk of pulmonary edema, heart failure, and/or cardiac arrhythmia increases in the third month. Because cardiac output peaks at 28 weeks of gestation, the client who has completed the seventh month of pregnancy without cardiac difficulty has a decreased chance of severe complications.

Congenital cardiac anomalies include atrial septal defect, patent ductus arteriosus, ventricular septal defect, pulmonary stenosis, and coarctation of the aorta.

Medical management

At least 50 percent of all cardiac disease diagnosed during pregnancy was not suspected by the client beforehand. Thus, the primary responsibility of the health care team is diagnosis. It has been emphasized that any organic heart disease will exhibit some of the following signs or symptoms:[6]

Diastolic murmur.
Cardiac enlargement (on x-ray).
Systolic murmur of at least grade III (on a scale of VI) intensity.
Presence of severe arrhythmia.

Once diagnosis is made, it is important to classify both the cause (RHD vs. congenital defects) and the functional capacity (Table 15-9).

A plan of management is usually the joint responsibility of the obstetrician and the cardiologist. Certain overriding concerns are para-

TABLE 15-9

Classification of Cardiac Disease

Class	Characteristics
I	Heart disease with no symptoms of any kind and no signs of fatigue, palpitations, dyspnea, or anginal pain with exertion.
II	Comfortable at rest, but symptomatic with ordinary physical activity.
III	Comfortable at rest, but symptomatic with less than ordinary effort.
IV	Symptomatic at rest.

Adapted with permission from New York Heart Association, Inc. Diseases of the Heart and Blood Vessels — Nomenclature and Criteria for Diagnosis. Little, Brown & Co., Boston. 1964. Sixth edition.

mount in the care of the cardiac client with either RHD or a congenital defect:

Decreased physical and emotional activity in order to prevent fatigue, dyspnea, or palpitations.

Frequent evaluation in clinic (weekly for symptomatic clients) with special evaluation after week 28.

Decreased sodium intake (1,000 milligrams). This requires omission of salty foods and salt at the table and when cooking.

Prevention of infection (upper respiratory infection [URI] and urinary tract infection [UTI]) to avoid increasing the metabolic rate.

Prophylaxis against bacterial endocarditis (1.4 million units of procaine penicillin intramuscularly and 1 gram of streptomycin sulfate intramuscularly 1 hour before delivery and twice daily for 3 days).

Adequate analgesia for pain relief during delivery.

Shortening of the second stage of labor to avoid the Valsalva's effect during pushing.

Intensive fetal and maternal monitoring during labor, delivery, and postpartum because two-thirds of all maternal deaths occur during these periods.

Nursing actions

1. Explain the anatomic and physiological bases of the problem to the client.

2. Allow the client to verbalize her feelings and fears concerning cardiac disease.
3. Review the client's activities of daily living and sleep requirements. Decreasing physical stress decreases the amount of work the damaged heart must do.
4. Review the client's emotional and social milieu. Emotional stress will tax the heart.
5. Evaluate the signs of dyspnea with or without exertion. This must be differentiated from the hyperventilation that results normally from pregnancy (*see* Chapter 2).
6. Observe for onset of orthopnea, anginal pain, cough, hemoptysis, tachycardia, or increasing edema — all signs of heart failure.
7. Observe for changes in heart rate or rhythm.
8. Teach the client to seek medical attention immediately if signs of UTI or URI occur.
9. Discuss dietary regimen:
   a. Avoidance of excessive weight gain.
   b. Sodium restrictions as ordered.
10. Emphasize the importance of good nutrition during pregnancy.
11. Review with the client the purpose and dosage of medications as ordered (cardiac drugs, diuretics, antibiotics, etc.).
12. Strongly urge the client to attend natural childbirth classes. A prepared client is not fearful and anxious. Thus, her blood pressure, pulse, and respirations will remain stable. However, the client should avoid practicing pushing or strenuous exercises.
13. Coordinate care with delivery room nurses so that they will expect the client and be prepared to provide for constant emotional support and continuous monitoring of her physical condition.

During labor, the nurse should do the following:

1. Place the client in a semi-Fowler's position.
2. Have oxygen ready at the bedside.
3. Coach the client with breathing and relaxation techniques.
4. Avoid using scopolamine hydrobromide because it may cause tachycardia or agitation.
5. Anticipate forceps or vacuum extraction to shorten second stage and to avoid the Valsalva's effect.

During the immediate postpartum period, the nurse should do the following:

1. Observe for cardiac failure and shock. (This is the most critical period.)
2. Avoid using ergot preparations because they are vasopressors and result in elevated blood pressure.

HYDATIDIFORM MOLE

Definition

Hydatidiform mole is a developmental placental abnormality of the trophoblastic cells that causes the chorionic villi to become swollen and degenerate into grapelike clusters. A retained, blighted ovum may sometimes be found.

The etiology is unknown, but the incidence is increased with age and parity. Women over 40 years of age with three or more pregnancies have a greater risk of molar pregnancy. In the United States, this dysplasia occurs in 1 per 2,000 pregnancies. In parts of Asia and the South Pacific, the incidence may run as high as 1 per 500 pregnancies.[7]

Although, in itself, the mole is a benign condition, it is the most common condition preceding choriocarcinoma. In women over 40 years of age, the incidence of choriocarcinoma secondary to a mole exceeds 30 percent.

Medical management

Hydatidiform mole should be suspected in the following conditions:

Severe nausea and vomiting in the first trimester.
Elevated human chorionic gonadotrophin (HCG) levels 100 days or more after the last normal menstrual period. (HCG should peak at the 10th week of gestation and remain at low levels after the 14th week of gestation.)
Persistent vaginal bleeding, sometimes associated with passage of grapelike vesicles.
Signs and symptoms of toxemia before the 20th week of gestation.
Absence of fetal heart tones and inability to palpate fetal parts.

Diagnosis is confirmed with ultrasonography.

If the woman does not wish to have any more children, a hysterectomy is the treatment of choice because of the risk of choriocarcinoma. If the woman does desire another pregnancy, the uterus is evacuated with suction curettage, with a sharp curettage performed 1 or 2 weeks later.

The intensive medical management after termination of a molar pregnancy has been detailed:[7]

Prevention of future pregnancy — preferably with oral contraceptives.

Evaluation with a 24-hour urine collection for quantitative HCG until titers are negative.

Evaluation monthly for 6 months after titers are negative for 3 weeks.

Cessation of choriocarcinoma screening after titers remain negative for 6 months. The client may then discontinue oral contraceptives if she wishes to become pregnant.

Initiation of intensive chemotherapy if titers level off or rise, and/or if metastasis occurs.

Nursing actions
1. Explain the physiological basis of the dysplasia.
2. Help the client work through grieving over the loss of the pregnancy.
3. Observe for weight loss, ketosis, or electrolyte imbalance resulting from hyperemesis.
4. Observe for signs and symptoms of toxemia.
5. Evaluate hematocrit levels and observe for signs of anemia because continuous vaginal bleeding may deplete iron stores.
6. Emphasize the importance of follow-up after surgery.
7. After curettage, review signs and symptoms of uterine infection (e.g., cramping, foul-smelling discharge, and fever).
8. Make sure the client understands the importance of avoiding pregnancy until HCG levels are normal.
9. When the client discontinues oral contraceptives, review with her the importance of avoiding pregnancy for at least 6 months.
10. Make sure the primary caregiver discusses the possibility of malignancy and provides the client with explicit information concerning follow-up and drug therapy.
11. If chemotherapy is required, review the treatment schedule with her and the specific side effects, such as gastritis, anorexia, and alopecia.

HYDRAMNIOS

Definition
The normal amount of amniotic fluid is from 800 to 1,200 milliliters. After 35 weeks of gestation, this amount may drop slightly.

Hydramnios occurs when there is more than 2,000 milliliters of amniotic fluid. The true incidence of this disorder is not known. It has been estimated to occur in 1 per 1,000 pregnancies. Maternal conditions associated with hydramnios include DM, toxemia, severe Rh disease, and multiple gestation. Fetal conditions associated with the problem include spina bifida, anencephaly, hypoplastic lung disease, or any esophageal malformation.

Medical management

Clinical diagnosis of hydramnios may not occur until levels of 3,000 milliliters or more are reached. Clients with diabetes, Rh disease, or twin gestation should be screened by ultrasonography for excessive amounts of amniotic fluid. Treatments depend on maternal symptoms. Bed rest and mild sodium restriction may suffice. Complaints of nausea, vomiting, or shortness of breath are managed by hospitalization and removal of excess fluid through amniocentesis.

The most frequent maternal complications are placental abruption, dysfunctional labor, and postpartum hemorrhage. Fetal complications include prematurity and cord prolapse. With DM, Rh disease, and central nervous system anomalies as predisposing etiologies, the perinatal mortality rate for hydramnios may be as high as 50 percent.

Nursing actions

1. Explain the definition of hydramnios to the client — causative factors vary and may not be known.
2. Explain sodium restriction, if necessary.
3. Observe for dyspnea, nausea, and vomiting. Teach the client to seek medical attention if these occur.
4. Reinforce the need for bed rest.
5. Observe for signs of dependent edema and institute relief measures (*see* Chapter 6).

HYPEREMESIS GRAVIDARUM

Definition

Hyperemesis gravidarum has been defined as a condition in which intractable vomiting and disturbed nutrition lead to an alteration of electrolyte balance, loss of weight (5 percent or more), ketosis, and acetonuria, leading ultimately to neurological damage, retinal hemorrhage, and renal disease.[8]

The etiology is unknown, and the incidence ranges from 3 per 1,000 to 10 per 1,000. Some investigators feel that high levels of

HCG contribute to hyperemesis. This theory may be correct because other conditions with high HCG levels (e.g., hydatidiform mole or multiple gestation) predispose the client to nausea and vomiting. Psychogenic causes (such as change in body image, loss of independence, or change in role from daughter to mother) are also thought to be possible etiologies.

Nausea and vomiting become pathological at the point when weight loss and ketosis are present. Left untreated, hyperemesis is a lethal condition.

Medical management

All other causes of persistent nausea and vomiting must be ruled out (Table 15-10). Treatment involves hospitalization to correct dehydration and electrolyte imbalance. Drug therapy includes parenteral vitamin supplementation, potassium replacement, and antiemetic drugs. Prochlorperazine is the antiemetic of choice. A psychiatrist should evaluate the client's mental status. The social worker must coordinate the care of any other children in the home and any economic concerns.

TABLE 15-10
Causes of Nausea and Vomiting During Pregnancy

Secondary to pregnancy	Not secondary to pregnancy
Simple nausea and vomiting in pregnancy	Acute gastroenteritis
Hyperemesis gravidarum	Cholecystitis, cholangitis, and biliary obstruction
Hydatidiform mole	Hepatitis
Multiple gestation	Pancreatitis
Reflux vomiting of late pregnancy	Peptic ulcer
Hydramnios	Intestinal obstruction
Preeclampsia	Pyelonephritis
Labor	Uremia
Pica	Diabetic ketoacidosis
Ptyalism	Appendicitis
	Peritonitis
	Twisted ovarian cyst
	Increased intracranial pressure

Adapted from Midwinter, A. Vomiting in pregnancy. *Practitioner* (January 1971). 743.

Nursing actions

1. Explain the possible causes to the client.
2. Explore her feelings about this pregnancy.
3. Evaluate her mental status.
4. Outpatient nursing responsibilities:
   a. Carefully evaluate complaints of nausea and vomiting.
   b. Schedule any client complaining of nausea and vomiting for weekly clinic visits.
   c. Carefully evaluate weekly weights and urine for signs of weight loss and/or ketosis.
   d. Review with the client the nursing relief measures for nausea and vomiting during pregnancy (*see* Chapter 6).
5. Inpatient nursing responsibilities:
   a. Coordinate health team.
   b. Maintain nutrition and hydration status.
   c. Work with dietitian to provide the following for the client: hot food that is hot, and cold food that is cold; an attractive arrangement of food; small portions; trays removed immediately after meals; and assignment of the client to a room where food smells will not be pervasive.

INTRAUTERINE GROWTH RETARDATION

Definition

A newborn is considered growth retarded if his birth weight is below the 10th percentile for his gestational age (Fig. 15-1). Multiple causes of growth retardation have been identified:

Poor maternal nutritional status, with associated inadequate weight gain and/or anemia.
Drug abuse.
Chronic vascular or renal disease.
Toxemia.
Pregnancy at high altitude.
Multiple gestation.
Fetal infection.
Fetal anomaly.

Medical management

Identification of predisposing factors alerts the clinician to clients at risk. A fetal growth pattern of 2 weeks or more smaller than gestational age is a prime indicator that the fetus has fallen behind in

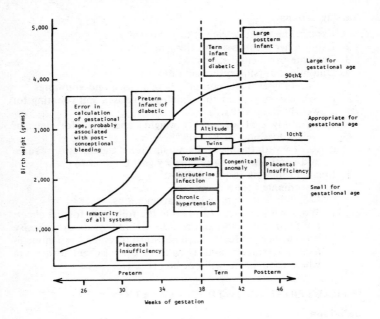

Figure 15-1. Representation of birth weight relationship to gestational age, with associated conditions. Note that a newborn is considered growth retarded if his birth weight is below the 10th percentile for his gestational age. *Adapted from* Lubchenco, L. O., C. Hausman, and L. Backstrom. Factors influencing fetal growth. *In* Nutricia Symposium: Aspects of Prematurity and Dysmaturity. H. E. Stenford Kroese B. V., Leiden, The Netherlands. 1968.

growth. (Techniques for assessing fundal height are described in Chapter 1.)

Definite diagnosis is made by ultrasonography. Bed rest, adequate nutrition with 100 grams of protein daily, and treatment of specific maternal complications may reduce the fetal risk. Non-stress testing monitors the fetal condition. A severely compromised fetus may need to be delivered by cesarean section.

The outcome of growth retarded infants presents an unclear prognosis. Weight below the 10th percentile alone is not necessarily a predictor of subsequent delay in neurological or intellectual develop-

ment. Delayed head growth before the third trimester (as documented by serial ultrasound) is associated with slow growth and neuro-
logical/intellectual impairment.

Nursing actions

1. Explain the condition to the client.
2. Emphasize the role of good nutrition during pregnancy.
3. Emphasize the importance of a high-protein diet and discuss the
   use of specific high-protein foods with the client. The goal is ingestion of 100 grams of protein per day (*see* Chapter 5).
4. Encourage bed rest. The working client may need to discontinue employment, and the mother with young children may
   need homemaker services.
5. Evaluate the client weekly to monitor weight gain and uterine
   growth.
6. Assess for the presence of anemia.
7. Allow the client to verbalize concerns about fetal outcome.
8. Teach the client about ultrasonography and other test measures
   that are used for diagnosis of fetal status.

MATERNAL RESPIRATORY DISORDERS

Two common respiratory disorders seen in pregnancy are
tuberculosis and asthma.

Definition

Tuberculosis. Tuberculosis (TB) is an infectious disease caused
by the tubercle bacillus. It is characterized by inflammatory
infiltrations, formation of tubercles, caseation necrosis, abscesses,
fibrosis, and calcification. Infection is acquired from contact with an
infected person or animal, or through drinking contaminated milk.
Recently, the incidence of TB has increased in urban areas, and it is
becoming a significant public health problem.

The prognosis for the pregnant client with TB is excellent,
provided that she follows her medication regimen. No increased
incidence of abortion or prematurity has been documented with
infants of treated mothers.

Medical management

A careful history is necessary to identify the client at risk:

A previous history of TB.
Known tuberculin conversion.

Pleural effusion.
Contact with known TB clients.
Chronic liver disease.
Presence of DM.
Severe psychological stress.

Tuberculosis should be suspected in clients who present with the following signs and symptoms:

Positive tine or purified protein derivative of tuberculin test (PPD) results after a known negative result within a 24-month period.
Suspicious chest x-ray.
Complaint of hemoptysis, weight loss, fatigue, malaise, night sweats, or chronic productive cough.
Localized chest pain accompanied by fever and malaise.

Positive diagnosis is confirmed by positive cultures for acid-fast bacteria. (At least three cultures should be obtained to complete an adequate evaluation.) The most effective antitubercular chemotherapy involves a combination of two of the following drugs: isoniazid, rifampin, ethambutol, or streptomycin (Table 15-11). There is little clinical data on these drugs with respect to teratogenesis. It is known that streptomycin may cause deafness in the newborn.

Nursing actions

1. Explain the causative factors of the disease to the client.
2. Explain the importance of compliance with the medication regimen.
3. Emphasize the excellent prognosis for client and infant, if the drug regimen is followed.
4. In active or suspected active cases, teach the client the importance of covering her nose and mouth while coughing, sneezing, or laughing.
5. Explore social, psychological, and economic milieu to discover undue stress or strain.
6. Emphasize the importance of good nutrition during pregnancy.
7. Report active cases to the local Board of Health for treatment of all contacts.
8. Stress the importance of continuation of medications during the postpartum period and check that postpartum hospital and discharge medication orders are written.

TABLE 15-11
Antitubercular Drugs

Drug	Daily dose	Maternal toxicity
Isoniazid	300-mg single dose (oral).	Hepatitis, neurological, hematopoietic, and induced lupus syndromes.
Rifampin	600-mg single dose (oral).	Hepatitis (rare), leukopenia (rare), and purpura (rare). Intermittent use may produce systemic reactions, such as hemolysis, renal failure, and severe pancreatitis.
Ethambutol	15 mg/kg (oral).	Optic neuritis (rare at this dose).
Streptomycin	15 mg/kg single dose, not to exceed 1 g daily for 3 mo (parenteral).	Vestibular and renal.

Reprinted with permission from Burrow, G. N., and T. F. Ferris. Medical Complications During Pregnancy. W. B. Saunders Co., Philadelphia. 1975. p. 576.

Definition

Asthma. Asthma — dyspnea secondary to varying degrees of bronchial constriction — is characterized by diffuse inspiratory and expiratory wheezes. The disease may be chronic or acute. Severe acute bronchial asthma — status asthmaticus — may be a life-threatening condition.

In pregnancy, the prognosis for clients with asthma follows the "rule of thirds." One third of the clients get better, one third stay the same, and one third deteriorate. Prematurity and intrauterine growth retardation have been reported only in severe asthmatic disease — probably as a result of hypoxia.

Medical management

Treatment for asthma depends on the severity of the symptoms. It is important to note that asthma may have its primary onset during pregnancy. Any client complaining of shortness of breath should be evaluated for the presence of wheezes.

The aim of treatment is to provide a wheeze-free state. Bronchodilators, corticosteroids, and antibiotics are used in combination in order to prevent bronchospasm, to remove excessive secretions, and to prevent infection. Antihistamines are generally not used because they tend to harden bronchial plugs or casts and make them difficult to remove.

Nursing actions
1. Explain the physiological basis of the disease.
2. Discuss the medication regimen with the client and explore her use of other, over-the-counter medications. These should be discontinued during pregnancy.
3. Urge the client to discontinue smoking, if applicable.
4. Stress the importance of seeking medical attention if the asthmatic condition worsens.
5. Urge the client to return for treatment at the first sign of a URI.

POSTMATURE PREGNANCY

Definition

An infant that is born after the 42nd week of gestation is classified as postmature. The factors that influence the onset of labor at any time during gestation are unclear (*see* Chapter 9). The factors that delay the onset of labor are even more obscure.

Fetal jeopardy occurs when placental functioning begins to be compromised. The supply of oxygen and nutrients may be decreased, thus causing fetal distress. The fetus will lose body weight, especially subcutaneous fat — giving the postmature newborn the typical wrinkled appearance. Meconium — a sign of fetal distress — may be found in the amniotic fluid. If aspiration of meconium occurs at delivery, a severe pneumonitis or even death may occur.

On the other hand, if the placenta continues to function well, the fetus may continue to grow. A large fetus increases the likelihood of cephalopelvic disproportion and the need for a cesarean section.

Medical management

The obstetrician will first recalculate the gestational age to make sure that the pregnancy is definitely postdate (*see* Chapter 7). Management centers around careful evaluation of placental functioning and fetal well-being. Placental functioning is assessed by urine or plasma estriol levels and/or serum lactogen levels (specifically, human placental lactogen). Fetal status is assessed by non-stress testing and amnioscopy to rule out the presence of meconium.

A vaginal examination is performed weekly, starting at the 42nd week, in order to establish a base line of cervical dilation and effacement and to judge whether the cervix is favorable for labor induction (*see* Chapter 16).

During labor or oxytocin induction, careful evaluation and continuous electronic monitoring of fetal heart rate and uterine contractions provide the optimum care for a potentially compromised fetus.

Nursing actions

1. Explain all testing procedures to the client.
2. Emphasize the importance of attending the clinic weekly.
3. Counsel the client to take a daily walk, which may help to stimulate the onset of labor.
4. Allow the client to voice her concerns and feelings about prolonged pregnancy. Most clients are just "tired of being pregnant" at this point.

Rh DISEASE

Definition

The Rh factor is an antigen that is present in the red blood cells of 85 percent of the white and 93 percent of the black population in the United States. If the antigen is absent, the client is Rh-negative. The Rh factor is a recessive genetic factor. If the mother and father are both Rh-negative, the baby will also be Rh-negative and will have no problem. If not, because the mother must be homozygous for absence of Rh factor, the infant's genetic makeup depends on whether the father is homozygous or heterozygous for the positive trait. If the father is homozygous, the infant will always be heterozygous for the positive trait. If the father is heterozygous, the infant has a 50 percent chance of being Rh-negative. When both the mother and father are heterozygous for the positive trait, the infant has a 25 percent chance of being Rh-negative (Fig. 15-2).

These genetic patterns demonstrate two important principles. Incompatibility does not always endanger fetal outcome, and Rh-positive parents may produce an Rh-negative infant.

Rh disease arises when an Rh-negative woman and an Rh-positive man produce an Rh-positive infant. Positive fetal cells cross over into the maternal bloodstream at birth and cause maternal antibody production. These antibodies cross through the placenta in subsequent pregnancies and attack fetal red blood cells. The destruction of fetal red blood cells causes anemia that may be severe enough to produce generalized edema and circulatory collapse (hydrops fetalis). The

		Rh factor			Rh factor	
A	Mother	-	-		-+	-+
				= Newborn		
	Father	+	+		-+	-+

		Rh factor			Rh factor	
B	Mother	-	-		+-	--
				= Newborn		
	Father	+	-		+-	--

		Rh factor			Rh factor	
C	Mother	+	-		++	+-
				= Newborn		
	Father	+	-		-+	--

Figure 15-2. Genetic composition and fetal outcome. (A) An Rh-negative woman and a homozygous man produce a heterzygous Rh-positive infant. (B) An Rh-negative woman and a heterozygous man have a 50 percent chance of producing an Rh-negative infant. (C) A heterozygous Rh-positive woman and man have a 25 percent chance of producing an Rh-negative infant.

level of bilirubin — a breakdown product of the red blood cells — rises and may result in jaundice. High bilirubin levels (18 mg/100 ml) may damage brain cells (kernicterus) (Fig. 15-3).

Medical management

The obstetrician carefully monitors maternal antibody titers and levels of fetal bilirubin in the amniotic fluid by means of the indirect Coombs's test. Rising titers and elevated bilirubin levels indicate fetal jeopardy. If the fetus is able to survive outside the uterus, a cesarean section is performed. If the fetus is too small or if the fetal lungs are immature, fetal anemia may be reversed by transfusing Rh-negative, type O packed cells directly into the fetal peritoneal cavity in utero.

If the infant is born with severe anemia, a complete exchange transfusion is performed immediately after birth. The jaundiced infant may require phototherapy, which reduces unconjugated, indirect bilirubin into a harmless, water-soluble compound.

Needless to say, the best treatment is the prevention of isoimmunization. Rh_o (D) immune globulin (RhoGAM) prevents development of maternal antibodies. Every Rh-negative woman who has an Rh-positive child, a miscarriage, a therapeutic abortion, or a transfusion should be evaluated. RhoGAM may be administered on a routine basis antenatally or prophylactically to Rh-negative women after amniocentesis (*see* Appendix A).

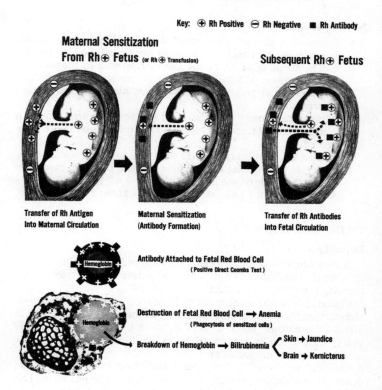

Figure 15-3. Erythroblastosis fetalis caused by transplacental transmission of maternal antibody, which is usually evoked by maternal and fetal blood group incompatibility. *Reprinted with permission from* Ross Laboratories, Columbus, Ohio.

The Coombs's test. The indirect Coombs's test measures the amount of antibodies present in maternal serum. This is the test used during pregnancy to evaluate the degree of antibody production. The direct Coombs's test is collected from cord blood and measures the number of fetal cells that are coated with maternal antibodies. This test is used to determine the need for RhoGAM administration to the mother after delivery.

Nursing actions

1. Explain the physiological basis of the problem to the client. Specifically, the client should understand the following points:
   a. The meaning of Rh factor and its relevance to pregnancy.
   b. The purpose of RhoGAM during pregnancy and its administration after pregnancy, miscarriage, abortion, and amniocentesis.
2. Explain diagnostic procedures (e.g., amniocentesis and Rh titers) or special treatment, such as fetal transfusion in utero, as needed.
3. Discuss the possibility of early delivery.
4. Facilitate the meeting of the client and the pediatric care team before the birth of the infant.
5. Allow the client to discuss her concerns about fetal outcome.

TWIN GESTATION

Definition

A logarithmic relationship exists between orders of multiple births in a large population. Twins occur at a rate of 1 per 89 births; triplets, 1 per 89^2, and quadruplets, 1 per 89^3.

Fraternal twinning is the result of fertilization of two separate ova. Heredity, race, maternal age, and parity all influence its incidence. A grand multiparous, black woman between the ages of 35 and 39 years, with a family history of twins, is most likely to conceive double ovum or dizygotic twins.

Identical twins result from the fertilization of a single ovum, producing monozygotic twins of the same sex and appearance. This type of twinning is not affected by any predisposing factors.

Medical management

Diagnosis may be suspected when the uterine size is at least 3 weeks ahead of the gestational date. Palpation of two heads or two breeches may be conclusive. Auscultation of two distinct fetal heart rates in two separate abdominal quadrants may alert the clinician to the possibility of twins. Antenatally, twinning is positively diagnosed through ultrasonography. Finally, at birth, if the clinician had estimated one large baby (4,000 grams), and a much smaller one (2,000 grams) is delivered, this may be the first indication of twins. Many twin gestations are diagnosed only at birth.

Several antenatal complications are associated with multiple gestation. Because of the high levels of HCG, nausea and vomiting may be severe during the first trimester. Anemia is common because the iron requirements for two fetuses may exceed 1,000 milligrams. The incidence of prematurity is higher, possibly because of the initiation of labor caused by an overdistended uterus. Toxemia of pregnancy occurs more frequently, and placental implantation may be low.

The management of twin or multiple gestation involves certain overriding concerns:

Control of nausea and/or vomiting.

Frequent screening for signs and symptoms of toxemia.

Prevention of premature labor.

Supplementation of iron and folic acid stores.

Evaluation of fetal well-being and growth through ultrasonography.

Careful conduct of labor and delivery.

Diagnosis of postpartum hemorrhage.

Nursing actions

1. Explain the physiological basis of the condition to the client.
2. Stress the importance of good nutrition during pregnancy.
3. Make sure that iron supplementation is increased and that folic acid is also added to the regimen.
4. Emphasize the importance of bed rest in the left lateral position to enhance placental perfusion and to prevent the onset of labor.
5. Review the signs of labor and counsel the client to seek medical attention if they occur.
6. Monitor carefully for signs or symptoms of toxemia.
7. Help the client to cope with the economic, psychological, and practical implications of mothering two newborns at once.

During the labor, delivery, and postpartum periods, the following procedures should be performed:

1. Monitor both twins with continuous external fetal monitoring.
2. Be sure that two units of whole blood are typed and cross-matched for the client.
3. Coach the client and significant other(s) on breathing and relaxing techniques.
4. Ensure that the delivery area is equipped with two sets of cord clamps, infant warmers, resuscitation equipment, and infant identification tags and papers.
5. Alert the pediatric team.
6. Observe carefully for postpartum hemorrhage.
7. Consider visiting nurse referral as supportive therapy for the client.

URINARY TRACT INFECTION

Definition

During pregnancy, anatomic changes in the urinary tract predispose the client to UTI. The growing uterus compresses both ureters, thereby impeding flow to the bladder. Dilation of the renal collection structures produces hydronephrosis during pregnancy. Dextrorotation of the uterus causes compression of the right kidney and ureter, making these changes more pronounced on the right side. The most common organism associated with UTI is *Escherichia coli*.

UTI may ascend into the kidneys, causing pyelonephritis. Although pyelonephritis occurs in only 2 percent of pregnancies, it is a major cause of hospitalization during pregnancy.

These infections may also be responsible for the onset of premature labor. Good obstetric management dictates that any client complaining of premature labor should be evaluated for UTI.

Sickle cell trait and anemia during pregnancy predispose the client to asymptomatic bacilluria. These clients should be screened once during each trimester. Every client should be evaluated at the first prenatal visit with a clean-catch, midstream-voided urine microanalysis and a urine culture and sensitivity test. The clean-catch microanalysis can be as much as 90 percent accurate, if the client understands exactly how to collect the specimen.

Medical management

The obstetrician and/or the nurse should ask the client at each prenatal visit if she has any signs or symptoms of UTI (Table 15-12). If these are present, a clean-catch urine microanalysis and a urine culture and sensitivity test should be ordered. The urine microanalysis results are usually available immediately. Those clients with results indicating the presence of bacteria and five or more white blood cells are treated. Ampicillin, 250 to 500 milligrams four times a day orally, is the treatment of choice while the client is waiting for the results of the urine culture and sensitivity test. In 48 hours, the treatment can then be changed to the antibiotic most likely to destroy the infecting organism (*see* Appendix B).

Nursing actions

1. Explain the cause of the infection to the client.
2. Review the method of obtaining the clean-catch, midstream-voided urine.
3. Review the medication schedule and emphasize the importance of completing the full course of treatment. (*Recheck drug allergies.*)

TABLE 15-12

Signs and Symptoms of Urinary Tract Infection

Signs	Symptoms
Foul-smelling or dark urine	Malaise
Concurrent vaginitis (especially trichomoniasis)	Suprapubic tenderness
Low-grade fever	Dysuria
Urine microanalysis containing:	Urgency
Bacilluria	Frequency
Red blood cells	Bladder spasm
White blood cells (5 or more per high-power field)	
Urine culture containing bacterial count of 100,000/ml	

Adapted from Neeson, J. D., and C. R. Stockdale. The Practitioner's Handbook of Ambulatory Ob/Gyn. John Wiley & Sons, Inc., New York. 1981.

4. Encourage the client to increase fluid intake, thus avoiding urinary stasis.
5. Urge the following dietary regimen:
   a. A source of vitamin C daily to promote healing.
   b. A large glass of cranberry juice at bedtime to acidify urine.
   c. Foods high in iron.
   d. Avoidance of bladder irritants (coffee, tea, alcohol, and spices).
6. Review the client's hematologic status. The client may need increased iron or folic acid supplementation.
7. Counsel the client to empty her bladder frequently and to never ignore the urge to void.
8. Teach the client to cleanse her perineal area from front to back in order to avoid contamination with *E. coli.*
9. Make sure the client is recultured in 2 weeks, after a full course of antibiotic therapy. For that test *only,* the client should be instructed to decrease fluid intake for at least 8 hours so that a concentrated specimen can be obtained.

VAGINITIS

Definition

Increased estrogen secretion during pregnancy causes more production of cervial mucus. These acidic secretions favor growth of organisms that cause vaginitis — inflammation of the vagina.

Medical management

Management depends on causative factors (Table 15-13).

Nursing actions

1. Explain the cause of the infection to the client.
2. Teach vaginal hygiene measures:
   a. Wear cotton underwear.
   b. Avoid tight clothing, such as blue jeans and panty hose.
   c. Avoid rubbing or scratching the labia.
   d. Discontinue vaginal hygiene sprays and colored or scented toilet paper.
   e. Bathe daily.
3. Teach the client the medication schedule and make sure she understands that she should use all of the medications.
4. Counsel the client to refrain from intercourse during treatment or to have her partner use a condom.
5. Reinforce the fact that douching is contraindicated during pregnancy.

VENEREAL DISEASE

Definition

Infections that are transmitted through sexual contact are called venereal diseases. The three most common venereal diseases in pregnancy are gonorrhea, syphilis, and herpes.

Sexually transmitted diseases also include some forms of vaginitis, such as trichomoniasis and hemophilus (*see* Table 15-13).

Medical management

Management depends on the type of infection detected. Various causative agents, their signs and symptoms, and their treatment modalities are listed in Table 15-14.

Nursing actions

1. Explain the causative factors of the infection.
2. Emphasize the importance of complying with the entire medication regimen.
3. Allow the client to discuss her feelings and concerns regarding the impact of the disease on her body, on her relationship with her partner, and on her infant.
4. Review general supportive measures for any infectious process:

a. Rest.
b. Increased fluids.
c. Good nutrition.
d. Increased intake of vitamin C.

5. Counsel the client to refrain from intercourse until retesting confirms that the infection has been eradicated.

6. Review general hygiene measures (e.g., hand washing after voiding or cleaning vulvar wounds) to prevent the spread of infection.

7. Review vaginal hygiene measures (*see* Chapter 6).

8. Explain that syphilis and gonorrhea must be reported to the local Board of Health so that contacts may be found and treated.

9. As a general rule, make sure that the following screening is completed:
   a. All clients with vaginal infections or complaints of leukorrhea should have a cervical culture for gonorrhea.
   b. All clients with herpes should be evaluated for the presence of a secondary vaginal infection.
   c. All clients with gonorrhea should be evaluated for syphilis, and clients with syphilis should be cultured for gonorrhea.

10. The specific relief measures for herpes are as follows:
   a. Advise a sitz bath with Aveeno Oilated or 2 tablespoons of Aveeno in a jar of warm water patted onto the affected area with a clean cloth four times a day to soothe and cleanse.
   b. Encourage high quality protein intake from meat, poultry, fish, and eggs. Not only will this enhance the client's general nutritional status, but it will also increase the amount of the essential amino acid, lycine, which is believed to suppress herpes infections.
   c. Teach the client to relieve dysuria by increasing fluid intake to dilute urine and/or by pouring water over the vulva when voiding or by voiding while in a sitz bath.
   d. When herpetic lesions are present in the third trimester, help the client understand the need for repeated cultures.
   e. Teach the client to tell the labor and delivery staff about ongoing infections and to seek immediate medical attention if labor ensues or the membranes rupture.
   f. If appropriate, refer the client to a self-help group that has been formed to support herpes sufferers:
   HELP
   P. O. Box 100
   Palo Alto, Calif. 94302

TABLE 15-13
Common Vaginal Infections

	Candida albicans	Trichomonas vaginalis	Hemophilus vaginalis
Clinical symptomatology			
Appearance of discharge	Cheesy and curdy, with white patches on vaginal mucosa and cervix.	Frothy, thin, and yellow-green. Copious amounts.	Minimal, creamy, yellow-gray.
Odor of discharge	"Yeasty."	Malodorous.	Usually none; may be malodorous.
Symptoms	Intense vulvar pruritus, vulvar edema/redness, and dyspareunia.	Pruritus, dyspareunia, or dysuria.	Usually no pruritus.
Microscopic findings	Filaments with budding spores.	Motile, colorless, flagellated trichomonads.	Clue cells (epithelial cells surrounded by the gram-negative Hemophilus bacilli).
Treatment	Nystatin vaginal suppositories bid for 14 days. Monistat vaginal cream qd for 7 days. Clotrimazole vaginal suppositories qd for 7 days. Gentian Violet vaginal preparation bid for 14 days.	Flagyl (Use during pregnancy is controversial. Contraindicated in first half of pregnancy.) Sulfa vaginal cream qd for 10 days.	Ampicillin, 500 mg PO qid for 10 days. Sulfa vaginal cream bid for 14 days.

Adapted from Varney, H. Nurse Midwifery. Blackwell Scientific Publications, Inc., Boston. 1980.

VIRAL INFECTIONS

Definition

Viruses can cross the placental barrier at any time during the pregnancy. Fetal exposure in the first trimester may result in miscarriage or fetal anomalies. In the second and third trimesters, intrauterine growth retardation and/or postnatal infection may occur.

Medical management

The medical management depends on the causative organism. Various viral infections, their possible fetal effects, and their current medical management procedures are listed in Table 15-15.

Nursing actions

1. Provide an opportunity for the client to discuss the prognosis for her baby with an obstetrician and a genetic counselor.
2. When and if appropriate, discuss the option of therapeutic abortion.
3. When appropriate, alert the delivery room nursing staff and the pediatric team to the birth of a potentially infected baby.
4. Explain any medications, treatment, or tests of fetal status to the client.
5. Evaluate the need for vaccination in the postpartum period.

REFERENCES

1. Benson. 803.
2. Pritchard and MacDonald. 741.
3. Pritchard and MacDonald. 740.
4. Dickason and Schultz. 119.
5. Cameron. 677.
6. Burrow and Ferris.
7. Neeson and Stockdale. 40-41.
8. Pritchard and MacDonald. 760.

TABLE 15-14

Venereal Disease During Pregnancy

	Gonorrhea	Herpes	Syphilis
Causative agent	*Neisseria gonorrhoeae* gram-negative diplococcus	Herpesvirus hominis	*Treponema pallidum* spirochete
Incubation period	1–14 days	≤14 days	10–90 days
Diagnostic test	Cervical, rectal, and/or throat culture.	Viral culture or Papanicolaou test of weeping lesion for giant body cells. (If herpes is suspected in the 3rd trimester, weekly or biweekly cultures are indicated.)	VDRL: if positive, confirm with FTA-ABS.
Signs and symptoms	Usually none; leukorrhea and arthritis.	Indurated vesicles or ulcers on vulva, vagina, or cervix. Severe pain. Itching and burning. Viremia with first infection. If lesions are on cervix, no symptoms may be present.	Chancre. Rash and/or influenza-like symptoms occurring 3 wk after appearance of chancre. Rash occurs on palms of hands or soles of feet.
Treatment	4.8 million U of procaine penicillin IM 30 min after 1 g of probenecid PO.	No effective treatment. If herpes is present at onset of labor, a cesarean section is performed.	2.4 million U of benzathine penicillin IM weekly for 5 wk.

Effects on fetus

Untreated: newborn infection or blindness.

Pneumonia, viremia, or death.

Untreated: peg-shaped teeth (Hutchinson's teeth); absence of nasal bridge; nasal snuffles rhinitis infected with spirochetes. Other sequelae: hepatitis, pneumonia, and death.

FTA-ABS, fluorescent treponemal antibody absorption; VDRL, Venereal Disease Research Laboratories.

TABLE 15-15

Viral Infections During Pregnancy

Disease	Incubation	Possible fetal effects	Incidence of fetal damage with maternal infection	Current management
Rubella	*days* 14-21	Cardiac anomalies. Deafness. Microcephaly. Meningoencephalitis. Cataracts. Intrauterine growth retardation. Spontaneous abortion.	1st trimester: 30-50%. 2nd trimester: 6.8%. 3rd trimester: 5.3%.	Gamma globulin reduces maternal symptoms but does *not* change fetal risk. Follow with rubella titers. Discuss the option of therapeutic abortion.
Rubeola	10-14	Congenital defects. Spontaneous abortion. Infant born with measles.	45-76% spontaneous abortion or early labor.	No specific treatment. Secondary infections respond to antibiotics.
Mumps	12-26	Spontaneous abortion. Stillbirth. Congenital defects.	15% spontaneous abortion or stillbirth. 16% congenital anomalies.	No specific treatment. Discuss the option of therapeutic abortion. Mumps vaccine available but not routinely administered to adults.
Chicken pox (varicella)		Chicken pox. Scars or varicella pneumonia at birth.	Very unusual.	No specific treatment. Be aware of the chance of neonatal pneumonia.

Hepatitis				
A	14-50 (avg. 28)	Prematurity. Neonatal hepatitis. Biliary agenesis.	High incidence of abortion. Prematurity.	Gamma globulin (0.02 ml/kg). Hospitalization.
B	30-150 (avg. 75)			Gamma globulin *not* proven effective. Hospitalization.
Cytomegal-ovirus	14-18	Prematurity. Intrauterine growth retardation. Congenital anomalies. Hydrocephalus. Blindness. Seizures.	A primary infection is needed to affect the fetus. This is almost always asymptomatic. Diagnosis is made after birth of the severely affected baby.	No effective therapy.

Adapted from Monif, G. Infectious Disease in Obstetrics and Gynecology. Harper & Row, Publishers, Inc., New York. 1974.

CHAPTER 16

INTRAPARTUM DEVIATIONS

Suzanne M. Smith

Although labor and delivery are normal physiological processes, certain deviations occur with sufficient frequency to warrant further discussion of them. It is imperative that the obstetric nurse be familiar with, and have a thorough understanding of, these deviations. Common deviations, their effect (if any) on labor, the expected fetal outcome, and recommendations for specific nursing interventions are presented in this chapter.

CESAREAN SECTION

Definition

Cesarean section is the delivery of the fetus by means of a surgical incision through the abdomen and uterus.

Indications

Cesarean section may be performed for either maternal or fetal indications. The following list contains the indications for cesarean section:

Previous cesarean section or uterine surgery (*see* p. 413).
Medical complications of pregnancy.

401

Uncontrollable third-trimester bleeding.
Placenta previa.
Pelvic obstruction.
Failure of labor progress.
Fetopelvic disproportion.
Malpresentation.
Fetal distress.

Nursing interventions

Regardless of whether the cesarean section is a scheduled or emergency procedure, the client must be prepared for surgery. Emotional support, reassurance, and information are provided according to individual needs. Nursing care includes monitoring fetal and maternal well-being before the surgery, and monitoring the mother's recovery postoperatively. The specific anesthetic route used, the estimated blood loss, the medical condition of the mother and her infant, etc., all determine the particular nursing care required (*see* Chapter 19).

HYPERTONIC UTERINE CONTRACTIONS

Definition

Hypertonic uterine contractions are those in which either the pressure gradient pattern is disrupted, the basal (resting) tone of the myometrium is elevated, or both. In cases in which the pressure gradient is disrupted, it appears that either the midsection, rather than the fundus, develops the greatest tone, or that areas of hypertonicity occur throughout the uterus. Alternatively, the gradient pattern may appear normal, but the uterus may not properly relax between contractions. Hypertonic contractions usually begin during the latent phase of labor.

Hypertonic labor is a relatively rare condition. It is sometimes seen in excessively anxious nulliparas. In addition, it may be iatrogenically caused by the improperly monitored use of oxytocin stimulation.

Effect on labor

Women experiencing hypertonic contractions complain of severe discomfort, apparently disproportionate to the intensity of the contractions. Exhaustion and anxiety are common. Because of the lack of uterine coordination, cervical change is hampered and labor is prolonged, which results in an increased risk of infection and postpartum hemorrhage.

Fetal outcome

Because the myometrial pressure is elevated, oxygen perfusion to the placenta may be reduced, leading to uteroplacental insufficiency, late decelerations, and severe fetal distress.

Nursing interventions

Prompt recognition of the abnormal labor situation is of greatest importance in the care of women with hypertonic uterine contractions. Often, the initial management is sufficient sedation or analgesia (barbiturates and/or morphine) to cause the client to sleep for several hours. If successful, she generally awakens with a normal labor pattern and progresses appropriately. The risk of fetal distress is sufficient to warrant continuous monitoring until normal labor is established. It is possible that cesarean section may be indicated if significant fetal distress develops.

HYPOTONIC UTERINE CONTRACTIONS

Definition

Hypotonic uterine contractions are those in which there is insufficient intensity to effect change in the cervix. Consequently, there is failure of progress in cervical dilation in the first stage of labor and/or of fetal descent in the second stage. In addition, hypotonic contractions often decrease in frequency and/or become uncoordinated in their pattern. The tone or intensity of normal contractions in labor is greatest at the fundus and weakest in the lower uterine segment and cervix. In hypotonic contractions, this pressure gradient retains the same pattern, but the rise in pressure is insufficient to cause any progress in labor. Even at the peak of a contraction, it is possible to indent the uterine wall by palpation.

Often, the cause of hypotonic contractions is not diagnosed. Among the possible causes are fetopelvic disproportion; malposition; prolonged maternal dehydration, nutrition deprivation, or electrolyte imbalance; and excessive maternal anxiety. Other factors associated with inefficient labor are intrauterine infection, placental abruption, and, perhaps, early or excessive use of analgesia or regional anesthesia.

Effect on labor

Women who develop hypotonic contractions have fewer complaints of discomfort during contractions and frequently sleep or rest. Unless this condition is corrected, labor will be prolonged, which, as with hypertonic contractions, leads to an increased risk of intra-uterine infection, maternal exhaustion, and postpartum hemorrhage.

Fetal outcome

Prolonged labor, as stated above, increases the risk of intrauterine infection, which may affect the fetus as well as the client. In addition, because the cause of hypotonic contractions may be fetal malposition or malpresentation, or fetopelvic disproportion, other problems may result from improper diagnosis or management of the dysfunction.

Nursing interventions

Conscientious, routine nursing observation of contractions and labor status (as described in Chapter 9) is essential to prompt identification of hypotonic contractions. As with any dysfunctional labor, nursing recognition and documentation of changes in contraction pattern and intensity, as well as in maternal perceptions of labor, are of paramount importance. The management of hypotonic contractions that do not result from fetopelvic disproportion involves the reestablishment of normal labor. Nursing care supports normal physiology — including maintaining maternal hydration and nutrition, encouraging position changes and/or ambulation, and preventing exhaustion — and will be of benefit in avoiding or correcting hypotonic contractions. The decision regarding an amniotomy and/or the use of oxytocin stimulation obviously has an impact on the continued nursing care provided (*see* p. 410). If hypotonic contractions are the result of fetopelvic disproportion, or if oxytocin stimulation does not correct the labor pattern, a cesarean section is indicated. An explanation of the need for a cesarean section and the fetal condition, the provision of information and support, and normal pre- and post-operative nursing care are required.

INSTRUMENTAL DELIVERY

Definition

An instrumental delivery refers to the delivery of the fetus through the vagina with the aid of forceps or a vacuum extractor.

Indications

With the increased fetal and maternal safety available with a cesarean section, many women who would previously have had a forceps delivery are now managed by cesarean section. The following are indications for instrumental delivery:

Fetal distress, with vaginal delivery more expedient than cesarean section.

Maternal exhaustion in the second stage, or an inability to push effectively.

Medical conditions, such as cardiac disease or hypertension, that do not require surgical intervention, but in which a shortened second stage is advisable.

Lack of progress in the second stage.

Elective (outlet) forceps for prophylaxis rather than for a specific indication.

Prematurity, to protect the fetal head.

Nursing interventions

The care of the client during an instrumental delivery is similar to the care of a client in labor who delivers spontaneously (*see* Chapter 10). The client, however, may require additional support and/or information to understand why the instrumental assistance is indicated. Postpartum care remains essentially the same; but perineal discomfort is sometimes increased as a result of the greater trauma and/or manipulation. Careful observation of the integrity of the perineal repair and of the amount of postpartum bleeding will aid in prompt recognition of a hematoma. Complaints of pain during urination, identification of hematuria, and/or recognition of an excessive delay in the return of micturition after delivery suggest the possibility of urethral trauma from the instrumental delivery (*see* Chapter 19).

MALPRESENTATION

Definition

Malpresentation refers to any presentation other than the vertex. In a cephalic presentation, the specific presentation depends on the degree of flexion of the baby's head:

Vertex presentation: well flexed.
Military vertex presentation (military attitude): neither flexed nor extended.
Brow presentation: partially extended.
Face presentation: completely extended.

There are also four types of breech presentation:

Frank breech: the buttocks present, with the thighs flexed and the knees extended.

Complete breech: the buttocks and feet present, with both the knees and the thighs flexed.

Footling breech: the leg(s) present(s), with the knee(s) and the thigh(s) extended.

Kneeling breech: the knee(s) present(s), with the thigh(s) extended and the knee(s) flexed.

A shoulder presentation results from a transverse lie of the fetus.

Effect on labor

A military presentation is often transitory, with flexion occurring as the head descends. On occasion, extension to a brow or face presentation may occur. Thus, progress may be slower, and the incidence of arrest of labor may be increased.

A brow presentation most often changes during the course of labor, either flexing and converting to a vertex, or extending into a face presentation. Fetal anomalies, tumors, or multiple nuchal cord loops may contribute to its occurrence. Labor in a brow presentation is often prolonged, and spontaneous delivery may not occur. Significant lacerations often accompany vaginal delivery of a brow presentation. Manual or forceps conversion to either a vertex or a face presentation may aid in the delivery, although a cesarean section may be required.

A face presentation may result in prolonged labor because of the decreased effectiveness of the face as a dilating wedge. In addition to the possible causes given for a brow presentation, prematurity may cause a face presentation. Anencephalic fetuses often present by the face. Consequently, labor discomfort and the incidence of vaginal lacerations are increased. Posterior positions of face presentations cannot deliver spontaneously, and attempted vaginal delivery generally results in a difficult forceps delivery with increased postpartum morbidity. Cesarean section is the safest means of delivery of a posterior position of face presentation.

A breech presentation may also result in a longer labor because of the poor dilating wedge. Lacerations of the cervix and vagina may occur with the delivery of the head, the largest and last part to deliver. Postpartum hemorrhage is more likely to occur. A cesarean section may be indicated as the means of delivery. Fetopelvic disproportion caused by a large fetus, a contracted pelvis, or hydrocephaly may predispose to breech presentation. Other maternal factors include fundal placental location, fibromyomas, and placenta previa. Fetal factors include prematurity, multiple gestation, and hydramnios.

Unless it converts spontaneously to a longitudinal lie (cephalic or breech), a shoulder presentation (transverse lie) cannot deliver vaginally except in extreme prematurity or intrauterine fetal demise. A cesarean section is mandatory for safe delivery. Uterine or pelvic anomalies, placenta previa, or pelvic mass may predispose to transverse lie. Fetal anomalies and prematurity may contribute to the cause of the transverse lie.

Fetal outcome

There is an increased risk of fetal mortality in a brow presentation. Delivery by brow presentation results in extensive molding and possible brain damage.

A face presentation results in edema and bruising, secondary to the forces of labor against the face. The baby must be observed for respiratory distress secondary to trauma to the larynx. In posterior face presentations, the airway is more extensively traumatized because of the length of time required to rotate or because of the difficult forceps birth.

A breech presentation occurs more frequently in premature infants. Congenital anomalies are also increased in breech presentations. Asphyxia, brain or head injuries, internal trauma, and fractures of the neck, clavicle, humerus, or femur may all result from the delivery technique or a difficult birth.

A shoulder presentation, unless converted to a longitudinal lie or delivered by cesarean section, will result in fetal death.

Nursing interventions

In all cases of malpresentation, preparation should be made for the possibility of a cesarean section. In addition, because the labor is likely to be longer and more uncomfortable than usual, the client will require more physical and emotional support. Careful monitoring of both maternal and fetal status will aid in the prevention of serious complications.

MECONIUM STAINING

Definition

Meconium staining of the amniotic fluid results from the passage of meconium in utero. The significance of meconium staining depends on the presentation of the fetus. In a breech presentation, it may have no significance because it may result from compression of the breech and abdomen during contractions. In cephalic presentations, however, meconium staining is considered to be a sign of fetal distress. It is believed that the fetal rectal sphincter relaxes in response to hypoxia.

Effect on labor

Meconium passage has no direct effect on the labor. However, close monitoring for evidence of continued or additional fetal distress is essential. Intervention to effect delivery is not indicated if meconium staining is the only sign of distress. However, preparation for a cesarean section should be made in the event that distress recurs or worsens.

Fetal outcome

In the presence of meconium staining, there is a greater need for resuscitation of the newborn. The incidence of perinatal morbidity and mortality is increased. It is uncertain whether this is a result of the meconium or whether the meconium is a sign of another cause of morbidity.

Aspiration of meconium-stained fluid, a serious complication of the newborn, contributes to various types of respiratory distress, including pneumonia.

Nursing interventions

Fetal well-being must be closely monitored throughout labor. An explanation of the situation to the client and support person(s) should ensure cooperation and understanding. Because the use of electronic monitoring requires limitation of mobility, additional comfort measures may be required.

At the time of delivery, the attendant or an assistant should be prepared to suction the newborn's mouth and nose to remove any meconium, which may otherwise be aspirated. Suctioning should be performed when the head is delivered in order to avoid allowing the first breath to occur before suctioning is complete. In addition, the vocal cords of the newborn must be inspected with a laryngoscope to ensure that meconium was not aspirated. The trachea should be suctioned, if indicated.

MULTIPLE GESTATION

Definition

Multiple gestation is a pregnancy that results from the conception of more than one fetus. Twin gestation may be either dizygotic (fraternal) as a result of the fertilization of two ova, or monozygotic (identical) as a result of the fertilization of one ovum, which subsequently divides. Fraternal twins may be of either the same or opposite sex. Identical twins must be of the same sex. Triplets, quadruplets, quintuplets, etc., may be all fraternal, all identical, or any combination of these.

Effect on labor

Premature labor is a frequent complication of multiple gestation. In addition, dysfunctional contractions, placental abruption, abnormal presentation, prolapsed cord, and postpartum hemorrhage may occur. The decision regarding a planned vaginal delivery or a cesarean section is based on maternal and fetal factors, including presentations, number of fetuses, gestational age, and well-being.

Fetal outcome

Multiple gestation often results in a higher risk of malformations, increased perinatal mortality, prematurity, and decreased birth weight for gestational age.

Nursing interventions

Close monitoring of all fetuses during labor is essential. Staff and equipment should be available for an immediate cesarean section. Pediatric attendance at the birth is advised because of the increased risk of newborn depression.

During the postpartum period, the mother will probably need and appreciate some extra instruction and support regarding the well-being of her babies, newborn care, normal development, hints on how to manage and cope with more than one infant, etc. Sometimes the client does not know before the birth that she is carrying twins. Such a client will have many adjustments — both psychological and practical — to make in her plans and expectations. Referral to a "mother of twins" club is recommended. Many mothers might also benefit from referrals to the visiting nurse service and social service.

OXYTOCIN INDUCTION AND AUGMENTATION OF LABOR

Definition

Induction of labor is the establishment of effective uterine contractions by artificial means. Augmentation of labor (stimulation) is the use of artificial means, after labor has already been established, to cause the uterine contractions to resume effectiveness. The most common methods for either induction or augmentation of labor are artificial rupture of membranes and the use of synthetic oxytocin (Pitocin).

Effect on labor

If successful, the use of oxytocin results in progressive cervical effacement and dilation, descent of the presenting part, and delivery. The likelihood of successful induction of labor can be determined by using the Bishop score (Table 16-1).[1]

Neither induction nor augmentation of labor may be considered a benign procedure. Thus, the use of oxytocin for the "convenience" of the mother or the attendant is contraindicated. Other contraindications include previous uterine surgery, transverse lie, significant risk of fetopelvic disproportion, placenta previa, and significant fetal distress. Induction is contraindicated if fetal maturity is not certain, unless there are complications that outweigh the risk of prematurity. Relative contraindications include grand multiparity and breech presentation.

Some indications for the induction of labor are medical complications of pregnancy that can no longer be safely managed: severe preeclampsia or eclampsia, intrauterine fetal demise, Rh incompatibility, postmaturity, and evidence of fetal compromise.

The maternal risks associated with the use of oxytocin include uterine rupture, amniotic fluid embolism, and failure of induction (resulting in either repeated attempts at induction or the need for a cesarean section).

Fetal outcome

In appropriately selected cases, the fetus will have a better outcome after induction or augmentation of labor than would have occurred otherwise. The risks to the fetus include fetal distress, prolapsed umbilical cord, infection, and iatrogenic prematurity.

Nursing interventions

The use of oxytocin requires continuous monitoring of both maternal and fetal well-being. It is generally considered safest to use the electronic fetal monitor for maternal uterine contractions as well as for fetal heart rate. The use of external or internal modalities, or a combination of the two, will depend on the specific situation. Factors to consider include the availability of each mode, the legibility of the tracing obtained, and the safety of performing artificial rupture of membranes in order to use internal modalities. When elec-

TABLE 16-1
*Bishop Score**

Factor	Score			
	0	1	2	3
Dilation, *cm*	Closed	1-2	3-4	≥ 5
Effacement, %	0-30	40-50	60-70	≥ 80
Station	-3	-2	$-1/0$	$+1/+2$
Consistency	Firm	Medium	Soft	—
Cervical position	Posterior	Mid-position	Anterior	—

*The probability of successful induction of labor increases as the total score increases.
Adapted from Bishop, E. H. Pelvic scoring for elective induction. *Obstetrics and Gynecology* (August 1964). 267. *Reprinted with permission from* the American College of Obstetricians and Gynecologists, Washington, D. C.

tronic monitoring is not available, the nurse should auscultate the fetal heart tones during and after every contraction, and careful palpation and recording of uterine contractions should be performed. The use of an oxytocin infusion requires the continuous presence of a nurse or physician who is skilled in recognizing appropriate or inappropriate uterine contractions and normal or abnormal fetal heart tones. The infusion should be slowly and carefully titrated to obtain effective contractions at the lowest possible concentration (dosage) of oxytocin. An electronic infusion pump provides the greatest accuracy in concentration regulation. The concentration of the infusion is generally increased every 15 to 30 minutes until contractions are occurring every 2 to 3 minutes with a duration of 45 to 60 seconds.

The increased efficiency of the contractions may necessitate additional physical and emotional comfort and support measures. An explanation of the procedure and of the indications for the use of oxytocin should be provided to the client and her support person(s).

If fetal distress occurs, the infusion should be discontinued immediately, the client positioned on her left side, and nasal oxygen administered. The physician must be notified immediately of the distress. Further use of oxytocin would require careful assessment of the cause of the distress and reevaluation of the need for induction or augmentation when weighed against fetal and maternal well-being. If hypertonic contractions or other abnormal contraction patterns occur, the oxytocin should be discontinued and the physician should be notified.

PREMATURE RUPTURE OF THE MEMBRANES

Definition

Premature rupture of the membranes (PROM) is the spontaneous rupture of the amniotic sac before the onset of effective uterine contractions. The time span between rupture of membranes and the onset of labor, which determines the diagnosis of PROM, varies among institutions. This time span may range from 12 hours or greater to only minutes or even seconds, as long as the rupture of membranes occurred before the first contraction. The membranes are considered ruptured even in those cases in which leakage of the amniotic fluid occurs while the membranes are palpable in front of the presenting part. The cause of the rupture is unknown. In approximately 80 percent of all women near term, labor begins spontaneously within 24 hours of PROM.

If active labor begins within 12 to 24 hours, there is generally no deviation in normal labor management (depending on practitioner and/or institutional policy) unless additional problems develop. If labor has not started spontaneously within this time period, the management will depend on the length of gestation, maternal and fetal well-being, "ripeness" of the cervix for induction, and practitioner preference. Management decisions may involve either continued observation or the initiation of oxytocin induction.

Effect on labor

The incidence of amnionitis increases if the delivery is prolonged beyond 24 hours after the membranes rupture. If signs of infection develop, expeditious delivery is essential. If attempts at induction are unsuccessful, a cesarean section is required.

Fetal outcome

The primary complications that affect the fetus after PROM are umbilical cord prolapse, prematurity, and infection. The initial assessment, in addition to determining PROM, the cervical status, and assigning a Bishop score, must also rule out the presence of both obvious and occult cord prolapse (*see* p. 414).

Prematurity, with its resultant respiratory and developmental complications, is in itself a threat to the newborn. Unless signs of infection develop, it is preferable to continue close monitoring of the client and her fetus and to avoid induction of labor until maturity is established. The development of infection, however, is a great hazard to both premature and term infants, and, in those cases in which amnionitis is suspected, immediate delivery is essential.

Nursing interventions

After PROM is documented, nursing care is directed toward monitoring maternal and fetal well-being, recognizing signs of possible infection (such as increased maternal temperature, malodor of the fluid, etc.), and identifying the onset of labor. Hospitalization and bed rest — if the presenting part is not well applied to the cervix — are standard precautions that are used to reduce the risk of infection. In premature gestation, some practitioners allow the client to go home, if the leak has sealed. The client must then be instructed in the danger signs of infection, the technique of taking and recording her temperature, and the safeguards that minimize the risk of infection.

PREVIOUS CESAREAN SECTION

Definition

Previous cesarean section refers to the delivery of a previous pregnancy by means of a cesarean section of any type. Most women who have previously undergone a cesarean section will be delivered by repeat cesarean section. However, an increasing number of women are requesting the opportunity to attempt a vaginal birth after a cesarean (VBAC). The situations in which a trial of labor may be considered are specified in most institutional or departmental policies that permit such a trial. The considerations for a trial of labor include low transverse incision through the lower uterine segment, a nonrepetitive indication for the past cesarean, the number of previous cesareans, the postoperative course, the antepartal course in the current pregnancy, the fetal presentation and well-being, and the informed consent and client desire to attempt vaginal delivery.

Certain factors are felt to absolutely contraindicate attempted vaginal delivery. These include classical uterine scar or extension of a low transverse scar, two or more previous cesareans of any type, and recurrence of the indication (or identification of another indication) for a cesarean.

Effect on labor

The presence of the uterine scar has not, in itself, been shown to influence the course of labor. However, the risk of spontaneous rupture of the uterus is increased because of the presence of the scar. Whereas certain practitioners prohibit the use of oxytocin during labor for clients with a previous cesarean, others use it if no additional contraindications exist.

Fetal outcome

In cases of both a VBAC and a repeat cesarean delivery, there has been no report of any change in the perinatal morbidity or mortality, with the exception of an increased risk if uterine rupture ensues.

Nursing interventions

Continuous electronic monitoring of the client and her fetus for signs of distress or deviation from normal labor is essential. Preparation for an emergency cesarean section must include the availability of operating room facilities, pediatric assistance, anesthesia, and blood and fluid replacement.

PROLAPSED CORD

Definition

Prolapse of the umbilical cord is the presence of the umbilical cord in the pelvis ahead of the presenting part. In the presence of intact membranes, the cord may still present below the presenting part, although the diagnosis may not be evident. Occult cord prolapse is the presence of the umbilical cord alongside, not below, the presenting part.

Cord prolapse is most likely to occur in situations in which the presenting part does not fit firmly against the cervix. Situations that predispose to prolapsed cord include transverse lie, breech presentation (particularly a single or double footling or a complete breech), prematurity, multiple gestation, and hydramnios.

If a vaginal examination, performed because the membranes have ruptured in the clinic or other setting, reveals any of the situations that predispose the client to cord prolapse (but there is no current presence of prolapse), the client should be kept lying down. A stretcher should be used to transport the client to the hospital or birthing facility, and the physician should be notified immediately of the situation.

Effect on labor

Cord prolapse is an obstetric emergency. It is because of the danger of prolapse that a vaginal examination must be performed immediately when the membranes rupture spontaneously in labor. If the vertex is already known to be engaged, many practitioners check the fetal heart tones first in order to avoid an unnecessary vaginal examination. If the cord is located either at the introitus or in the vagina or cervix, the presenting part must be supported off the cord to avoid compression of the vessels and interruption of fetoplacental circulation. If the fetus is viable, immediate delivery is mandatory. Delivery must be by a cesarean section, unless vaginal delivery is imminent.

Fetal outcome

Except in rare instances, cord prolapse that occurs outside of the hospital or that is misdiagnosed or mismanaged in the hospital, will result in fetal death. The likelihood of significant fetal distress is great even with appropriate management.

Nursing interventions

Whoever diagnoses the prolapsed cord, whether by vaginal examination or by seeing the cord outside the introitus, must immediately lift the presenting part out of the pelvis and keep his or her hand in the vagina until the fetus is safely delivered abdominally. If the cord is outside the body, it must either be kept moist with a sterile towel and normal saline or be placed back into the lower vagina. The nurse should help the mother into a position that will reduce the risk of cord compression to the greatest possible extent (knee-chest or all fours). Other members of the staff should alert the obstetric team and prepare for a cesarean section. Oxygen should be administered to the client by mask or nasal cannula to increase oxygenation of the fetus. An explanation of the situation and its severity to the client and her support person(s) is essential.

TRANSVERSE ARREST

Definition

Transverse arrest refers to the failure of the occiput to complete internal rotation to either an occiput anterior (OA) or an occiput posterior (OP) position. There are two primary causes of transverse arrest. First, hypotonic uterine contractions (see p. 403) may develop, thus reducing the force necessary for rotation. Second, certain pelvic architectures, particularly platypelloid and android types, decrease the anterior-posterior diameter of the midpelvis and predispose to transverse arrest.

Effect on labor

Labor will be prolonged until the arrest of internal rotation is resolved. Before a vaginal delivery is attempted, however, it is essential to perform clinical and/or radiological evaluation of the pelvis in order to determine its adequacy for delivery. If the arrest is a result of hypotonic contractions, the use of oxytocin augmentation may be sufficient to cause completion of rotation. Alternatively, manual rotation to the OA position during a vaginal examination is often successful. A forceps delivery, including rotation to the OA or OP position, may be conducted. Finally, if the attempts to rotate the head are unsuccessful, or if fetopelvic disproportion is diagnosed, a cesarean section may be performed.

Fetal outcome

With accurate diagnosis and intervention, there is no increased fetal morbidity. However, if the transverse arrest continues for some length of time, extensive molding results, with or without the formation of caput succedaneum. If a vaginal delivery is attempted in the case of fetopelvic disproportion, the risk of fetal injury and morbidity is great.

Nursing interventions

Position changes (to the lateral, squatting, or knee-chest) and encouragement in effective pushing during the second stage may aid in the internal rotation of the head. The client may become exhausted and/or uncomfortable because of the length of the labor and the fetal position. It would then be necessary to institute comfort and support measures in order to provide the optimal conditions for resolution of the arrest.

SUMMARY

Each of these deviations is potentially serious for the client and/or the fetus. It is the nurse's responsibility to provide optimal nursing care and to recognize signs of any deviation from the norm at the earliest possible moment. By careful attention to detail and continuous caregiving, the nurse can provide the client and her baby with the safest possible outcome.

REFERENCE

1. Bishop.

CHAPTER 17

OBSTETRIC EMERGENCIES

Susan Papera

The discussion of obstetric emergencies presented in this chapter is by no means an exhaustive one. It confines itself to those emergencies that the practitioner is most likely to encounter and for which he or she would need a reference for immediate management.

BLEEDING DISORDERS

Abortion, ectopic pregnancy, placenta previa, abruptio placentae, and third-stage and postpartum hemorrhage can be associated with severe hemorrhage and shock and are true obstetric emergencies. Because of the many commonalities among them, the nursing assessments and interventions will be presented after the discussion of this group of obstetric problems.

Abortion

Spontaneous abortion is the premature expulsion of a nonviable fetus.

Classification. The following is a list of the four classifications of abortion (Fig. 17-1), with an explanation of each:

1. Threatened: The pregnancy is in jeopardy but may continue without further problems.
2. Imminent or inevitable: The pregnancy is in jeopardy without hope of salvage.

417

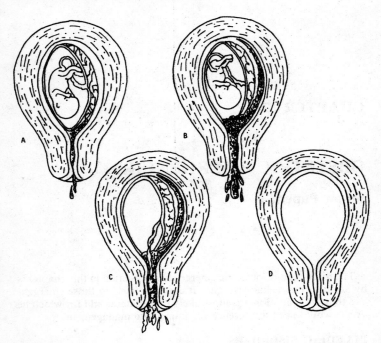

Figure 17-1. The four classifications of spontaneous abortion. (A) Threatened, (B) imminent, (C) incomplete, and (D) complete.

3. Incomplete: The products of conception have been partially expelled.
4. Complete: The entire products of conception have been expelled.

Etiology and predisposing factors.   The causes of abortion are divided into three categories:

1. Fetal:
   a. Abnormal ovum development.
   b. Chromosomal abnormalities incompatible with life.
   c. Abnormal placental development.
2. Maternal:
   a. Systemic infections.
   b. Nutritional factors.
   c. Abnormalities in the reproductive system.

    d. Endocrine disorders.
    e. ABO blood group incompatibility.
    f. Radiation or trauma.
    g. Psychogenic factors.
3. Unknown:
    a. Thought to be a combination of both fetal and maternal factors.

Signs and symptoms.

1. Uterine cramping.
2. Lower back pain in early gestation.
3. Vaginal bleeding.
4. Passage of part or all of the products of conception.

Ectopic pregnancy

Ectopic pregnancy is the abnormal implantation of the fertilized ovum outside of the uterine cavity. Most frequently, implantation occurs in some portion of the fallopian tube, but it may also occur within the ovary, the broad ligament, the abdominal cavity, or the cervix (Fig. 17-2).

Etiology and predisposing factors. Any factor that affects tubal patency, tubal ciliary action, tubal contractility, or sperm motility can predispose to ectopic pregnancy.[1] Three such factors are listed below:

1. Partial tubal occlusion secondary to inflammation.
2. The use of an intrauterine contraceptive device.
3. The use of oral contraceptives composed solely of progesterone.[2]

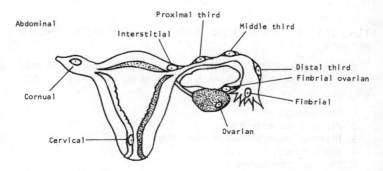

Figure 17-2.   The sites of ectopic pregnancies.

Signs and symptoms.

1. Amenorrhea (with or without irregular vaginal bleeding).
2. Subjective feelings of early pregnancy (e.g., fatigue, nausea, and breast discomfort).
3. Lower abdominal pain.
4. Lower back pain in early gestation.
5. Referred shoulder pain.
6. Hemoperitoneum and shock with a ruptured ectopic pregnancy.

Placenta previa

Placenta previa is the abnormal implantation of the placenta in the lower portion of the uterus.

Classification.   The following is a list of the three classifications of placenta previa (Fig. 17-3), with an explanation of each:

1. Total: The placenta totally covers the internal cervical os.
2. Partial: The placenta partially covers the internal cervical os.
3. Low-lying: The placental edge is near the internal cervical os but is not encroaching on it.

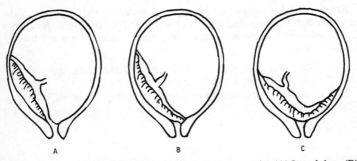

Figure 17-3.   The three classifications of placenta previa. (A) Low-lying, (B) partial, and (C) total.

Etiology and predisposing factors.   The exact cause of placenta previa is unknown. The following is a list of the most common predisposing factors:

1. Multiparity.
2. Previous placenta previa.
3. Previous lower uterine segment scar.
4. Short maternal stature.
5. Uterine abnormalities.

Signs and symptoms.   The only symptom of placenta previa is painless, bright red vaginal bleeding in the third trimester of pregnancy. The bleeding is caused by the tearing of the placental vessels during the latter part of pregnancy and during labor with the development of the lower uterine segment.

Abruptio placentae

Abruptio placentae is the premature separation of the placenta from the wall of the uterus.

Etiology and predisposing factors.   The exact cause of abruptio placentae is unknown. The following is a list of the most common predisposing factors:

1. Short umbilical cord.
2. Trauma.
3. Precipitous labor.
4. Uterine anomalies or tumors.
5. Sudden decompression of the uterus.
6. Chronic hypertension.
7. Pregnancy-induced hypertension.
8. Folic acid deficiency.
9. Compression of the inferior vena cava.

Signs and symptoms.

1. Vaginal bleeding (in some cases).
2. Localized or generalized uterine tenderness. (Pain is often out of proportion to the palpatory signs.)
3. Uterine irritability and hypertonicity.
4. Absence of fetal heart tones (in severe cases of abruptio placentae).
5. Variable signs of maternal hypovolemia.

Bleeding may be either apparent or concealed, mild or severe. Vaginal bleeding is thought to result from bleeding into the decidua with retroplacental clot formation and subsequent shearing of a segment of the placenta from the anchoring decidua (Fig. 17-4). The degree of fetal and maternal compromise depends on the extent of the separation and on the amount of blood loss (Table 17-1).

Third-stage and postpartum hemorrhage

Third-stage hemorrhage is acute blood loss before the delivery of the placenta, secondary to its partial separation. Immediate post-

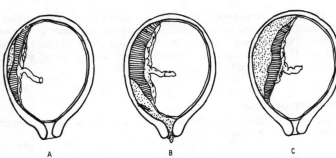

Figure 17-4.   The three types of abruptio placentae. (A) Internal (concealed) hemorrhage, (B) external hemorrhage, and (C) complete separation.

TABLE 17-1
Placental Separation

Factor	Mild	Moderate	Severe
Degree of separation	≤ 1/6.	1/6-2/3.	> 2/3.
Blood loss, *ml*	< 500.	500-1,000.	> 1,000.
Uterine pain and irritability	Slight pain. Uterus relaxes between contractions.	Increased pain and irritability.	Severe pain and irritability.
Maternal effect	No hemodynamic compromise.	Hypotension.	Shock, renal failure, and coagulopathy.
Fetal effect	No compromise.	Signs of compromise.	Severe compromise. Fetal death.

Adapted from Aladjem, S., editor. Obstetrical Practice. C. V. Mosby Co., St. Louis. 1980. p. 462.

partum hemorrhage, often described as a blood loss of greater than 500 milliliters, has the following five etiologies:

1. Partial separation of the placenta.
2. Uterine atony.
3. Lacerations of the cervix, vagina, and perineum.
4. Retained placental tissue.
5. Blood dyscrasias (e.g., afibrinogenemia and hypofibrinogenemia).

The predisposing factors and the signs and symptoms of third-stage and postpartum hemorrhage are listed below.

Predisposing factors.

1. Mismanagement of the third stage of labor.
2. Overdistention of the uterus:
   a. Hydramnios.
   b. Large fetus.
   c. Multiple gestation.
3. Prolonged labor.
4. Precipitous labor.
5. Oxytocin induction or stimulation.
6. History of uterine atony with previous births.
7. Grand multiparity.
8. Maternal exhaustion.
9. Excessive use of analgesics or anesthetics.
10. Abruptio placentae.
11. Placenta previa.
12. Instrumental delivery (e.g., forceps).

Signs and symptoms.

1. Heavy vaginal bleeding in the third stage of labor or within the first 24 hours postpartum.
2. Variable signs of maternal hypovolemia.

Outcomes

The immediate consequences of all of these bleeding disorders are maternal hypovolemia and shock, both of which may lead to renal damage and disseminated intravascular coagulation. Significant bleeding during the prenatal and intrapartum periods has the added consequence of causing fetal distress and neonatal morbidity. The ultimate possible results are maternal and fetal death.

Nursing assessment and intervention

Nursing assessment and intervention should be based on the following information and procedures:

1. Historical data:
   a. Obstetric history.
   b. Present pregnancy history.
   c. Onset, duration, and severity of symptoms (e.g., abdominal pain and vaginal bleeding).
   d. Predisposing factors.

2. Physical examination:
   a. General appearance.
   b. Blood pressure, pulse rate and quality, and respiratory rate and quality.
   c. Abdominal palpation for labor status, presence and degree of pain, and uterine tone.
   d. Presence and amount of bleeding.

Nursing intervention should consist of the following actions:

1. Estimate and record blood loss.
2. Maintain the client in a supine position.
3. Closely monitor blood pressure, pulse rate and quality, respiratory rate and quality, skin color, and temperature.
4. Evaluate and record the presence and degree of abdominal pain.
5. Monitor labor status.
6. Monitor fetal status.
7. Inform the client and her support person(s) of any necessary procedures and their rationales.
8. Maintain fluid and/or blood replacement. Use a large-bore plastic cannula for intravenous infusion. Two lines may be necessary.
9. Monitor urinary output:
   a. Insert Foley catheter.
   b. Record and report the hourly output.
   c. Measure and record the specific gravity.
10. Measure and record the central venous pressure.
11. Administer oxygen via face mask at 4 to 7 liters/min.
12. Update laboratory data:
   a. Draw client's blood for type and cross-match, hemoglobin and hematocrit levels, and a coagulation profile.

FETAL DISTRESS

Fetal distress describes a situation in which the well-being of the fetus is compromised. This occurs when maternal-fetal gas exchange is disturbed within either the umbilical cord or the placenta.

Etiology and predisposing factors

The following is a list of the maternal and fetal conditions that can cause fetal distress. Any of these conditions, when coupled with the stress of uterine contractions, may lead to acute fetal distress.

1. Maternal conditions:
   a. Chronic hypertension.
   b. Preeclampsia-eclampsia.
   c. Diabetes.
2. Fetal conditions:
   a. Prematurity.
   b. Intrauterine growth retardation.
   c. Umbilical cord problems (abnormal insertion, true knot, or atresia).
3. Any other condition that interferes with placental circulation (e.g., cord compression or maternal hypotension).

The fetal heart is very sensitive to the effects of disturbed gas exchange (hypoxia). Therefore, both the fetal heart rate and the heart rate patterns are indicators of the fetal condition.

Although careful auscultation of the fetal heart with a fetoscope is an accurate assessment tool, electronic monitoring is indicated in the presence of any predisposing factors or audible abnormalities (*see* Chapter 18).

Proper interpretation of a fetal heart monitor is based on the following data:

1. The base-line fetal heart rate.
2. The heart rate variability.
3. Any periodic heart rate changes (*see* Chapter 18).

Signs and symptoms

1. Base-line tachycardia (heart rate of greater than 160 beats/min).
2. Base-line bradycardia (heart rate of less than 110 beats/min).
3. Decreased or absent variability.
4. Persistent and deep variable decelerations.
5. Repetitive late decelerations.

Variability of the fetal heart rate represents the short-term fluctuations from the base line and is indicative of a mature and functioning fetal nervous system. A decrease in this variability (*see* Chapter 18) may be seen with fetal immaturity and congenital anomalies, the administration of maternal medications, and fetal hypoxia and acidosis.[3]

Outcomes

Fetal hypoxia and acidosis have been implicated in the etiology of mental retardation, cerebral palsy, and fetal death.

PREECLAMPSIA-ECLAMPSIA

Preeclampsia is a progressive hypertensive disorder that only occurs in pregnancy. It is characterized by elevation of blood pressure, proteinuria, and generalized edema. Physiologically, the primary aberration is peripheral arteriolar vasoconstriction and vasospasm, leading to alterations in many maternal organ functions. Vasospasm in the arterioles leads to an increase in blood pressure and, ultimately, to a decrease in uterine blood flow.[4]

The most characteristic alteration caused by preeclampsia occurs in the kidneys. Renal vascular lesions, glomeruloendothelioses, cause a decrease in renal blood flow, a decrease in the glomerular filtration rate, and, consequently, proteinuria.

Changes in the central nervous system may include cerebral edema, leading to headaches and visual disturbances. As the preeclampsia progresses, hyperactivity of the deep tendon reflexes ensues. Hepatic alterations include enlargement of the liver and tension on the liver capsule, resulting in epigastric pain.

Eclampsia, the continuation of this process, results in generalized seizures.

Etiology and predisposing factors

Even though our understanding of preeclampsia has increased markedly, the exact cause is still unknown. Many theories have been developed (for an in-depth review, the reader is directed to a standard obstetric textbook and the Bibliography).

The following is a list of the most common predisposing factors:

1. A client of less than 20 or greater than 35 years of age.
2. Parity. (Although this is known as a disease of first pregnancies, it is also seen in the multiparous client, especially in the presence of other risk factors.)
3. Preexisting renal disease.
4. Diabetes.
5. Multiple gestation.
6. Hydatidiform mole. (Preeclampsia generally occurs after the 20th week of pregnancy but is seen earlier with a molar pregnancy.)
7. Socioeconomic factors (e.g., limited access to prenatal care and poor nutrition).

Signs and symptoms

1. Rise in base-line blood pressure. (Defined as 30 mmHg systolic and 15 mmHg diastolic, although more subtle changes should be noted.)

2. Generalized edema. (Reflected in a sudden, excessive weight gain of greater than 2 pounds in 1 week. Most significant is edema other than dependent: i.e., that of the hands, face, and abdomen.)
3. Proteinuria (1 + or greater in a clean-catch specimen).
4. Hyperreflexia.
5. Visual disturbances (e.g., blurring, double vision, and scotoma).
6. Headache.
7. Epigastric pain.
8. Nausea and vomiting.
9. Hemoconcentration.
10. Oliguria.
11. Convulsions.

Outcomes

Severe preeclampsia and eclampsia have been associated with such serious complications as cerebral edema and cerebrovascular accident, acute renal failure, abruptio placentae, disseminated intravascular coagulation, and fetal and maternal death. Worldwide, maternal and fetal mortality rates have been said to range from 0 to 17 percent and from 10 to 37 percent, respectively.[4]

Nursing assessments and interventions

Bed rest and a minimization of external stimuli are the cornerstones of nursing management of preeclampsia-eclampsia. The preferred maternal position is a lateral one. (This is thought to increase renal blood flow and placental perfusion.) The nurse should note any existing predisposing factors and explain the disorder, the therapeutic regimen, and its rationale to the client.

Magnesium sulfate is the drug most widely used to prevent seizures in severe preeclampsia. Although this drug may be mildly antihypertensive, it is primarily used for its depressive effect on the central nervous system and its inhibitory effect on the neuromuscular junction.

Magnesium sulfate can be administered either intramuscularly or intravenously. A loading dose of 3 to 4 grams is administered intravenously, followed by a dose of 1 g/hr.

Magnesium sulfate is excreted primarily by the kidneys, and, if there is a decrease in renal functioning, the dose must be carefully adjusted to avoid toxicity. Associated hypertension may be controlled by the use of hydralazine hydrochloride or another antihypertensive agent. (For further information about the pharmacological agents used, *see* Appendix A.)

Outpatient management

1. Stress the importance of bed rest in the lateral position.
2. Review the danger signs of preeclampsia, and advise the client to seek medical attention if they occur.
3. Review diet instructions. Encourage the client to maintain a high protein intake and to avoid decreasing sodium or fluid intake.
4. Review the use, effects, and side effects of any medications (e.g., phenobarbital) that may be ordered by the physician.
5. Stress the importance of regular and frequent clinic appointments.
6. Coordinate the efforts of the health care team to enhance maternal and fetal well-being.

Inpatient management

1. Maintain a quiet environment.
2. Monitor blood pressure, pulse, and respirations every 15 minutes, if medications are in use.
3. Monitor biceps, patellar, and ankle reflexes every 15 minutes and/or before administration of magnesium sulfate.
4. Check for clonus (the rapid, involuntary, and rhythmical contraction and relaxation of a muscle as it is stretched sharply).
5. Monitor the degree and location of edema.
6. Insert a Foley catheter, if indicated.
7. Record intake and output hourly.
8. Monitor the fetus, using a continuous electronic fetal monitor, if available.
9. Investigate and record the client's subjective and somatic complaints (e.g., headache, visual disturbances).
10. Obtain laboratory data as ordered (e.g., quantitative urinary protein, or blood chemistries: blood urea nitrogen, creatinine, uric acid, liver enzymes, hematocrit and hemoglobin, and coagulation profile).
11. Observe for signs of fibrinogen depletion (e.g., bleeding gums or oozing from the intravenous site).
12. Maintain seizure precautions (i.e., emergency drugs and equipment, including tongue blade, at the bedside; padded side rails).
13. Alert pediatric and anesthesia personnel to the client's condition.
14. Be prepared for emergency cesarean section, if maternal or fetal condition deteriorates.

15. The client receiving magnesium sulfate needs special precautions:
    a. Monitor for signs of toxicity (e.g., flushing, muscle flaccidity, and depressed reflexes).
    b. Have calcium gluconate (the specific antidote to magnesium sulfate) near the bedside.
    c. Monitor blood pressure, respirations, and reflexes every 15 minutes.

PREMATURE LABOR

Premature labor is a process that may lead to the expulsion of a viable fetus between the 26th and 38th week of gestation. It is a situation with many associated factors and no known cause.

Etiology and predisposing factors

1. Low socioeconomic status.
2. Maternal medical conditions (e.g., acute systemic infections).
3. Urinary tract infection.
4. Genetic factors.
5. Premature rupture of the membranes.
6. Placenta previa.
7. Abruptio placentae.
8. Multiple gestation.
9. Hydramnios.
10. Previous premature birth.
11. Uterine anomalies.
12. Incompetent cervix.
13. Uterine myomas.
14. Closely spaced pregnancies.
15. Surgery during the pregnancy.

Signs and symptoms

The hallmark of premature labor is regular uterine contractions that lead to cervical effacement and/or dilation. The following is a list of common symptoms:

1. Menstrual-like cramps.
2. Low backache.
3. Pelvic pressure.
4. A change in the character of vaginal secretions.[5]

A client who presents with these complaints, especially in the presence of one or more of the factors associated with premature labor, is considered at risk and is in need of astute medical and nursing care.

Once labor has been diagnosed, treatment consists of bed rest, hydration, fetal and maternal monitoring, and determination and treatment of the underlying problem, if possible.

If the cervix is dilated less than 4 centimeters and the membranes are intact, and if there are no maternal or fetal contraindications, glucocorticoids (to hasten fetal lung maturity) and tocolytic agents (to forestall birth) may be administered. Some examples of tocolytic agents are alcohol (rarely), magnesium sulfate, isoxsuprine hydrochloride, ritodrine hydrochloride, and terbutaline sulfate. (For further information, *see* Appendix A.)

Outcomes

Neonatal problems that are associated with prematurity include respiratory distress syndrome as a result of immature lungs; hyperbilirubinemia; hypocalcemia; and hypoglycemia. Premature infants are also more prone to the development of infections.

Because of the nature of the intensive care that is required for some premature infants, the disruption in the development of parent-newborn attachment is an important consideration (*see* Chapter 14).

That the neonatal death rate in the United States has decreased from 20.5/1,000 in 1950 to 9.4/1,000 in 1978 is, in large part, the result of the fact that more preterm infants survive.[6] Nevertheless, prematurity remains the leading cause of perinatal morbidity and mortality today.[5]

Nursing assessments and interventions

1. Reinforce the medical regimen and its rationale to the client and her family.
2. Provide emotional and psychological support. Help the client and her family prepare for an early birth.
3. Assess the client's and family's coping mechanisms, and support and build on their strengths.
4. Maintain close observation of both the maternal and fetal conditions by monitoring and recording maternal vital signs and labor status and by monitoring and recording fetal status.
5. If drug therapies are used, administer appropriate doses at the proper time. Do not hesitate to question an unclear or improper order. Monitor the client for signs of toxicity.
6. If long-term hospitalization is required, maintain contact with the client and her family in order to build on the relationship that began in the labor area.

SHOULDER DYSTOCIA

Shoulder dystocia (difficulty in delivering the infant's shoulders) occurs when either one or both shoulders fail to pass through the pelvis after the birth of the head.

Etiology and predisposing factors

In this situation, the shoulders (bisacromial diameter) enter the pelvis in the anterior-posterior diameter instead of in the more favorable oblique diameter. The anterior shoulder becomes impacted above the symphysis pubis while the posterior shoulder passes the promontory of the sacrum and enters the pelvis.

The following is a list of the most common predisposing factors:

1. Large fetus.
2. Maternal diabetes.
3. Maternal obesity.
4. An estimated fetal weight of at least 1 pound greater than the client's largest previous infant.

Outcomes

Shoulder dystocia may lead to a variety of maternal and infant complications. Extensive vaginal and perineal lacerations are common. In addition, as a result of the traumatic delivery and/or infant damage, there may be a mild to severe emotional reaction by the client. Brain damage, Erb's palsy, and a fractured clavicle often result from shoulder dystocia. Ultimately, it may lead to intrapartum or neonatal death.

Nursing assessments and interventions

The following is a list of the relevant nursing assessments and interventions for shoulder dystocia:

1. Note any predisposing factors and anticipate potential problems.
2. Inform the client and support person(s) of the situation and help them to work with the attendant (i.e., pushing and positioning).
3. Have a pediatrician in attendance, if possible, and prepare for infant resuscitation.
4. Apply suprapubic pressure as directed (see below).
5. Visit the client during the postpartum period to allow her to air any questions or feelings that she may have regarding the delivery.

It should be noted that fundal pressure, which does not relieve shoulder pressure, should not be used. Fundal pressure will only lead to further impaction of the shoulders. Suprapubic pressure is applied by placing a fist or both hands in the midline, above the symphysis pubis, and exerting downward pressure. Greater force can be attained by standing on a stool or kneeling on the delivery bed or table. Suprapubic pressure brings the anterior shoulder into and through the pelvis.

SUMMARY

The nurse can play a significant role in reducing the morbidity and mortality that are associated with these obstetric emergencies. It is often through the astute observations of the nurse that the problem is initially recognized and appropriate treatment is begun. Every nurse who is responsible for providing care to pregnant women must be able to recognize these problems and begin the nursing process without delay.

REFERENCES

1. Clausen et al. 687.
2. Bolton et al.
3. Oxorn. 252.
4. Zuspan and Zuspan.
5. Queenan et al.
6. Pritchard and MacDonald. 929.

CHAPTER 18

FETAL MONITORING

Kathleen Buckley

PHYSIOLOGY OF FETAL HEART RATE CHANGES

The placenta and the autonomic nervous system modulate fetal heart rate (FHR) changes.

The major function of the placenta is to provide for fetal oxygen and carbon dioxide exchange. Any malfunction will decrease the amount of oxygen available to the heart muscle and directly slow the FHR. This condition is known as placental insufficiency.

The parasympathetic and the sympathetic branches of the autonomic nervous system can also change the FHR. Stimulation of the parasympathetic nerve (cranial nerve 10 — the vagus nerve) causes a decrease in the FHR. For example, pressure on the fetal head during a vaginal examination may stimulate the vagus nerve and decrease the FHR. Atropine, on the other hand, blocks the neurohormone secreted by the cranial nerve ending and, consequently, increases the FHR. Branches of the sympathetic nervous system are found in the heart muscle itself, the aorta, and the carotid sinuses. Any increase in the carbon dioxide level or decrease in the oxygen level causes a compensatory increase in blood pressure and FHR.

BASE-LINE FHR CHANGES

Base-line FHR changes are those that occur in the absence of, or in between, contractions. The normal base-line range of beats per minute is 120 to 160, with a short-term variability of 6 to 10. The specific changes to note are tachycardia, bradycardia, and decreased variability.

Tachycardia

Etiology. The most common cause of tachycardia (above 160 beats/min) is maternal fever.[1] Other maternal causes include anxiety, dehydration, and hyperthyroidism. Fetal causes include infection, hypoxia, and cardiac arrhythmias.[1] In addition, certain drugs produce fetal tachycardia (*see below*).

Nursing actions.

1. Check the client's temperature.
2. Investigate the client's hydration status. (Review history of nutrition and excretion, intake and output records, patency of intravenous infusion, if applicable, and urine specific gravity.)
3. Position the client on her left side to enhance placental perfusion.
4. Assess the emotional status of client and significant other(s).
5. Check the client's medications. (Ritodrine hydrochloride, isoxsuprine hydrochloride, atropine, and scopolamine cause increased FHR.)
6. Notify the physician.

Bradycardia

Etiology. The most common cause of bradycardia (below 110 beats/min) is fetal hypoxia, which is a sign of fetal distress. Maternal hypothermia and fetal heart block also decrease the FHR.[1]

Nursing actions.

1. Discontinue any intravenous infusion of oxytocin, if applicable.
2. Notify the physician.
3. Position the client on her left side to enhance placental perfusion.
4. Check the client's temperature.
5. Anticipate the following procedures:
   Vaginal examination.
   Oxygen, via face mask at 8 liters/min.
   Fetal scalp blood sample (FSBS) (*see* p. 440).
   Cesarean section, if condition worsens or if fetal pH is 7.2 or lower.
6. The FHR may decrease just before birth. If the client is fully dilated and pushing and the FHR suddenly drops, be sure to check the perineum. Birth may be imminent.

Variability

Etiology. A healthy fetal autonomic nervous system causes the FHR to be slightly irregular or variable. Short-term variability is the most important factor in assessing fetal well-being. Decreased variability (less than 6 beats/min) may be a sign of fetal hypoxia. On the other hand, a normal, healthy, sleeping fetus may seem to have decreased variability. However, the normal fetal sleep cycle is short, lasting for approximately 20 minutes. Narcotics, barbiturates, tranquilizers, and anesthetics all decrease FHR variability. If the client is administered any of these substances, it will be difficult to ascertain whether the fetus is hypoxic or just under the depressive influence of the analgesia/anesthesia.

Nursing actions.

1. Position the client on her left side to enhance placental perfusion.
2. If it is thought that the fetus is asleep, perform an abdominal examination. (Gently jiggle the fetal head and rump to wake the fetus up. Variability should return.)
3. Check the client's chart to assess the administration of analgesia/anesthesia within the past 3 to 6 hours. (Note: Intravenous analgesia should be cleared from maternal-fetal circulation within 1 hour. Intramuscular analgesia should be cleared within 3 hours. The time required for barbiturates, tranquilizers, and anesthesia varies.)
4. Notify the physician.
5. Anticipate the following procedures:
   Oxygen, via face mask at 8 liters/min.
   FSBS (*see* p. 440).
   Cesarean section, if condition worsens or if fetal pH is 7.2 or lower.
6. Carefully observe for the appearance of late decelerations, which indicate a severely jeopardized fetus (*see below*).

PERIODIC FHR CHANGES

In 1967, the American College of Obstetricians and Gynecologists developed standard terminology to describe FHR changes that occur with contractions. Three types were identified: early, late, and variable decelerations (Fig. 18-1).

Early decelerations

Etiology. Early decelerations coincide with uterine contractions. The onset and recovery of the FHR variation mirror the uterine contraction. Compression of the fetal head stimulates the vagus nerve,

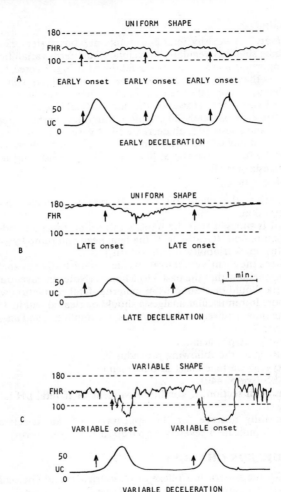

Figure 18-1. Classification of periodic fetal heart rate (FHR) changes in relation to uterine contractions (UC). (A) Early decelerations, secondary to pressure on the fetal head, are uniform and mirror the UC. (B) Late decelerations, secondary to uteroplacental insufficiency, are uniform and reflect the shape of the UC. (C) Variable decelerations, secondary to umbilical cord compression, are not uniform and do not reflect the UC.

and the FHR drops to within a range of 100 to 140 beats/min. Early decelerations are not a sign of fetal distress.

Nursing actions.   Just before the delivery of the fetal head, early decelerations are common and more pronounced. If pronounced early decelerations occur, the nurse should check the client's perineum.

Late decelerations

Etiology.   In late decelerations, the onset of the FHR deceleration occurs after the uterine contraction. The cause is fetal hypoxia as a result of insufficient oxygen and carbon dioxide exchange via the placenta. Decreased oxygen levels directly affect the myocardium and slow the fetal heart. This is the most ominous FHR pattern, and it is associated with fetal mortality and morbidity. In addition, it is insidious because the FHR range is usually within the normal limits (120 to 160 beats/min).

Nursing actions.

1. Discontinue any intravenous infusion of oxytocin, if applicable.
2. Position the client on her left side to enhance placental perfusion.
3. Notify the physician.
4. Anticipate the following procedures:
   Vaginal examination.
   Oxygen, via face mask at 8 liters/min.
   FSBS (*see* p. 440).
   Cesarean section, if condition worsens or if fetal pH is 7.2 or lower.

Variable decelerations

Etiology.   Variable decelerations are caused by compression of the umbilical cord. The onset can occur at irregular or "variable" times during the uterine contraction. Arterial and venous flow are temporarily decreased, causing the FHR to fall. The causes of cord compression include cord prolapse, true knot, and nuchal or body cord. Variable decelerations are associated with asphyxiated newborns only when the pattern is severe or prolonged.

Nursing actions.   For mild variable decelerations, a change of position (from supine to lateral, or from lateral to lateral) is usually all that is needed to relieve the compression. For severe or sudden profound variable decelerations, the following nursing actions apply:

1. Notify the physician.
2. Perform a vaginal examination to assess the possibility of cord

prolapse. Variable decelerations may be more pronounced just before the delivery of the fetal head, if a nuchal cord is present.

3. Discontinue any intravenous infusion of oxytocin, if applicable.
4. Change the client's position. (Turn her to the left side first. If that does not alleviate the decrease in FHR, turn her onto her right side. If the cord is prolapsed or if the lateral positions are not effective, have the client immediately assume the knee-chest position.)
5. Anticipate the following procedures:
   Vaginal examination.
   Oxygen, via face mask at 8 liters/min.
   FSBS (see p. 440).
   Emergency vaginal delivery or cesarean section, if condition worsens, cord has prolapsed, or fetal pH is 7.2 or lower.

NURSING RECORDS

Each obstetric nursing service has its own criteria for the recording of nursing observations and assessments. It is important to remember that the monitor strip itself is a legal document and remains with the client's chart. The procedures and the client's vital signs must be charted on the strip as well as in the nurse's notes.

The following guidelines have been adapted from a large obstetric tertiary care unit:[2]

1. Label each new strip with the client's name, the unit number, the date, and the Roman numeral I. Label each subsequent strip with the name, unit number, date, and the appropriate Roman numeral (e.g., II, III, IV, etc.).
2. Record the time and blood pressure every 30 minutes.
3. Record a full set of vital signs every hour.
4. Note all major obstetric events:
   a. Time, route, and dosage of any drug.
   b. Continuous use of a drug at an unchanged dosage every 30 minutes.
   c. Time and results of the vaginal examination.
   d. Time and type (artificial vs. spontaneous) of rupture of membranes, and character of amniotic fluid.
   e. Time and change of maternal position.
   f. Unusual functioning (e.g., vomiting).
   g. Treatments (e.g., time and results of FSBS, regional anesthesia, etc.).
   h. Time and name of obstetrician called in by nurse to evaluate suspicious tracing.

i. Time and type of monitoring used (e.g., external vs. internal, application of fetal scalp electrode, application of uterine catheter, etc.).

METHODS FOR MONITORING INTRAPARTUM FETAL HEALTH

The traditional technique for counting the FHR involves listening with a fetoscope. This is an intermittent evaluation because a mere sample of the FHR is used to make an assessment about fetal health.

Two types of electronic fetal monitoring — external and internal — enable a continuous readout of both the FHR and the uterine contraction pattern. The fetus at risk is a candidate for continuous electronic monitor evaluation (Table 18-1). The external monitoring

TABLE 18-1
Criteria for Electronic Monitoring

Prenatal factors	Intrapartum factors
Toxemia.	No prenatal care.
Maternal weight of <45.4 kg (<100 lb) or >90.7 kg (>200 lb), or a weight gain of <7.7 kg (<17 lb).	Gestational age <37 or >42 wk, or small for gestational age.
	Toxemia.
Rh-sensitized pregnancy.	Hydramnios or oligohydramnios.
Maternal age <17 or >35 yr.	Premature rupture of membranes of >12 hr.
Drug or alcohol abuse.	Failure to progress in labor.
Anemia.	Use of medication (magnesium
Metabolic disease (diabetes, thyroid condition, etc.).	sulfate, oxytocin, narcotics, etc.).
Cardiac disease.	Meconium staining.
Renal disease.	FHR abnormalities.
Chronic hypertension.	Abnormal presentation or lie.
Maternal obstetric history (previous stillbirth, neonatal death, premature infant, previous cesarean section, etc.).	Grand multiparity.
Seizure disorder.	
Suspicious or positive NST or OCT.	
Falling estriol levels.	

FHR, fetal heart rate; NST, nonstress test; OCT, oxytocin challenge test.
Adapted from Hobel, C. Prenatal and intrapartum high risk screening. *American Journal of Obstetrics and Gynecology* (September 1973). 1-9.

system (EMS) involves placing an ultrasound transducer on the maternal abdomen to pick up the motion of the fetal heart valves. A simple pressure gauge transducer anchored on the abdomen records uterine contractions. The use of the internal monitoring system (IMS) involves placing a cardiac electrode on the fetal presenting part to obtain an FHR tracing. A strain gauge is inserted directly into the uterine cavity to measure the intensity of uterine contractions.

It is important to note that the EMS has some drawbacks. The beat-to-beat base-line FHR variability and the uterine contraction strength cannot be accurately assessed. Fetal movement, maternal position, and bowel sounds may interfere with an adequate reading.

IMS, the most invasive monitoring technique, is the most accurate. All labor and fetal measurements may be accurately quantified. However, fetal scalp abscess and postpartum uterine infection have been reported with the use of IMS.

FSBS

A normal FHR tracing is always associated with a healthy newborn outcome in the absence of birth with trauma, airway blockage, congenital anomalies, or other unexpected events. However, the converse is not true. Suspicious or even totally abnormal tracings are associated with a poor outcome in only about one half of all cases.

For the purpose of diagnosing fetal jeopardy, a new technique — FSBS — has been developed. A small amount of blood is taken directly from the fetal scalp and measured for pH. Obviously, this technique can be employed only if the membranes are ruptured and the fetal head is low and fixed in the pelvis.

Whereas abnormal FHR tracings have a poor correlation with fetal outcome, FSBS is a strongly positive indicator of outcome. A normal pH (above 7.25) is *always* associated with a good outcome. The converse is also true: a low pH (below 7.2) is *always* associated with a poor outcome.[3] For this reason, FSBS is a necessary adjunct to continuous fetal monitoring.

Controversy over electronic fetal monitoring

As many as 70 percent of all births in the United States are continuously monitored. Although the obstetric community extols the virtues of these techniques, more and more clients are demanding that normal birthing be returned to the family: in the home, birth center, or hospital birthing room.

Although it is true that continuous monitoring decreases perinatal mortality in high-risk clients, there is no research to document the efficacy of these techniques with normal laboring clients. In fact, some studies have documented that intermittent monitoring is a safe alternative, especially when undertaken by specially trained obstetric nurses.[4]

Future research must resolve the following questions:

1. Effects of ultrasound (EMS) on maternal and fetal outcomes.
2. Incidence of morbidity and mortality with IMS.
3. Safety of intermittent monitoring in medically and obstetrically normal births.

Without answers to these questions, clients and caregivers will only become increasingly more polarized and divided in their opinions about electronically controlled childbirth.

The National Institute of Child Health and Human Development has adopted the following guidelines for nurses, nurse-midwives, and physicians in order to promote family-centered care regardless of the modality of fetal assessment:[5]

1. Neither electronic fetal monitoring (EFM) nor any other technology should ever be used as a substitute for clinical judgment. EFM is only one parameter of fetal assessment.

2. The proper use of both intermittent auscultation and continuous EFM in both high- and low-risk clients should, at the onset, include a discussion with the client of her wishes, concerns, and questions concerning the benefits, limitations, and risks of fetal monitoring. Women should have the opportunity to discuss the use of all forms of monitoring during the course of prenatal care, and again upon admission to the labor suite. The use of all forms of monitoring should be accompanied by supportive and knowledgeable personnel who are attentive to the client's expectations regarding the conduct of her labor. Hospital personnel should be cognizant of the potential impact of EFM on family-centered childbirth.

3. Periodic auscultation of the FHR (for 30 seconds every 15 minutes during the second stage, immediately after a contraction) is an acceptable method for assessing fetal distress. Interpretation of auscultated FHR data should include an understanding of the relationship of FHR changes to uterine contractions.

(Although the weight of current evidence does not show any benefit in EFM use in low-risk clients, under certain circumstances, clients or physicians may choose to use EFM in such cases.)

4. The use of EFM should be strongly considered in high-risk clients. Some of the high-risk situations may include (*a*) low birth weight, prematurity, postmaturity, and intrauterine growth re-

tardation; (b) medical complications of pregnancy; (c) meconium staining of the amniotic fluid; (d) intrapartum obstetric complications; (e) the use of oxygen in labor; and (f) the presence of abnormal auscultatory findings. The medical record should reflect careful consideration of the benefits and risks to each individual, including a discussion of the indications for EFM.

5. Because unexpected risk factors may arise during labor in clients without prior evidence of risk, all hospitals and birth centers that provide maternity care should have the necessary trained staff and equipment to assess carefully the status of each fetus in labor and to take appropriate actions.

6. For EFM to be used appropriately, the health care professions should encourage, through their various educational modalities, a thorough understanding of the principles and procedures of intrapartum FHR assessment by all personnel responsible for the care of pregnant women. Special attention should be given to the benefits, limitations, and risks of each mode of assessment. Acquisition of expertise in the use of continuous FHR and intrauterine pressure data requires the opportunity for supervised practical training in the interpretation of monitor tracings, the use of FSBS, and the integration of such data into the clinical setting.

7. The use of FSBS pH determination is strongly encouraged as an adjunct to EFM.

8. Attention to the known potential hazards of EFM should accompany its use. The placement of the fetal scalp electrode and intrauterine pressure catheter should be performed with attention to aseptic and atraumatic technique. The client should avoid staying in the supine position for prolonged periods, and maternal mobility should not be unnecessarily limited.

9. Hospital personnel should be cognizant of the potential impact of EFM on family-centered childbirth. Family-centered care and indicated intrapartum fetal monitoring are not mutually exclusive. Maternity services should be encouraged to integrate the concepts of family-centered care with the care of women who are electronically monitored.

Women's response to electronic monitoring

It has been documented that all women who were electronically monitored expressed a need for the nurse to remain with them.[6] It has also been found that women with a history of poor obstetric outcomes are more accepting of electronic monitoring, whereas women who are medically and obstetrically normal view it as an interference and an invasion of privacy.[6]

REFERENCES

1. Hon. 28.
2. Columbia Presbyterian Medical Center.
3. Petrie and Pollack.
4. Haverkamp.
5. National Institute of Child Health and Human Development. III165-167.
6. Shields.

REFERENCES

1. ...
2. ...
3. ...
4. ...
5. ...

CHAPTER 19

THE POSTPARTUM PERIOD

Smriti Panwar

The postpartum period is a time of rapid physiological and psychological changes: the mother's body quickly returns to the non-pregnant state, and the family begins to incorporate its new member into its system. This chapter discusses the normal adaptations as well as some common deviations from the norm that occur during the first 6 weeks after delivery. Nursing assessments, nursing actions, and anticipatory guidance for the postpartum family are also included.

ANATOMIC ADAPTATION

Breasts

During pregnancy, the breasts undergo marked changes as a result of increased levels of estrogen and progesterone (which are secreted by the ovary and placenta). Elevated progesterone levels promote the gradual development of breast lobules and alveoli. The increased level of estrogen stimulates the proliferation and development of breast ducts. The high levels of both of these hormones produce an inhibitory effect on prolactin secretion, which results in no milk secretion during pregnancy.

Colostrum — a thin, yellowish premilk fluid — may be expressed from the nipples after the first few months of pregnancy. Colostrum continues to be secreted for the first 3 to 5 days after delivery, gradually changing to milk. Colostrum is richer in protein, minerals, vitamin A, and inorganic salts, but has less sugar and fat, than mature breast milk. It also contains fat globules and high levels of immunoglobulin A.

Delivery results in a sudden drop in estrogen and progesterone levels and a simultaneous rise in the secretion of prolactin by the anterior pituitary. Prolactin stimulates the alveolar cells of the breasts and, thus, promotes milk production. Oxytocin, a posterior pituitary hormone, increases the contractility of the myoepithelial cells that surround the walls of the mammary ducts and stimulates the "let-down reflex," i.e., ejection of milk from the alveolar sacs (Fig. 19-1).

The breasts usually become engorged by the third or fourth post-partum day, mainly as a result of lymphatic and venous stasis, which are normal precursors of lactation. The skin appears shiny and red, and feels warm to the touch, although no fever accompanies this process. The woman may experience a throbbing sensation in her breasts, and breast-feeding may be difficult. Sometimes the glandular breast tissue in the axilla becomes engorged and filled with milk. This engorgement usually lasts for 24 to 48 hours. Thereafter, the breasts are heavy but not uncomfortable. The hard mass in the axilla, if present, gradually disappears, and the milk dries up if the mother is not breast-feeding.

Nursing actions.

1. Explain the possible causes of the discomfort to the client and significant other(s).
2. Reassure her about the limited nature of the discomfort.
3. Encourage the use of support bras, a daily bath, and cleansing of the nipples. Apply lanolin ointment or vitamin E to the nipples.
4. Teach the client arm and upper trunk exercises (Fig. 19-2).

Non-breast-feeding mother:

1. Apply cold packs to the breasts for comfort.
2. Administer analgesics as ordered, if necessary.
3. Teach the mother to avoid stimulating the breasts or expressing milk.

Breast-feeding mother:

1. Encourage regular and frequent feeding. This is the most important measure for relieving pain and establishing lactation.
2. Ensure privacy and a restful feeding environment. Provide emotional support by positive feedback and encouragement.

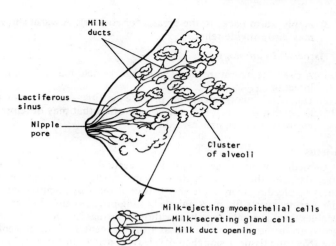

Figure 19-1. Cross section of milk-producing structures in the human breast. The release of oxytocin from the pituitary gland causes the myoepithelial cells to contract and release milk from the gland cells into the milk ducts. *Adapted from* Jensen, M. D., R. C. Benson, and I. M. Boback. Maternity Care. The Nurse and the Family. C. V. Mosby Co., St. Louis. 1981. Second edition. p. 664.

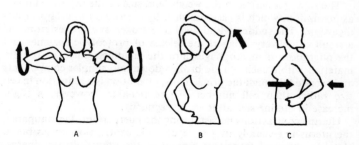

Figure 19-2. Arm and trunk exercises. (A) With hands on shoulders and elbows raised to shoulder height, the client should slowly rotate her elbows in wide circles (to a maximum of 10 rotations). (B) With left hand on hip and right arm raised over the head, the client should bend at the waist to the left and return. Repeat on opposite side (several times on each side). (C) With both hands on hips, the client should push her elbows and shoulders back as far as possible, return to starting position, and repeat several times.

3. Apply warm packs to the breasts for comfort. A warm shower may also provide relief.

Associated pathology.

1. A rise of temperature along with engorgement may be a sign of infection.
2. Unilateral engorgement may precede mastitis — an infection of the breast — which is a rare complication that may develop in mothers who are breast-feeding.

Uterus

Immediately after delivery, the placental site is raised and irregular, and about 8 to 9 centimeters in diameter, with open venous sinuses. Bleeding from large vessels is controlled by compression of the uterine muscle fibers. A unique healing process called exfoliation enables the placental site to heal without scarring. Endometrial tissue grows from the margins as well as from the center of the placental site. Necrotic tissue is sloughed off, leaving a smooth surface. Thus, future pregnancies may implant in any portion of the uterus, and are not limited by scarring.

After delivery, the uterus undergoes a rapid reduction in size and weight. Immediately after delivery, an average uterus weighs about 1,000 grams (2.2 pounds). This decreases to 500 grams (1.1 pounds) 1 week later, and to 350 grams (11 to 12 ounces) 2 weeks after delivery. The rate and amount of reduction vary with parity and the size of the pregnant uterus.

The rapid reduction in the weight and size of the uterus is known as involution, which is accomplished by a process of autolysis (self-digestion). The sudden withdrawal of estrogen and progesterone, as a result of delivery, triggers the release of proteolytic enzymes and the migration of macrophages into the endometrium. The protein materials within each cell are broken down into simpler components and excreted through the urine. Thus, involution is a reduction in cell size rather than cell number. There remains, however, a slight increase in uterine size after each pregnancy.

Uterine contractions persist during the puerperium. In primiparas, the uterus is generally in a state of tonic contraction unless blood clots or placental fragments remain in the uterus. In multiparas, however, the uterus has lost some of its tone. Rather than maintaining a constant state of sustained contractions, the uterus relaxes and contracts at intervals. These may be experienced as marked cramping sensations, which are often called "afterpains." Afterpains are more prominent during suckling of the infant.

Immediately after delivery, the uterus is usually situated approximately 2 centimeters below the umbilicus. On external palpation, it feels firm and about the size of a grapefruit. Within 12 hours after delivery, the fundal height rises to one fingerbreadth (1 centimeter) above the umbilicus. On each succeeding postpartum day, the size of the fundus should reduce by one fingerbreadth. By the end of the first postpartum week, it is palpable at the symphysis pubis. By the end of 2 weeks, it is no longer palpable abdominally (Fig. 19-3).

Nursing actions.

1. Explain the physiological basis of the afterpains. Assess progression of involution.
2. Reassure the client about the limited nature of the discomfort.
3. Teach the client the relief measures for afterpains:
   Teach her to massage her uterus to keep it in a state of sustained contraction.
   Encourage her to lie on her abdomen.
   Encourage her to keep her bladder and bowels empty.
   Reassure her that analgesics are available if she needs them.

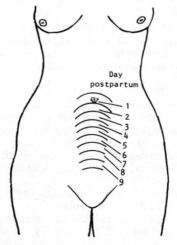

Figure 19-3. Immediately after delivery, the uterus is usually situated approximately 2 centimeters below the umbilicus. Within 12 hours, it rises to one fingerbreadth (1 centimeter) above the umbilicus. It then descends at a rate of 1 cm/day. By the end of the first week, it is palpable at or above the symphysis pubis. By the end of 2 weeks, it is no longer palpable abdominally.

Lochia.

Lochia rubra: The discharge from the uterus immediately after delivery is dark red and present from delivery through the fourth postpartum day. It contains blood and placental and decidual debris. Persistent lochia rubra after the first 4 days may indicate retained placental fragments.

Lochia serosa: The uterine discharge from approximately the 4th until the 10th postpartum day is pinkish, thin, and serosanguineous in consistency. It is composed of serous exudate, shreds of degenerating decidua, erythrocytes, leukocytes, cervical mucus, and numerous microorganisms.

Lochia alba: Lochia alba is creamy white and contains leukocytes and cellular debris. It begins at about the 10th postpartum day, and may last for up to 2 weeks. Continued lochia serosa and/or lochia alba accompanied by fever, pain, and tenderness may indicate endometritis.

Lochia has a fleshy, menstrual odor. An offensive odor usually indicates infection. The amount varies from woman to woman, and with activity. The daily average is between 251 and 271 grams during the first 5 to 6 postpartum days.[1] The amount is gradually reduced to about 2 to 5 g/day.

Nursing actions.

1. Assess the lochia for color, amount, consistency, and odor.
2. Teach the client about the normal amount, color, consistency, and odor, and the progression of lochia.

Associated pathology.

1. Early postpartum hemorrhage (blood loss of 500 milliliters or more during the first 24 hours) may result from uterine atony.
2. Continuous seepage of blood in conjunction with a firm fundus may be indicative of cervical or vaginal lacerations.
3. Late postpartum hemorrhage, occurring after the first 24 hours, is usually a result of retained placental fragments or subinvolution.
4. Foul-smelling lochia accompanied by fever and/or uterine tenderness is indicative of infection.
5. Subinvolution of the uterus is usually caused by infection or retained placental fragments. Occasionally, however, the cause is unknown.

Cervix, vagina, and perineum

After delivery, the *cervix* is spongy, soft, and floppy. By the fifth postpartum day, it has regained its shape. By the end of the first week, the external os is contracted and admits only one fingertip.

The *vagina* appears edematous and bruised, and the introitus gapes when intra-abdominal pressure is increased. Rugae are not present immediately after delivery, but they begin to reappear by the third postpartum week.

The pelvic floor muscles are overstretched and weak. The soft tissues in and around the *perineum* may be edematous and bruised. If an episiotomy was performed, it may be painful because of edema or tension on the sutures. Even if an episiotomy was not performed, the client may experience perineal discomfort.

Nursing actions.

1. Review or teach perineal care. Explain the importance of cleanliness and hand washing before and after perineal care. The client should be taught to wipe from front to back after using the toilet, to apply perineal pads from front to back, and to change perineal pads frequently. If the client had an episiotomy, she should be taught to use the spray bottle to cleanse the perineum, and to pat dry from front to back.
2. Teach the client to tighten her buttocks before sitting to avoid direct trauma to the perineum. The lateral position is also helpful.
3. Apply an ice pack to the perineum for the first 24 postpartum hours to reduce edema and promote comfort.
4. Provide moist heat by means of a sitz bath after the first 24 hours to increase circulation and to promote healing.
5. Use dry heat in the form of heat lamps, if sitz baths are not available.
6. Administer pain medication or topical analgesics (such as witch hazel pads or benzocaine [Dermoplast] spray) as ordered, if necessary.
7. Teach and encourage perineal-tightening exercises. The Kegal exercise, which increases the tone of the pubococcygeal muscle, may be started immediately after delivery. The client is instructed to tighten the muscles of her vagina. (She can learn to contract the correct muscle by stopping and restarting her flow during urination.) She is encouraged to continue the exercise to the count of 10 and to practice it several times a day.

Associated pathology.   Perineal pain that is accompanied by bruising, induration, redness, swelling, and/or a poorly approximated suture line, may indicate infection or hematoma.

Ovulation and menstruation

On average, menstruation returns in non-breast-feeding women within 6 to 8 weeks after delivery. In lactating women, however, menstruation may not begin until the infant is weaned. The first menstrual period is much heavier than normal, and it may be anovulatory. Although the onset of menstruation is no reason to discontinue breast-feeding, lactating women should be reminded that ovulation precedes menstruation, and that a woman may become pregnant while lactating. Hence, contraception should be discussed (*see* Chapter 20).

Nursing actions.

1. Explain to the client when ovulation and menstruation can be expected to occur.
2. Discuss contraception as appropriate.

SYSTEMIC ADAPTATION

Circulatory system

The average blood loss during a vaginal delivery is approximately 400 to 800 milliliters. It is approximately 700 to 1,000 milliliters in a cesarean section. Total blood volume continues to be high during the first week of the puerperium, but, by the third week after delivery, the hypervolemia characteristic of pregnancy has resolved.

Laboratory blood values should approximate prepregnancy values within 1 week postpartum. During the first week of the puerperium, the leukocyte count and sedimentation rate remain high. By the end of the first week, they return to normal. Hemodynamic changes occur rapidly in the first 3 days postpartum, and hemoglobin and hematocrit levels may be unreliable indicators of red blood cell status.

The hormones of pregnancy increase the activation of blood coagulation factors — an effect that persists during the postpartum period. Immobility, sepsis, and trauma further predispose the client to thromboembolitic disease. Superficial varicosities that developed during pregnancy will persist and continue to require special attention. However, with the decrease in blood volume, the decrease in progesterone, and the decrease in venous stasis caused by uterine compression, there will be some improvement in the varicose veins after childbirth.

Diaphoresis in the form of night sweats and heavy sweating during the day is frequent and may continue for as long as 3 weeks after delivery. Diaphoresis is one mechanism of eliminating the excess fluid accumulated during pregnancy.

Nursing actions.
Diaphoresis:

1. Explain the possibility of postpartum diaphoresis occurring.
2. Reassure the client about the limited nature of her discomfort.

3. Teach the client to stay out of drafts and wear adequate clothing.
4. Assist the client with her daily bath and frequent clothing and bed linen changes.
5. Ensure that the client maintains adequate fluid intake.

Varicose veins and the prevention of thromboembolism:

1. Explain the possible causes of varicose veins and the prognosis for improvement.
2. Encourage ambulation.
3. Encourage the client to rest her feet firmly on the floor or on a chair while sitting on her side of the bed. Encourage her to avoid dangling her feet or sitting with her legs crossed.
4. Encourage the client to elevate her legs while lying down.
5. *See* Chapter 6.

Associated pathology.

1. The increased activation of clotting factors, together with immobility, trauma, and/or sepsis, predispose the client to thromboembolism. Signs and symptoms of thromboembolism include redness, pain, warmth, a cordlike sensation, and a positive Homans's sign.
2. A significant drop in hemoglobin and hematocrit levels indicates abnormal blood loss. A four- to five-point drop in hematocrit represents 1 pint of blood loss.
3. A persistently elevated leukocyte count, together with a rise in temperature, indicates infection.

Gastrointestinal system

The client may be hungry after delivery and may enjoy a light meal. Postpartum bowels are sluggish because of (1) decreased gastrointestinal motility, which may be a result of the stress of labor and delivery or of the analgesia/anesthesia administered during labor; (2) relaxed abdominal muscles; (3) an empty bowel, as a result of a cleansing enema, if used, and a lack of solid food intake during labor; (4) dehydration; and/or (5) perineal pain. Hemorrhoids are varicose veins of the rectum. They frequently develop in late pregnancy from the pressure on the veins below the level of the uterus. Pushing during the second stage of labor may exacerbate this condition.

Nursing actions.
Constipation:

1. Explain the possible causes of the discomfort to the client. Reassure her about the integrity of the perineum, as appropriate.

2. Reassure her about the limited nature of the discomfort.
3. Encourage the client to prevent constipation and gas by increasing fluids.
4. Encourage the client to eat a diet high in roughage and natural laxative foods.
5. Encourage ambulation and postpartum exercises (Fig. 19-4).
6. Administer laxatives or an enema as ordered, if necessary.

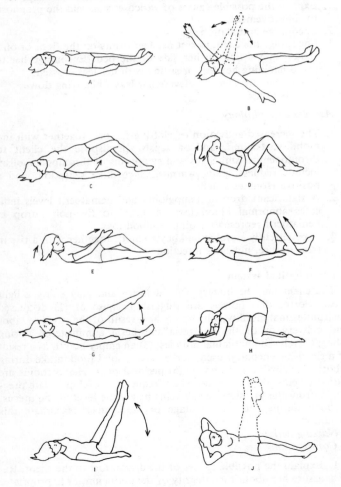

Hemorrhoids:

1. Explain what hemorrhoids are and their possible causes.
2. Reassure the client about the limited nature of her discomfort.
3. Teach measures to prevent and/or relieve constipation (*see* Chapter 6).
4. Apply a cold compress (e.g., a cold witch hazel compress) to reduce swelling.
5. Encourage the client to take sitz baths with the water temperature maintained at about 38 °C (100 °F) for 20 minutes.
6. Teach the client how to replace the hemorrhoids in the ano-rectal canal. Encourage the client to repeat the replacement procedure after bowel movements, or as necessary.
7. Encourage Sims's or the prone position while the client is in bed.
8. Administer analgesics as ordered, if necessary.

Associated pathology.   A client who has had a fourth-degree perineal laceration (laceration through the rectal mucosa) should not receive any rectal treatments, e.g., enema, rectal temperature, or suppository. She should have at least one bowel movement before being discharged from the hospital.

Urinary system

Diuresis occurs during the first 12 to 24 hours postpartum and may last as long as 5 days. The urinary output is up to 3,000 ml/day. This

---

Figure 19-4. Postpartum exercises. (A) Day 1: Breathe deeply, expanding the abdomen. Slowly exhale and draw in the abdominal muscles. (B) Day 2: Assume a supine position with legs slightly parted. Place arms at right angles to torso and slowly raise them, keeping the elbows stiff. Gradually return to original position and repeat. (C) Day 3: Assume a supine position with arms at the side. Draw knees up slightly and arch back. (D) Day 4: With knees and hips flexed, lift head and pelvis upward and contract buttocks. (E) Day 5: With legs straight, raise head and left knee slightly. Reach for, but do not touch, knee with right hand. Repeat with other leg and hand. (F) Day 6: On back, flex one knee and thigh toward abdomen. Lower foot toward buttocks, then straighten and lower the leg. (G) Day 7: In supine position, with toes pointed and knees straight, raise one leg and then the other as high as possible, using abdominal muscles to slowly lower. (H) Day 8: On elbows and knees, keep elbows and lower legs together. Hump back upward (cat position), contracting buttocks and drawing in abdomen. Relax and breathe deeply. (I) Day 9: Same as for day 7, but lift both legs at once. (J) Day 10: In supine position, with hands clasped behind head, sit up and lie back slowly. (Feet may be hooked under furniture, at first.)

mechanism, whereby tissue fluid is eliminated, is also referred to as the reversal of the water metabolism of pregnancy. It is important to differentiate between frequent urination (associated with increased urinary output) and urinary frequency (associated with urinary tract infection). Urinary frequency accompanied by suprapubic or costo-vertebral angle pain, fever, urinary retention, hematuria, or dysuria often signifies urinary tract infection and indicates the need for urine analysis, urine culture, bacterial sensitivity tests, and, probably, wide-spectrum antibiotic therapy. Postpartum diuresis is increased in women with preeclampsia-eclampsia, hypertension, and/or diabetes. Hematuria secondary to bladder trauma may occur. Acetonuria may be present in clients with a prolonged labor, dehydration, or diabetes. Proteinuria is present in approximately 40 percent of all women after delivery, and it may persist for 3 days.

The dilation of the ureters and the renal pelves resolves by the end of the fourth postpartum week. Urinary retention may occur after delivery, and the bladder is usually edematous and hyperemic. Other contributing factors are in increased bladder capacity secondary to an increased intra-abdominal capacity; a decreased sensitivity to fluid pressure as a result of analgesia/anesthesia administration; swelling and bruising of the tissues around the urethra secondary to birth trauma; and an inability to void in the recumbent position.

Nursing actions.
Diuresis:

1. Explain the possible causes of the discomfort to the client.
2. Reassure her about the limited nature of the discomfort.
3. Check her bladder frequently, and encourage the client to empty her bladder when it is full (usually within the first 2 hours). Encourage her to empty her bladder frequently thereafter.
4. Encourage ambulation and fluid intake.
5. Maintain a record of intake and output until the client is able to completely empty her bladder with each voiding.

Urinary retention:

1. Observe for signs of bladder distention and residual urine.
2. Use nursing measures to encourage voiding.
   Encourage voiding while in a warm shower or sitz bath, or while running warm water over the perineum.
   Encourage the client to void while blowing bubbles through a straw in a glass of water.
   Place peppermint oil in her bedpan.
   Encourage the client to void while listening to the sound of running water.

Assist her to the bathroom to void.
Place her hands in a pan of warm water.
3. Encourage ambulation and fluid intake.
4. Catheterize the client, if necessary. A urine specimen may be obtained and sent for culture and sensitivity to rule out bacilluria.

Associated pathology.

1. With urinary stasis, there is an increased incidence of urinary tract infection. Symptoms of urinary tract infection include dysuria, hematuria, suprapubic or costovertebral angle pain, and fever.
2. A full bladder reduces uterine contractility and, therefore, increases blood loss and the possibility of postpartum hemorrhage.

Weight loss

Immediately after delivery, the client's weight will have decreased by approximately 4.5 to 5.4 kilograms (10 to 12 pounds), which is accounted for by the weight of the baby, the placenta, and the amniotic fluid. A loss of an additional 2.3 kilograms (5 pounds) occurs during the early puerperium as a result of diuresis.

During pregnancy, the body stores 2.3 to 3.2 kilograms (5 to 7 pounds) of fat — 14,000 to 24,000 calories — for lactation needs. A lactating mother will gradually utilize this fat store over the first 4 to 6 months, and she will return to her approximate prepregnancy weight during this period. A nonlactating mother, however, without the demand of breast-feeding, tends to retain some of the excess weight gained during pregnancy.

Nursing actions.

1. Explain to the client the process of gradual return to prepregnant weight.
2. Encourage good dietary habits.
3. Encourage postpartum exercise (*see* Fig. 19-4).

Associated pathology.

1. Little or no weight loss may be due to fluid retention or poor dietary habits.
2. Extreme weight loss may indicate systemic illness or poor postpartum psychological adjustment, or it may reflect excessive dieting.

Endocrine system

During pregnancy, the placenta produces estrogen, progesterone, human chorionic gonadotrophin, human placental lactogen, human chorionic somatomammotrophin, and thyrotrophin. Placental hormones inhibit the production of prolactin and gonadotrophic hormones. Hormone production from the thyroid and adrenal glands is increased (see Chapter 2).

After delivery, with the source of placental hormones being gone, the levels of those hormones decrease. During the first postpartum day there is a reduction in human chorionic gonadotrophin and estrogen. During the first week, there is a reduction in the production of estrone, estradiol, and progesterone. During the second or third week there is a reduction in estriol levels.[2]

With the decrease in placental hormones, prolactin is allowed to increase immediately after delivery and gonadotrophic hormones increase within the first 3 to 4 weeks. Oxytocin production is stimulated by infant suckling in the breast-feeding client. The levels of thyroid hormone peak at delivery, fluctuate widely for the first few postpartum days, then gradually decrease to normal nonpregnant levels. The decrease in human placental lactogen and chorionic somatomammotrophin causes a relative deficiency in anti-insulin activity, which leads to low fasting plasma glucose levels, decreased insulin requirements in diabetic clients, and difficulty in interpreting the results of glucose tolerance tests. The levels of corticoid decrease immediately, and 17-ketosteroids decrease to normal levels within the first few days after delivery.

BREAST-FEEDING

Lactation

Lactation is a complex process. It is the end result of numerous interacting factors, including the health and nutrition status of the mother, the health status of the newborn, and the development of the breast tissue under the influence of estrogen and progesterone. The mechanism of milk production and ejection (let-down reflex) is controlled by secretions of the endocrine glands — particularly the pituitary hormones, prolactin and oxytocin — and is influenced by sucking and maternal emotions.

The establishment and maintenance of lactation are determined by the following factors (see Fig. 19-1):

1. The anatomic structure of the mammary glands and the development of alveoli.
2. The initiation and maintenance of milk secretion.
3. The ejection and propulsion of milk from the alveoli to the nipple.[3]

Stages of lactation

Milk initiation (lactogenesis). Lactogenesis begins during the latter part of pregnancy with the production of colostrum as a result of stimulation of mammary alveolar cells by placental lactogen, a prolactin-like substance. The amount of colostrum secretion may vary from 5 to 15 milliliters at each feeding during the first few days postpartum.

Colostrum is very high in immunoglobulin A (IgA), a type of antibody secreted by lymphocytes and plasma cells. Although the functions of IgA are not clearly understood, it seems to provide protection against infection of the respiratory and gastrointestinal tracts and the eyes. IgA does not cross the placental barrier, and, unlike other immunoglobulins, it is not affected by gastric action. Consequently, colostrum may be an important source of passive immunity for the breast-feeding infant. Early breast-feeding should be encouraged to provide the infant with passive immunity and to stimulate milk production.

Milk secretion. The secretion of milk is a process of extrusion of milk from acini cells. This process depends on two factors: sufficient production of the anterior pituitary hormone, prolactin, which is under the control of the hypothalamus (Fig. 19-5), and maternal nutrition. After lactation is initiated, continued lactation depends on suckling, which inhibits the release of prolactin-inhibiting factor. Thus, prolactin is produced and stimulates milk production.

The mother will need 20 grams of protein and 500 extra calories over nonpregnant dietary requirements. She needs approximately 3,000 milliliters of fluids each day to maintain adequate milk production. Vitamin and mineral requirements are also higher during lactation. For example, the breast-feeding mother needs approximately 50 percent more calcium, phosphorus, magnesium, and zinc. (Vitamin and mineral supplementation for the breast-feeding mother is common.) Complete recommended dietary allowances are listed in Table 19-1.

In addition, many medications are excreted in breast milk, whereas others affect the production of milk. For a complete discussion of the effects of medications during the breast-feeding and postpartum periods, *see* Appendix A.

Milk ejection. A neurohormonal mechanism (the let-down reflex) causes ejection of milk from alveoli where it is secreted through the milk ducts, to the lactiferous sinuses, and, finally, to the nipple (Fig. 19-6). Sucking on the nipple causes oxytocin to be released from the posterior pituitary, which causes increased contractility of the myoepithelial cells surrounding the alveoli and the

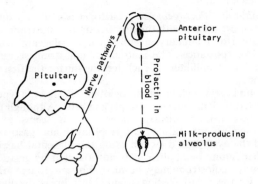

Figure 19-5. Simplifed illustration of suckling, leading to stimulation of the anterior pituitary, leading to the production of prolaction, resulting in the stimulation of milk-producing alveoli. *Adapted from* Jensen, M. D., R. C. Benson, and I. M. Bobak. Maternity Care. The Nurse and the Family. C. V. Mosby Co., St. Louis. 1981. Second edition. p. 665.

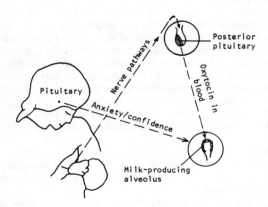

Figure 19-6. Simplified illustration of the let-down reflex. Sucking of the nipple causes oxytocin to be released from the posterior pituitary, which causes increased contractility of the myoepithelial cells (*see* Fig. 19-1), resulting in the production of milk. *Adapted from* Jensen, M. D., R. C. Benson, and I. M. Bobak. Maternity Care. The Nurse and the Family. C. V. Mosby Co., St. Louis. 1981. Second edition. p. 665.

TABLE 19-1

Nutrients in Breast Milk and Recommended Dietary Allowances

Nutrient	Estimated content in 850 ml of milk	Recommended dietary allowances		
		Woman (19-22 yr)	Lactating woman (19-22 yr)	Percentage increase
Calories	635	2,100	2,600	24
Protein, g	10	44	64	45
Calcium, mg	275	800	1,200	50
Phosphorus, mg	120	800	1,200	50
Iodine, μg	40	150	200	33
Iron, mg	0.4	18	*	*
Magnesium, mg	33	300	450	50
Zinc, mg	3	15	25	67
Vitamin A, μg RE	420	800	1,200	50
Vitamin D, μg	0.5	7.5	12.5	67
Vitamin E, mg α-TE	1.8	8	11	38
Ascorbic acid, mg	40	60	100	67
Folacin, μg	40	400	500	25
Niacin, mg	1.4	14	19	36
Riboflavin, mg	0.3	1.3	1.8	38
Thiamin, mg	0.1	1.1	1.6	45
Vitamin B6, mg	0.1	2.0	2.5	25
Vitamin B12, μg	0.2	3.0	4.0	33

RE, retinol equivalents; TE, tocopherol equivalents.

*Iron needs during lactation are not substantially different from those of the nonpregnant woman, but continued supplementation for 2 to 3 months postpartum is advisable.

walls of the mammary ducts and results in the ejection of milk. After lactation is established, psychological factors, such as the sound of the infant's cry, may stimulate the let-down reflex.

Other factors that may affect breast-feeding

Positive maternal emotions about and attitude toward breast-feeding are important considerations in achieving successful lactation. The client needs support from health care providers and her family while establishing breast-feeding. She may also benefit from an extended breast-feeding support network that she can contact, if problems with breast-feeding arise after discharge from the hospital.

Milk production is diminished by the repeated inhibition of the let-down reflex, by failing to empty the breasts frequently and completely, and by stress or other negative emotions. Frequent breast-feeding, every 2 to 3 hours, may restore lactation for mothers who have received drugs to suppress lactation.[4]

Variation in milk production

Colostrum is gradually replaced by milk. The beginning of milk production may coincide with, but is not the cause of, breast engorgement (see p. 446). In the primipara, milk production usually begins on approximately the third postpartum day. Multiparas who have breast-fed previously may start producing milk as early as 24 hours postpartum. Milk production is controlled by supply and demand. Mothers who feed early and more frequently may experience earlier milk production. The production of prolactin diminishes after several weeks of breast-feeding. The subsequent mechanism of milk production is not clear.

PARENT-CHILD ATTACHMENT

The attachment bond has been defined as a unique relationship between two people that is specific and endures through time.[5] Various theories have been expounded to explain the basis for attachment behavior. Freudian psychoanalytic theorists believe that the development of the bond between the infant and the mother is the result of the mother's desire to satisfy the innate needs of her infant; i.e., to socialize with another human being and to have the physical need for survival met.

According to other observers, the concept of attachment also includes the concept of mutuality, which has been described as a corresponding set of maternal behaviors in response to infant behaviors and characteristics. For example, signaling behaviors of the infant, such as crying, cooing, and smiling, usually result in the reduction of the discomfort of the mother (or the primary caretaker). Whereas other behaviors, such as rooting, sucking, grasping, and postural adjustment, encourage physical contact. (For an indepth discussion of maternal-infant attachment, *see* Chapter 14.)

MATERNAL CONCERNS OF THE POSTPARTUM PERIOD

The early postpartum days are a period of great social and psychological stress. The mother may be both happy about the baby's birth and concerned about the responsibilities of motherhood.

Taking-in phase

The taking-in phase is a time when the new mother "takes in" care and support from others. She is not yet ready to provide care for her baby — not until her own needs are met. In the postpartum period, the mother is initially preoccupied with her self, food, and sleep. The mother exhibits passivity and dependence, and is emotionally labile. She may be concerned about her mood changes and become tearful with the slightest provocation. Transient postpartum blues are a common occurrence because of the reduced physical reserves (low hemoglobin and hematocrit, poor nutrition, and inadequate rest), hormonal changes, and role-change adjustment. This phase lasts about 2 or 3 days.

Taking-hold phase

On the second or third day postpartum, the mother is ready to take charge of her life and is eager to succeed as a "good mother." This is the beginning of the taking-hold phase. She is now concerned about her bowel and bladder functions. A breast-feeding mother is concerned about the quality of her breast milk and her ability to successfully breast-feed her infant.[6]

Nursing actions.

1. Explain the possible causes of emotional stresses to the client and significant other(s).
2. Assess the maternal support systems and encourage rooming-in, if possible.
3. Reassure the significant other(s) about the limited nature of the mother's change of moods.
4. Provide a therapeutic environment and protect the client's privacy. Allow time for readjustment. Restrict or select visitors if necessary. Arrange a visit from her labor and delivery nurse.[6]
5. Create an unhurried atmosphere. Evaluate the client's readiness to talk, listen, and learn. Evaluate her readiness to assume responsibilities for personal and infant care.

6. Encourage and teach the parents to perform the actual care of the baby. Provide any necessary guidance and support, and demonstrate confidence in their abilities. Encourage and answer questions.
7. Enhance the client's physical reserves by providing a restful environment, good nutrition, and iron and vitamin supplementation, as ordered.
8. Observe for signs of excessive mood swings, sleeplessness, anorexia, frequent tearfulness, and a feeling of depression.

Associated pathology. Depression, frequent tearfulness, and persistent apathy toward the newborn may indicate postpartum psychosis or the possibility of child abuse in the future.

NURSING MANAGEMENT IN THE POSTPARTUM PERIOD

Immediate postpartum care

The initial objective of nursing care in the immediate postpartum period (after the fourth stage) is to safely receive the mother and her baby on the postpartum unit. The nurse should establish an initial physical and psychological data base, on which the nursing care plan will be based (Table 19-2). The mother should be oriented to the unit and introduced to any other mothers sharing the room. The call bell, unit routine, and bathroom privileges should be explained. The mother should be made comfortable, with analgesics provided as needed. At this time, the mother might feel refreshed by a bath. She may be hungry, or she may need to sleep. She may be anxious for an undisturbed period of time with her infant and/or significant other. The nurse's primary responsibilities are to promote establishment of the family unit, to assist the mother during her recovery process, and to observe for signs and symptoms of maladaptation.

Establishing a nursing data base. The nurse must obtain a complete data base on which to base her nursing care plan for the postpartum mother. The information needed for the data base comes from the client's history, physical examination, and laboratory data. The following nursing actions and information will help the nurse to establish a sound data base:

1. Receive report:
   Labor and delivery course: gravidity and parity, type of delivery, time of birth, complications during labor and delivery, administration of medications, type of analgesia/anesthesia, type and condition of episiotomy/lacerations, and blood loss.
   Postpartum course: nutrition and excretion status, treatments, physical examination findings (including breasts, abdomen, uterus, lochia, perineum, and vital signs).

Infant status: health of the baby, sex of the baby, and method of feeding planned.

Psychosocial status: support systems and reactions to the baby and parenting.

2. Review records:

History: family history, medical-surgical history, obstetric history, history of this antepartum course.

Physical examination: pertinent findings from antepartum or intrapartum physical examinations.

Laboratory data: rubella titer, blood type and Rh factor, and other pertinent data.

Psychosocial data: pertinent findings from antepartum or intrapartum course.

3. Perform an admission physical assessment:

General condition: color, affect, posture, energy level, and skin and mucous membrane status.

Vital signs: temperature, pulse, respirations, and blood pressure.

Uterus: consistency, size, location, and client's assessment of discomfort.

Lochia: amount, color, presence of clots, and odor.

Bladder: presence of distention.

Perineum: redness, edema, ecchymosis, discharge, and approximation.

Extremities: Homans's sign, edema, redness, tenderness, and increased skin temperature.

Breasts: examine both breasts for size, shape, masses, and tenderness. Examine the nipples for size, shape, and the presence of colostrum.

Pain and discomfort: degree of pain and discomfort.

4. Psychological assessment:

Client's general attitude.

Client's fatigue level, sense of satisfaction, and feeling of competence.

5. Chart findings.

Subsequent care during the hospital stay

After the client has been safely received on the postpartum unit, a nursing care plan should be developed. Nursing care should focus on (1) supporting the mother's return to the nonpregnant state during the recovery period, (2) observing and identifying deviations from the norm, and (3) educating the mother/family to prepare her/them for independent self-care and for baby care after discharge.

In order to support the mother both physiologically and psycho-

TABLE 19-2

Postpartum Nursing Care Plan

Assessment	Normal findings	Problems	Interventions	Teaching and guidance
Maternal vital signs. (Assess every 4-8 hr.)				
Temperature	36.2-37.6 °C (97.2-99.7°F).	Fever.	Record and report findings.	Encourage increased fluid intake.
Pulse	60-90 beats/min.	Tachycardia or bradycardia.	Record and report findings.	Encourage rest in bed.
Respirations	16-20 respirations/min.	Hyperpnea.	Record and report findings.	Encourage rest in bed.
Blood pressure	100/60-140/90.	Hypertension or hypotension.	Record and report findings.	Inform the client about orthostatic hypotension. Instruct her to sit down if she feels faint. Assist her during her first time out of bed.
Laboratory findings. (Assess on the second day.)				
Hemoglobin	2 mg less than on admission.	Blood loss.	Observe, record, and report signs of hemorrhage. Send blood specimen for cross-match, as ordered.	Explain therapeutic regimen, including bed rest, increased fluid intake, diet, and iron and vitamin supplementation.
Hematocrit	Less than a 3 ml/100 ml drop since admission.			

Urine (Findings for catheterized specimen.)	No red blood cells or bacteria. Specific gravity of 1.020. Glycosuria or acetonuria may be present in the first 3 days.	Urinary tract infection. Symptoms include the presence of bacteria, white blood cells, and a specific gravity of greater than 1.020.	Observe, report, and record laboratory findings or other symptoms of urinary tract infection to the clinician.	Explain the therapeutic regimen, including bed rest and increased fluid intake.
Nutrition. (Provide from soon after delivery onward.)	Light or regular diet tolerated.	Anorexia.	Observe, report, and record dietary intake. Elicit special nutritional needs or preferences of the client. Consult with dietitian and arrange for attractively served meals, in a calm atmosphere. Assess whether psychological factors are interfering with dietary intake.	Explain the importance of a balanced diet, fluids, and roughage. Emphasize the need for an additional 500 cal, 25 g of protein, and 200 mg of ascorbic acid for healing.
Rest and activity. (Assess individual need for rest.)	Rests for 6-8 hr after delivery. Gradually resumes activities of daily living.	Fatigue.	Evaluate individual rest needs. Organize daily activities to promote rest. Provide rest periods before breast-feeding. Encourage rooming-in client to rest while her baby sleeps. Initiate activities gradually. Encourage exercise.	Teach the client to evaluate and regulate her activities. (1) Adequate rest and exercise, (2) light housekeeping at home after first week, (3) moderate housekeeping after second week, and (4) full activity after postpartum examina-

Assessment	Normal findings	Problems	Interventions	Teaching and guidance
				tion. Resume employment after 4-6 wk. Encourage postpartum exercises (see Fig. 19-3). Assist in organizing her day for rest periods.
Body weight. After delivery	Loses 4.5-5.4 kg (10-12 lb).	Anorexia. Weight retention/weight gain.	Anorexia: see above. Weight retention/gain: take diet history, review activity patterns, assess whether psychological factors are interfering with dietary intake.	Discuss nutritional requirements. Teach and encourage postpartum exercises. Refer to support group for weight reduction. Encourage medical consultation before beginning any dietary restrictions.
First 3-4 days	Loses an additional 1.8-2.3 kg (4-5 lb).			
4-6 mo	Loses approximately 10.9-12.7 kg (24-28 lb) total.			
Elimination status. Bladder	Voids copious amounts.	Difficulty in elimination: bladder distention or residual urine.	Encourage voiding every 6-8 hr. Monitor intake and output. Evaluate bladder distention. Assist client	Encourage frequent bladder emptying, and explain importance of doing so. Encourage increased fluid intake.

			to bathroom. Pour warm water over her perineum and/or leave faucet running to encourage voiding. Catheterize, if necessary.	Encourage ambulation. Review relaxation techniques.
		Urinary tract infection. (Symptoms: frequency, urgency, dysuria, nocturia, fever, and increased pulse rate.)	Observe, record, and report to the physician. Send clean-catch or catheterized specimen to the laboratory for microscopic examination and culture and sensitivity. Institute antibiotic therapy and administer antispasmodic or analgesic agents on physician's order. Breast-feeding may be curtailed (depending on the choice of antibiotic).	Encourage increased fluid intake. Encourage the client to rest and maintain good nutritional status. (See nursing relief measures for urinary tract infection in Chapter 15.) Explain the rationale for decision regarding breast-feeding.
Bowels	Defecates spontaneously by the third day.	Constipation and/or flatulence.	Encourage normal bowel movement. Administer laxatives or enemas as ordered, if necessary.	Teach the importance of regular bowel habits. Encourage dietary intake of fresh fruits, roughage, and natural laxative foods. Encourage an increased fluid intake and ambulation.

Assessment	Normal findings	Problems	Interventions	Teaching and guidance
Breasts. (Assess daily for tenderness, redness, warmth, firmness, and lactogenesis.)	Increased secretion of colostrum, changing to milk.	Engorgement on second or third postpartum day. (Symptoms: fullness, tenderness, and prominent venous pattern.)	Provide appropriate relief measures. Breast-feeding clients: frequent feedings, warm compress, manual or mechanical expression of milk, support brassiere, and ointment and exposure to air for cracked nipple (see below).	Encourage rest and relaxation. Help the father or other support people to support the client in her efforts to breast-feed. Teach the client self-help comfort measures.
			Non-breast-feeding clients: medication to suppress lactation on physician's order, cold compress, avoidance of breast stimulation, avoidance of manual expression of milk, and administration of analgesics as ordered.	Reassure the client. Encourage ambulation and arm exercises. Teach the client self-help comfort measures.
		Sore or cracked nipples.	Provide measures for relief or prevention: proper breast hygiene (i.e., no harsh soap, alcohol, or iodine), change of position for nursing, exposure to air, and suckling on sore breast last.	Teach the client proper nursing techniques: to break suction correctly before removing the baby from the breast, to be sure that the baby grasps entire areola in his or her mouth, and to avoid suckling on an empty breast.

Uterine involution. (Assess size, location, consistency, and tenderness every 2 hr for the first 8 hr, and then every 8 hr.)	Fundus found in the midline, firm and well contracted.	Uterine atony. (Symptom: boggy, soft uterus.)	Observe, record, and report height and consistency of the fundus. Ascertain whether the client's bladder is empty. Gently massage the uterus until well contracted.	Explain the importance of frequent emptying of the bladder. Encourage ambulation. Encourage the client to keep her hand on her abdomen to help uterine contraction. Encourage the client to lie in the prone position.
		Afterbirth pains.	Check bladder for fullness. Expel clots from the uterus. Administer mild analgesics on physician's order, as necessary.	Explain the cause of the pains and reassure the client. Encourage the prone position and ambulation. Encourage breathing and relaxation exercises. Teach the client to massage her fundus to keep it well contracted.
Lochia. (Assess for color, amount, clots, and odor.)	Bright red, no clots, fleshy odor. No more than eight perineal pads saturated per day.	Hemorrhage with atonic uterus.	Observe, record, and report to the physician. Obtain blood pressure every 15 min. Encourage breast-feeding. Count perineal pads used. Evaluate size of clots. Administer continuous infusion of fluids and oxytocin on order. Administer intramuscular	Explain each procedure, with reassurance, as appropriate.

Assessment	Normal findings	Problems	Interventions	Teaching and guidance
			injections of methylergonovine maleate or ergonovine maleate as directed by the physician. Prepare the client for return to the surgical area for investigation for possible retained products of conception. Monitor vital signs.	
		Endometritis. (Symptoms: uterine tenderness, scanty lochia, and foul odor or lochia.)	Observe, record, and report position and consistency of the uterus and the characteristics of the lochia. Administer antibiotics on the physician's order. Monitor vital signs.	Explain to and reassure the client, as appropriate. Review hand washing and perineal hygiene. Encourage increased fluid intake, rest, and sleep. Teach the client to maintain a good nutritional status, including a source of ascorbic acid.
Perineum. (Assess every 8 hr. Assess episiotomy for REEDA.)	Tissue is approximated, with minimal edema.	Perineal trauma.	Apply cold pack during first 24 hr. Thereafter, apply heat. Provide analgesic spray such as Dermoplast. Perform a culture on indication. Monitor vital signs.	Encourage proper perineal care: wash hands before perineal care, cleanse from front to back, use blotting motion when drying the area, and perform perineal exercises.

Assessment	Normal findings	Deviations and nursing interventions	Health teaching
Legs. (Assess daily for warmth, tenderness, and Homans's sign.)	No complaints. Negative Homans's sign.	Hemorrhoids. — Observe, record, and report presence. Provide sitz baths, witch hazel pads, and ointment. Administer stool softener to prevent constipation as ordered.	Encourage prone position. Teach the client how to avoid constipation.
		Thrombosis. (Symptoms: pain, local warmth and redness, cordlike sensation, and positive Homans's sign.) — Observe, record, and report symptoms of thrombosis. Apply elastic bandages or support hose. Avoid administering estrogens to suppress lactation. Confine the client to bed with affected limb elevated on pillows. Administer medications as ordered.	Explain therapeutic regimen and rationale.
Immune system. (Evaluate rubella titer, blood type, and Rh factor.)	All findings are normal (see Appendix B).	Susceptible to rubella and/or Rh-negative blood type. — Observe, record, and report symptoms of allergies. Administer rubella vaccine if mother is not already immune. Administer RhoGAM within 72 hr of delivery, if appropriate (see Appendix A).	Emphasize the mandatory use of contraception for 3 mo after rubella vaccination. Teach the client the reason for RhoGAM administration and its implications for future childbearing.

Assessment	Normal findings	Problems	Interventions	Teaching and guidance
Psychological adjustment. (Assess daily for problem cues.)	Has visitors who are supportive, happy, or anxious. Willing to learn and provide care for herself and her infant. Concerned about bowel, bladder, and breast functioning. Positive mother-infant interaction. Experiences mood changes and transient postpartum blues.	Prolonged postpartum blues (depression). (Symptoms: excessive fatigue, excessive preoccupation with self, poor mother-infant interaction, low self-esteem, marital problems, lack of support system, and current family crisis.)	Observe, record, and report any abnormal findings. Refer the client to a public health (or other appropriate) agency. Support ventilation of maternal feelings. Discuss appropriateness of psychiatric referral with the physician.	Reassure the client that mood swings and negative feelings are normal in the immediate postpartum period.

REEDA, redness, edema, ecchymosis, discharge, and approximation (of the perineum) (*see* p. 465).

logically during the recovery period, the nurse must provide for rest, exercise, and graduated activities; for nutrition, hydration, and excretion; and for comfort (e.g., relief of pain and anxiety). To identify deviations from the normal postpartum course, the nurse must monitor the mother's and baby's physical and psychological status (see Table 19-2).

To assist the mother to prepare for her new responsibilities, the nurse must first provide opportunities for her to express feelings of anxiety related to the altered life-style she will assume. The nurse must also provide anticipatory guidance regarding the mother's self-care and care of the baby. Specifically, the nurse should provide the following information:

1. Self-care
    a. Review danger signs and symptoms:
        Fever/chills. (Make sure the client knows how to read a thermometer.)
        Redness and/or pain in breasts.
        Abdominal pain.
        Dysuria.
        Redness and/or pain at the episiotomy site.
        Redness and/or pain in the legs.
    b. Review breast-feeding techniques, if applicable.
    c. Encourage rest and gradual, progressive return to activities of daily living.
    d. Teach postpartum exercises (see Fig. 19-3).
    e. Discuss contraceptive methods with the client. The woman may resume intercourse in 2 to 3 weeks (when she feels comfortable and when any episiotomy repair has healed). Menses will begin in approximately 4 to 6 weeks if she is not breast-feeding.
    f. Help the client learn to assess and evaluate involutional changes in uterine size and characteristics of lochia.
    g. Review postpartum nutritional requirements, making sure that the breast-feeding mother understands the added requirements.
    h. Make sure the client has follow-up appointments for herself and her baby. She should also have telephone numbers to call in case of emergency.
2. Infant care
    a. Review feeding routines.
    b. Teach skin and cord care.
    c. Review patterns of elimination and diaper care.

    d. Teach the client infant activity patterns. She should know that a new baby sleeps as much as 20 hr/day. Infant crying spells usually signal hunger, wet diapers, or the need to be held.

Care of the postpartum client with deviations from normal

Many clients who are identified as being high risk during the prenatal or intrapartum course are no longer at risk once the baby is delivered. Others have deviations from the norm that require special nursing care during the postpartum period. Clients with deviations from the norm experience most of the same physiological and psychological changes that are experienced by normal clients. The nurse must remember to give complete nursing care for these clients — for the normal adaptations in the postpartum period as well as for the particular complication the client is experiencing.

Postoperative care of the client with a cesarean section. The immediate postoperative care of the client who has undergone a cesarean section is similar to the immediate postoperative care of any surgical patient. Vital signs must be taken frequently — every 15 minutes for the first 1 to 2 hours, then every hour — in order to identify deviations from the normal course. For clients who received general anesthesia, the nurse must pay careful attention to maintaining a patent airway. For clients with spinal or epidural anesthesia, the nurse must carefully monitor the return of sensation and motion to the lower extremities. With spinal anesthesia, it is important for the client to understand that she must remain flat in bed for 6 to 12 hours in order to prevent headache from leakage of cerebrospinal fluid. The client must be asked to turn, cough, and deep breathe frequently (as often as vital signs are taken) in order to prevent pooling of fluid in the lungs, which contributes to pneumonia. The nurse must check dressings and the bed beneath the client for evidence of hemorrhage. Intravenous fluids must be administered as directed by the physician, urinary catheter care must be provided, and intake and output must be monitored. The client's need for pain relief can be met by the use of comfort measures and analgesic medications ordered by the physician. Other medications, such as antibiotics, should be administered as indicated.

As the client progresses in her recovery, her needs will change. Activity should progress gradually, from turning from side to side, to sitting on the side of the bed, to sitting in a chair, to ambulation. Early ambulation should be encouraged. When the urinary catheter is removed (usually on the first postoperative day), the client must be assisted to the bathroom to urinate. The nurse should assess whether the bladder is being emptied by strict monitoring of intake and output and by palpating the bladder after urination. The client's need for pain relief will continue, but, after 24 to 48 hours, oral analgesics will probably suffice. Gastrointestinal motility tends to be sluggish after general anesthesia. When bowel sounds have returned (usually within the first 2 to 3 days), oral intake may resume. The intake will begin with clear fluids and progress within a few days to a full regular diet. Once oral intake is underway, intravenous fluids may be discontinued, unless the intravenous route is the preferred route for administration of medications.

In the first few hours after surgery, the mother may want to see her baby for a few minutes, or at least to be informed of the sex, weight, and health status of the baby. As she progresses, she will want to begin to feed and care for her baby. Unless the mother is breast-feeding, the nurse should administer analgesics, if needed, so that she will be as comfortable as possible when caring for her baby. Mothers who wish to breast-feed will be able to do so, and they should begin breast-feeding as soon as they are comfortable enough to do so.

Before discharge, the postoperative client will need anticipatory guidance about the gradual return to normal activity, the importance of good nutrition to promote healing, and the need to return to her physician or clinic for follow-up care.

Care of the client with an infection.   Infection may be diagnosed before delivery, or it may first become evident during the postpartum period. Not all postpartum temperature elevations are due to infection. In fact, a temperature elevation in the first 24 hours after delivery is most often due to dehydration. Puerperal morbidity is defined as a temperature elevation to 38 °C (100.4 °F) or higher, occurring on any 2 of the first 10 days postpartum after the first 24 hours. When infection is first suspected, cultures should be taken to ascertain (or confirm) the location of the infection as well as to identify the causative organism(s) and effective antibiotics. Cultures are usually taken of blood, urine, and lochia. Cultures may also be taken of the throat or sputum if symptoms indicate that the respiratory tract is a possible site. The most common site of postpartum infection is the urinary tract. Urinary stasis and bladder or urethral trauma during the birth are contributing factors. Other sites of infection include the endometrial lining and the perineal suture line.

Once infection has been diagnosed, the nurse should take vital signs frequently (at least every 4 hours). The nurse should encourage intake of oral fluids and administer intravenous fluids if necessary. Antibiotics and antipyretics should be administered as prescribed by the physician. The nurse should encourage the mother to maintain a good nutritional intake in order to promote healing.

Depending on the site and causative organism of the infection and the institutional protocol, the mother may not be allowed to see her baby for a short period of time in order to minimize the chance of spreading the infection to the newborn. The nurse should explain the reason for the separation to the mother, reassure her that it is only temporary, and give her as much information as possible about the status of her baby. A breast-feeding client should be encouraged to manually express her milk until breast-feeding is allowed.

Care of the preeclamptic client.   Preeclampsia is usually diagnosed in the prenatal or intrapartum period. Occasionally, however, it first becomes evident after delivery. For any client with preeclampsia, the nurse should check blood pressure, presence of edema, quality of deep tendon reflexes, and urinary output hourly. Each urine specimen should be checked for albumin. The respiratory rate should also be monitored hourly for clients receiving magnesium sulfate. Emergency medications and equipment (such as a tongue blade, suction equipment, and calcium gluconate) should be kept at the client's bedside. Medications should be administered as ordered. Magnesium sulfate is often administered during the first postpartum day, followed by sedatives for several days. The mother should be counseled to return to her physician or clinic for follow-up care and to have her blood pressure checked periodically since she is at risk for developing chronic hypertension later in life.

There is no need for the preeclamptic client to be separated from her baby. However, her medications may have a depressant effect and may interfere with her ability to care for her baby in the first few postpartum days.

Care of the client with twins.   The mother of twins will undergo normal postpartum physiological adaptations. She is at increased risk for postpartum hemorrhage as a result of overdistention of the uterus. Therefore, her blood loss must be carefully monitored. She will need a great deal of supportive guidance from the nurse about how to care for two infants at once (*see* Chapters 14, 15, and 22). Referral to a support group for mothers of twins might be helpful.

REFERENCES

1. Pritchard and MacDonald. 160.

2. Jensen et al. 561.

3. Jensen et al. 663.

4. Olds et al. 907.

5. Klaus and Kennell. 2.

6. Olds et al. 922.

CHAPTER 20

POSTPARTUM CONTRACEPTION

Nancy Kulb

Contraceptive counseling is an integral component of postpartum care. Although some clinicians ask clients to adhere to the rule, "No intercourse until after your 4- to 6-week postpartum examination," most clinicians currently believe that there is no reason to prohibit sexual intercourse once the lochia has ceased and the perineum has healed.[1] Many clients who are advised to abstain for 4 to 6 weeks admit at the time of the postpartum checkup that they have resumed intercourse. Because ovulation normally occurs by 10 weeks postpartum (often as early as 6 weeks), clients who resume intercourse before their scheduled postpartum examination run the risk of becoming pregnant again before they are physically or psychologically prepared. Close spacing of pregnancies is a risk to both the mother and the fetus because the mother is unable (1) to replenish the nutritional stores that were depleted in the previous pregnancy and (2) to complete full involution to the nonpregnant state. Clients who are lactating may not resume ovulation until much later, but, because ovulation may resume before menstruation, the client should not rely on lactation as a contraceptive measure.

It is not possible or desirable to initiate some methods of contraception in the immediate postpartum period before hormones and the anatomic characteristics of the uterus and vagina have returned to the nonpregnant state. Therefore, the concomitant use of spermicidal foam and condoms is frequently recommended as the method of choice until other methods are initiated at the 4- to 6-week postpartum examination. The postpartum client needs to have full information on the various contraceptive options that will be available to her at the time of the examination. She and her partner should consider the options and select the best one(s) for them from among those that are not medically contraindicated. Final selection may not be made until the postpartum examination. Full information includes information on all available options, how they work, what the client/couple must do to use them, side effects, possible sequelae, effectiveness, and the need for follow-up evaluation.

This chapter provides basic information about the common methods of birth control, with emphasis on points that are of particular importance to the postpartum client.

ORAL CONTRACEPTIVES

Definition

Oral contraceptives are tablets that contain estrogens, progestins, or, most often, both. Oral contraceptives are taken by the female to prevent conception.

Contraceptive action

The action of oral contraceptives is based on the contraceptive properties of estrogen and progestins. The following is a list of the contraceptive effects of estrogens:[2]

1. Inhibition of ovulation. Estrogen feedback to the hypothalamus suppresses secretion of the gonadotrophin-releasing factor, thus suppressing the release of follicle-stimulating hormone (FSH) and luteinizing hormone (LH) from the anterior pituitary. Ovulation is suppressed by oral contraceptives in approximately 95 percent of all cycles. In addition, other hormonal effects contribute to the efficacy of oral contraceptives.

2. Inhibition of implantation of the fertilized ovum. High doses of estrogen that are administered after conception alter the secretory endometrium, with areas of edema alternating with dense cellular areas.

3. Acceleration of ovum transport. The ovum is carried more quickly through the genital tract when estrogen is administered after conception.

4. Luteolysis. Degeneration of the corpus luteum and, therefore, loss of the source of progesterone required for the maintenance of early pregnancy may also occur.

The following is a list of the contraceptive effects of progestins:[3]

1. Hostile cervical mucus. Progestins encourage the production of hostile cervical mucus: i.e., scanty, thick mucus that inhibits sperm penetration, transport, and survival.
2. Inhibition of capacitation. Progestins alter cervical secretions, thus leaving the sperm unable to penetrate the cells surrounding the ovum.
3. Slowing of ovum transport. Progestins delay ovum transport through the genital tract when administered before fertilization. Note that the progestin effect on ovum transport is the opposite of the estrogen effect.
4. Inhibition of implantation. Implantation may be inhibited by alterations in FSH and LH, thereby causing a decreased progesterone production by the corpus luteum. Ultimately, after long-term progestin use, an atrophic endometrium that is unable to support pregnancy may result.
5. Inhibition of ovulation. Progestin feedback to the hypothalamus alters the release of FSH and LH that is required for ovulation to occur.

Types of oral contraceptives

There are four types of oral contraceptives:

1. The progestin-only "mini-pill" is a low-dose progestin that should be taken every day.
2. Diethylstilbestrol is the estrogenic postcoital "morning-after" pill.
3. Sequential pills are those in which estrogen alone is taken for 14 to 15 days, followed by a combination of progestin and estrogen for several days.
4. Combination pills, the most widely used oral contraceptives, consist of a combination of estrogen and progestin taken for 21 days, followed by 7 days of taking no hormone (either no pill at all or a placebo that serves to keep the woman in the habit of taking one pill each day).

Because the combination pill is by far the most widely used form of oral contraceptive, the following discussion will be limited to that type.

There are two estrogens used in combination pills: ethinyl estradiol and mestranol, both of which are synthetic estrogens. There are five progestins currently used, each one different in its estrogenic, anti-estrogenic, progestational, and androgenic potency. Therefore, the numerous oral contraceptives on the market vary according to which estrogen is combined with which progestin, and in what dose. The progestins currently in use and their characteristics are listed in Table 20-1. The significance of knowing the specific components of each pill is that an oral contraceptive can be chosen to complement a woman's hormonal profile, and that pills can be changed to minimize side effects, when necessary, according to the hormonal profile of the pills. (*See* Table 20-2 on identification and composition of oral contraceptives.)

Low-dose combination oral contraceptives have 20 to 35 micrograms of estrogen. Because of the potential serious side effects of oral contraceptives (*see below*), many clinicians believe that all women should be initiated on low-dose pills and switched to higher doses only if required to do so by side effects.

Effectiveness

Theoretically, the effectiveness rate for oral contraceptives is nearly 100 percent, with reports varying from 0.1 to 0.3 pregnancies per 100 woman-years of experience. In actual use, however, because of not taking the pills correctly, the rate is 5 to 10 pregnancies per 100 woman-years (*see* Appendix C). Therefore, women should be counseled about the importance of taking pills correctly, and they should be provided with a backup method in case they stop taking the pills for any reason. Finally, clients cannot be guaranteed that they will not get pregnant, even if they take the pills correctly.

Contraindications

The contraindications to the use of oral contraceptives are based on the effects of the hormones, primarily estrogen. The following is a list of absolute contraindications:

Thromboembolic disorders, or a history thereof.
Cerebrovascular accident, or a history thereof.
Impaired liver functioning.
Malignancy of the breast or reproductive system.
Pregnancy.

Relative contraindications to the use of the pill mean that there is risk involved. Women with these conditions (*see below*) should be counseled about the risks and, preferably, provided with other forms of contraception. However, there may be occasions when, based on assessment of a woman's total medical and psychosocial status, oral contraceptives are initiated with full knowledge of the risks, in the belief that the contraceptive benefits outweigh the risks. The following is a list of strong relative contraindications:[4]

TABLE 20-1

Relative Potency of Progestins Used in Oral Contraceptives

Progestin	Estrogenic effect	Anti-estrogenic effect	Androgenic effect	Progestational effect
Norethynodrel	2.08	0.00	0.00	0.10
Norethindrone	0.25	2.50	1.60	0.38
Norethindrone acetate	0.38	25.00	2.50	0.44
Ethynodiol diacetate	0.86	1.00	1.00	0.53
Norgestrel	0.00	18.50	7.60	1.00

Adapted from Hatcher, R. A., G. K. Stewart, F. Stewart, F. Guest, D. W. Schwartz, and S. A. Jones. Contraceptive Technology 1980-1981. Irvington Publishers, Inc., New York. 1980. Tenth edition. p. 27-28; and Dickey, R. P. Managing Contraceptive Pill Patients. Creative Informatics, Inc., Aspen, Colo. 1980. Second edition. p. 14-15.

TABLE 20-2

Composition and Identification of Oral Contraceptives

Name	Progestin	mg	Estrogen	µg	Manufacturer	Color (A/IA*)
Brevicon	Norethindrone	0.50	Ethinyl estradiol	35	Syntex	Bl/O
Demulen	Ethynodiol diacetate	1.00	Ethinyl estradiol	50	Searle	W/P
Enovid-E	Norethynodrel	2.50	Mestranol	100	Searle	P
Enovid 5	Norethynodrel	5.00	Mestranol	75	Searle	P
Enovid 10	Norethynodrel	9.85	Mestranol	150	Searle	P
Loestrin 1.5/30	Norethindrone acetate	1.50	Ethinyl estradiol	30	Parke, Davis	G/Br
Loestrin 1/20	Norethindrone acetate	1.00	Ethinyl estradiol	20	Parke, Davis	W/Br
Lo/Ovral	Norgestrel	0.30	Ethinyl estradiol	30	Wyeth	W/P
Micronor	Norethindrone	0.35	None		Ortho	G
Modicon	Norethindrone	0.50	Ethinyl estradiol	35	Ortho	W/G
Norinyl 1 + 50	Norethindrone	1.00	Mestranol	50	Syntex	W/O
Norinyl 1 + 80	Norethindrone	1.00	Mestranol	80	Syntex	Y/O
Norinyl 2	Norethindrone	2.00	Mestranol	100	Syntex	W
Norinyl 10	Norethindrone	10.00	Mestranol	60	Syntex	W
Norlestrin 1/50	Norethindrone acetate	1.00	Ethinyl estradiol	50	Parke, Davis	Y/W(Br)
Norlestrin 2.5/50	Norethindrone acetate	2.50	Ethinyl estradiol	50	Parke, Davis	P/Br
Norr-Q.D.	Norethindrone	0.35	None		Syntex	Y
Ortho-Novum 1/35	Norethindrone	1.00	Ethinyl estradiol	35	Ortho	O/G
Ortho-Novum 1/50	Norethindrone	1.00	Mestranol	50	Ortho	Y/G
Ortho-Novum 1/80	Norethindrone	1.00	Mestranol	80	Ortho	W/G
Ortho-Novum 2	Norethindrone	2.00	Mestranol	100	Ortho	W
Ortho-Novum 10	Norethindrone	10.00	Mestranol	60	Ortho	W
Ovcon-35	Norethindrone	0.40	Ethinyl estradiol	35	Mead Johnson	Pe/G

Ovcon-50	Norethindrone	1.00	Ethinyl estradiol	50	Mead Johnson	Y/G
Ovral	Norgestrel	0.50	Ethinyl estradiol	50	Wyeth	W/P
Ovrette	Norgestrel	0.07	None		Wyeth	Y
Ovulen	Ethynodial diacetate	1.00	Mestranol	100	Searle	W/P

*A/IA, 21 active/7 inactive or ferrous fumarate (Br) pills; Bl, blue; Br, brown; G, green; O, orange; P, pink; Pe, peach; W, white; Y, yellow.
Adapted from Dickey, R. P. Managing Contraceptive Pill Patients. Creative Informatics, Inc., Aspen, Colo. p. 12-13.

Migraine headaches.
Hypertension.
Full-term gestation terminated within the past 2 weeks.
Diabetes, prediabetes, or a strong family history of diabetes.
Gallbladder disease.
Postcholecystectomy.
History of cholestasia during pregnancy.
Acute phase of mononucleosis.
Sickle cell disease or sickle cell C disease.
Undiagnosed abnormal genital bleeding.
Fibrocystic breast disease.

The following is a list of other relative contraindications:[5]

Varicose veins.
Asthma.
Cardiac or renal disease.
Mental retardation.
Chloasma.
Uterine fibromyomas.
Epilepsy.
Depression.
Anovulation or fertility problems (e.g., late onset of menses and/or irregular, painless menses).
Lactation.
Thyroid disease.
Systemic lupus erythematosus.
Arthritis.
Surgery scheduled within 4 weeks.
Age (over 35 to 40 years old).
Smoking.

The immediate postpartum period is a strong relative contraindication to oral contraceptives. The reason is the hypercoagulability of the postpartum period, which predisposes women to blood clotting disorders. Because the estrogen component of the pill increases the risk of clotting disorders, the pill is contraindicated. Lactation is a relative contraindication. Oral contraceptives act to reduce milk production, and the hormones are excreted in breast milk with unknown effects on the infant. Therefore, in the immediate postpartum period, the mother should be counseled on the types of contraceptives available to her, their risks and benefits, and their effectiveness. If she chooses oral contraceptives, and if there are no other contraindications, she should be informed of the risks involved with taking the pill in the immediate postpartum period and given a backup method with instructions for use. She should also be given an appointment for an evaluation regarding the initiation of oral contraceptives at 4 to 6 weeks postpartum.

Danger signs

Table 20-3 lists the danger signs of oral contraceptives and the possible problems that they may represent. Clients who use oral contraceptives should be instructed to see a physician immediately if they experience any of these danger signs.

Side effects

The possible side effects of the pill are numerous, but, in most women, they are minor and/or not noticed at all. Most of the side effects are nonspecific to the pills and must be differentiated from other causes. Because the hormonal makeup of each woman is different, the same pill may cause different side effects in different women. Table 20-4 lists the underlying hormonal cause(s) of a number of side effects. With this information, it is possible to switch pills to minimize side effects. For example, a woman who is experiencing nausea and dizziness as a result of the pill is experiencing

TABLE 20-3
Aches and Pains That May Be Warnings of Serious Problems

Signal	Possible problem
Abdominal pain (severe).	Gallbladder disease, hepatic adenoma, blood clot, pancreatitis.
Chest pain (severe) or shortness of breath.	Blood clot in lungs or myocardial infarction (heart attack).
Headaches (severe).	Stroke or hypertension or migraine headache.
Eye problems: blurred vision, flashing lights, or blindness.	Stroke or hypertension or temporary vascular problem of many possible sites.
Severe leg pain (calf or thigh).	Blood clot in legs.

Reprinted with permission from Hatcher, R. A., G. K. Stewart, F. Stewart, F. Guest, D. W. Schwartz, and S. A. Jones. Contraceptive Technology 1980-1981. Irvington Publishers, Inc., New York. 1980. Tenth edition. p. 33.

TABLE 20-4
Pill Side Effects: Hormone Etiology

Estrogen excess	Progestin excess	Androgen excess	Estrogen deficiency	Progestin deficiency
1. Nausea, dizziness.	1. Increased appetite and weight gain (noncyclic).	1. Increased appetite and weight gain.	1. Irritability, nervousness.	1. Late breakthrough bleeding, spotting.
2. Edema and abdominal or leg pain with cyclic weight gain, bloating.	2. Tiredness, fatigue, weak feeling.	2. Hirsutism.	2. Hot flushes, vasomotor symptoms.	2. Heavy menstrual flow, clots.
3. Leukorrhea.	3. Depression, decreased libido.	3. Acne.	3. Uterine prolapse, pelvic relaxation symptoms.	3. Delayed onset of menses.
4. Increase in leiomyoma size.	4. Oily scalp, acne.	4. Oily skin, rash.	4. Early and midcycle spotting.	4. Dysmenorrhea.
5. Chloasma.	5. Loss of hair.	5. Increased libido.	5. Decreased amount of menstrual flow.	5. Weight loss.
6. Uterine cramps.	6. Cholestatic jaundice.	6. Cholestatic jaundice.	6. No withdrawal bleeding.	
7. Irritability.	7. Decreased length of menstrual flow.	7. Pruritus.	7. Decreased libido.	
8. Increased female fat deposition.	8. Hypertension?		8. Diminished breast size.	
9. Cervical exstrophy.	9. Headaches between pill packages.		9. Dry vaginal mucosa, atrophic vaginitis, dyspareunia.	
10. Contact lenses do not fit.	10. Monilia vaginitis, cervicitis.		10. Headaches.	
11. Telangiectasia.	11. Increase in breast size (alveolar tissue).		11. Depression.	
12. Vascular type headache.	12. Breast tenderness.			
13. Hypertension.	13. Decreased carbohydrate tolerance.			
14. Lactation suppression.	14. Dilated leg veins.			
15. Headaches while taking pills.	15. Pelvic congestion syndrome.			
16. Cystic breast changes.				
17. Breast tenderness.				

18. Increased breast size (ductal tissue, fatty tissue, fluid retention).
19. Thrombophlebitis.
20. Cerebrovascular accidents.
21. Myocardial infarction.
22. Hepatic adenoma.
23. Cyclic weight gain.

Reprinted with permission from Hatcher, R. A., G. K. Stewart, F. Stewart, F. Guest, D. W. Schwartz, and S. A. Jones. Contraceptive Technology 1980-1981. Irvington Publishers, Inc, New York. 1980. Tenth edition. p. 36-37.

symptoms of estrogen excess. Even if she is on a relatively low estrogen-effect pill, her body is experiencing it as excessive estrogen, and she needs an even lower estrogen-effect pill.

Whereas some side effects of the pill tend to be alleviated over time, others intensify. Table 20-5 provides a time framework with regard to side effects that result from the use of the pill.

Counseling

The postpartum client who is considering oral contraceptives should be provided with information on how to take the pill, how it works, effectiveness, danger signs, possible dangerous and minor side effects, types of oral contraceptives, the need for regular clinic appointments while taking the pills, the need for using a backup method until the pills have been taken for 1 month, and how to use the backup method she chooses. Instructions for taking the pill and managing missed pills are provided below:

Start taking the pills the Sunday after your baby is 1 month old. (Some clinicians prefer to wait until the woman has her first menstrual period after delivery. In that case, she should begin taking pills the Sunday after her period begins. Beginning the pills on Sunday will arrange her periods during the week rather than on weekends. Every subsequent pack of pills will also begin on Sunday.)

Take one pill every day, preferably at the same time each day. Try to associate taking the pill with some daily activity, such as brushing your teeth or after eating dinner.

You will take one pill a day for 21 days. If you are taking a 21-day pill, you will take no pills for 7 days and will begin a new pack the next Sunday. Your period will occur when you are not taking any pills. If you are taking a 28-day pack, you will continue to take one pill each day, but, during the last 7 days, you should take the pills of a different color. Your period will occur when you are taking these last seven pills. Begin your new pack of pills on Sunday, the day after you finish your old pack.

If you miss one pill, take it as soon as you remember it, and take your next pill at the regular time. You probably will not get pregnant, but you may want to use a backup method for the rest of the month, just to be sure. If you miss more than one pill, use another method of contraception and phone the clinic.

When you go to a physician for any reason, be sure to tell him or her that you are taking oral contraceptives.

INTRAUTERINE DEVICE

Definition

The intrauterine device (IUD) is an implement placed inside the uterus to prevent pregnancy (Fig. 20-1).

Contraceptive action

The exact mechanism of action of the IUD is not known. However, several theories have been proposed:[6]

1. Inflammatory response. A local inflammatory response in the endometrium may prevent implantation or may destroy the blastocyst.
2. Mechanical displacement. The IUD may dislodge the blastocyst from the uterine lining.
3. Increased motility of the fallopian tube. The IUD may cause the fertilized ovum to reach the uterus before the endometrium is optimally prepared for implantation.
4. Immobilization of sperm. The IUD may interfere with sperm motility.

Certain materials added to the IUD, such as copper or progesterone, increase the contraceptive effect by their local effect on the lining of the uterus.

Types of IUDs

IUDs are generally made of an inert plastic, and they are available in a number of shapes (Fig. 20-2). Some, such as the Lippes Loop and the Saf-T-Coil are available in different sizes. The addition of copper to the Copper 7 and the Copper T, and of progesterone to the Progestasert, increases their effectiveness while retaining a small, easy to tolerate shape. These three IUDs generally cause less bleeding and cramping. Copper 7 and Copper T must be removed and replaced every 2 to 3 years. Progestasert must be replaced every year.

Effectiveness

The effectiveness of the IUD varies, depending on such factors as the size and shape of the device, ease of insertion, skill and experience of the clinician, and rate of expulsion (especially expulsion undetected by the client). Overall, the theoretical effectiveness is approximately 95 to 99 percent. Because there is little opportunity for error in actual use (other than failure to detect expulsion), the actual effectiveness is similar: approximately 90 to 94 percent. Because expulsion is more probable in the first month after insertion than it is later, many clinicians advise clients to use a backup method such as foam and/or condoms for the first month after insertion.

Contraindications

The following is a list of the contraindications to insertion of an IUD:[7]

TABLE 20-5

Pill Side Effects: A Time Framework

Worse in first 3 months	Over time: steady-constant	Worse over time	Worse after discontinuation
1. Nausea, dizziness.	1. Headaches during 3 weeks that pills are being taken.	1. Headaches during week pills are not taken.	1. Infertility, amenorrhea, hypothalamic and endometrial suppression, miscalculation of the expected date of confinement.‡
2. Thrombophlebitis (venous): Leg veins. Pulmonary emboli.* Pelvic vein thrombosis.* Retinal vein thrombosis.	2. Arterial thromboembolic events, blurred vision, stroke.*	2. Weight gain.	
		3. Monilial vaginitis.	2. One form of acne.
3. Cyclic weight gain, edema.	3. Anxiety, fatigue, depression.	4. Periodic missed menses while on oral contraceptives.	3. Hair loss (alopecia).
4. Breast fullness, tenderness.	4. Thyroid function studies: Elevated PBI. Depressed T3 resin uptake.	5. Chloasma.*	4. Depression (in some women).
5. Breakthrough bleeding.		6. Myocardial infarction.*	
6. Elevated serum lipid levels even to the extent of pancreatitis.*	5. Susceptibility to amenorrhea after pill discontinuation.	7. Spider angiomas.	
		8. Growth of myoma.	
7. Abnormal glucose tolerance test.*	6. Decreased libido.	9. Predisposition to gallbladder disease.	
8. Contact lenses fail to fit because of fluid retention.	7. Autophony, chronic dilation of eustachian tubes rather than cyclic opening and closing.	10. Hirsutism.	
		11. Decreased menstrual flow.	
9. Abdominal cramping.	8. Acne.	12. Small uterus, pelvic relaxation, cystocele, rectocele, atrophic vaginitis.	
10. Suppression of lactation.			
11. Failure to understand correct use of oral contraceptives, pregnancy.		13. Cystic breast changes.	
		14. Photodermatitis (sunlight sensitivity with hypopigmentation).	

15. One form of hair loss
    (alopecia).
16. Hypertension.*
17. Focal hyperplasia of liver,
    hepatocellular adenomas.*

PBI, protein-bound iodine; T3, triiodothyronine.
*May be irreversible or may produce permanent damage.
†To avoid this complication in many patients who desire to be pregnant, discontinue pills 3 to 6 months before desired pregnancy. Another possible way to avoid this problem is to avoid prescribing pills for women with a history of very irregular menses.
Reprinted with permission from Hatcher, R. A., G. K. Stewart, F. Stewart, F. Guest, D. W. Schwartz, and S. A. Jones. Contraceptive Technology 1980-1981. Irvington Publishers, Inc., New York. 1980. Tenth edition. p. 35.

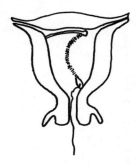

Figure 20-1. Placement of the intrauterine device within the uterus. *Adapted from* Martin, L. L. Health Care of Women. J. B. Lippincott Co., Philadelphia. 1978. p. 87.

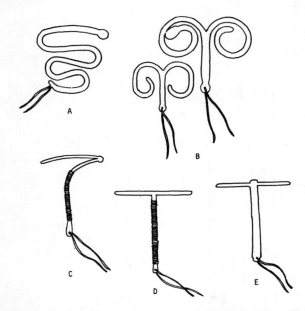

Figure 20-2. Types of intrauterine devices. (A) Lippes Loop, (B) Saf-T-Coil, (C) Copper 7, (D) Copper T, (E) Progestasert. *Adapted from* Hatcher, R. A., G. K. Stewart, F. Stewart, F. Guest, D. W. Schwartz, and S. A. Jones. Contraceptive Technology 1980-1981. Irvington Publishers, Inc., New York. 1980. Tenth edition. p. 54.

Pregnancy.
Active or chronic pelvic infection (pelvic inflammatory disease).
Cervical or uterine carcinoma (including undiagnosed abnormal uterine bleeding).
Blood dyscrasias, such as coagulopathy.
Uterine abnormalities that prevent insertion, including a small uterus (a uterine sound measurement of less than 4.5 centimeters), myomas, bicornuate uterus, etc.
History of ectopic pregnancy.
Allergy to copper (contraindication to a copper device).

The following is a list of the relative contraindications to insertion of an IUD:

Acute cervicitis.
Valvular heart disease.
Recurrent pelvic inflammatory disease.
Cervical stenosis.
Anemia.
Severe dysmenorrhea, excessive menstrual bleeding, or bleeding between periods.
Desire for future pregnancy in a nulligravida.
Multiple sexual partners.

Most clinicians prefer to insert the IUD during the client's menstrual period in order to rule out pregnancy and because the endocervical canal is open, thus making insertion easier. In addition, menses masks the bleeding and cramping that may result from insertion. However, because the endocervical canal is slightly open, there may be a greater chance of infection resulting from IUD insertion during menses. Many clinicians will insert an IUD at a client's 4- to 6-week postpartum checkup, regardless of resumption of menses, because the chances of pregnancy at that time are negligible. Others will wait until menses, and insert it at 8 to 12 weeks postpartum. After a cesarean section, some clinicians recommend that an IUD not be inserted until 3 months postpartum. However, individual practice may vary.

Danger signs and side effects

Although rare, some of the possible side effects of the IUD present life-threatening situations. The following is a list of some of these side effects:

Vasovagal syncope, cardiac arrhythmias, or cardiac arrest on insertion.
Severe or prolonged bleeding.

Pelvic infection.
Cervical or uterine perforation.
Ectopic pregnancy.
Septic abortion.

The symptoms of these serious side effects that the client may experience at home include fever, lower abdominal or pelvic pain, tenderness or cramping, and/or unusual vaginal bleeding. The client should be instructed to return to her physician or clinic at once if she experiences any of these symptoms.

Because of the danger of sepsis and septic abortion, it is recommended that if pregnancy occurs with the IUD in place, the IUD should be removed. Chances of a subsequent spontaneous abortion are approximately 25 percent, whereas chances of a spontaneous abortion are approximately 50 percent if the device is left in place.

The following is a list of some other side effects or complications of the IUD:

Spotting and/or cramping for a few days after insertion.
Dysmenorrhea, metrorrhagia, and menorrhagia (especially for the first 3 months after insertion).
Expulsion of the IUD, which is more probable in the first few months after insertion or with menses.
Pregnancy, either with the IUD in place or after expulsion.

Counseling

The postpartum client considering the IUD should be informed about how IUDs are thought to work, the types of IUDs available and their advantages and disadvantages, effectiveness, the possible complications and side effects, the need to keep regular clinic appointments for surveillance of the method, the need for a backup method during the first month after insertion and any time thereafter when expulsion is suspected, how to use the chosen backup method, and how to check the placement of the IUD.

The client should be provided with the following information on how to check that the IUD is in place:

Wash your hands. Insert your middle finger in the vagina in a backward and inward direction until you locate your cervix. Feel for a string coming out of the cervix. Feel for a hard tip (the end of the IUD) protruding out of the cervix. If you can feel the tip of the device or you cannot feel the string, consider the device to be out of place. Use a backup method of contraception and return to the clinic. Check the strings frequently during the first few months after insertion of the IUD and then after your period each month. Check sanitary napkins before discarding them to be sure that the device has not been expelled. Do not attempt to remove the device yourself.

VAGINAL DIAPHRAGM

Definition

The vaginal diaphragm is a dome-shaped cup with a circular metal spring in the rim. It is intended to hold a spermicidal jelly or cream, and it is placed over the cervix in the vagina (Fig. 20-3).

Contraceptive action

The primary and major contraceptive action of the diaphragm is the action of the spermicidal jelly or cream: the immobilization and killing of sperm. The diaphragm keeps the spermicide directly over the cervical os, thus preventing sperm from entering the cervix. Secondarily, the diaphragm itself may mechanically block the cervix; however, research has shown that the diaphragm moves about during intercourse.[8] The client should use the largest size diaphragm that fits comfortably in order to ensure that the cervix will remain covered during intercourse.

Types of vaginal diaphragms

There are three types of vaginal diaphragms. Their only difference is in the type of metal spring in the rim. Many clinicians use only one type — the arcing spring diaphragm — with good results. However, the other types can meet the needs of individual clients. The three types of diaphragms are listed below:

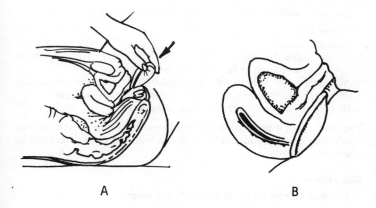

A   B

Figure 20-3. The diaphragm. (A) Manual insertion of the diaphragm. (B) The diaphragm in its proper position. *Adapted from* Martin, L. L. Health Care of Women. J. B. Lippincott Co., Philadelphia. 1978. p. 69.

Flat spring. A flat band of metal in the rim. It is used for women with a shallow pubic arch.

Coil spring. A metal coil-type spring. It is used for women with good vaginal tone, especially nulliparas.

Arcing spring. A firm rim, a combination of the springs used in the coil and flat spring diaphragms. It is characterized by an arced shape when the sides of the rim are compressed together. The arcing spring is used for women with poor vaginal tone; mild to moderate cystocele, rectocele, or uterine prolapse; or women whose cervix is in an unusual position, which might make proper insertion difficult with another rim type or allow a less firm rim to slip out of place during intercourse. Many clinicians use this type routinely, and it is likely that this is the type that postpartum clients will receive.

Effectiveness

The theoretical effectiveness of the diaphragm is quite high: three pregnancies per 100 woman-years, which is a rate comparable to that of the IUD. Because of inconsistent or improper use, the actual effectiveness is 20 to 25 pregnancies per 100 woman-years. Therefore, a highly motivated couple can rely on the diaphragm as an effective form of contraception, but it is a poor choice for a woman/couple who feel they may use it inconsistently.

Contraindications

The contraindications to the use of the diaphragm are few:

Severe uterine prolapse.
Severe cystocele.
Vesicovaginal fistulas.
Severe anteversion or retroversion of the uterus.
Allergy to the rubber of the diaphragm or to the spermicide (although alternative brands may not contain the allergen).
History of recurrent urinary tract infections.

The diaphragm is not a good method for women who are reluctant to touch their own genitals, or for those in whom a good fit cannot be achieved.

Side effects

The side effects of the diaphragm are rare:

Allergic reaction to the diaphragm or the spermicide.
Growth of microorganisms if the diaphragm is left in place too long.

Urinary tract infection, encouraged by the pressure of the rim on the urethra.

Counseling

The postpartum client who is considering the vaginal diaphragm as a means of contraception should be provided with information on how it works (pictures or a pelvic model may help her to visualize placement); effectiveness; possible side effects; the need for a backup method of contraception until she is comfortable using the diaphragm, and how to use the backup method; the need for a re-check of the diaphragm after it is fitted, followed by yearly visits; and how to use the diaphragm. She should be told that the diaphragm can be fitted at her 4- to 6-week postpartum examination, when her pelvic organs have returned to their nonpregnant state. Instructions for the use of the diaphragm are listed below:

Use only a spermicidal jelly or cream that is intended for use with a diaphragm. Use the spermicidal jelly or cream every time you use the diaphragm because it provides the primary contraceptive action. By itself, the diaphragm will *not* be very effective.

Wash your hands. Holding the diaphragm with the dome side down, squeeze from 1 teaspoon to 1 tablespoon of jelly or cream into the diaphragm. With your fingers, spread the spermicide evenly inside the dome and around the rim.

Insert the diaphragm as follows: Assume any position that will help you insert the diaphragm (lying down, squatting, standing with one foot on a chair, etc.). Spread your labia with one hand, and compress the sides of the diaphragm together with the other. With the dome side down, insert the diaphragm into the vagina in a backward and inward direction as far as it will go. Tuck the rim in the front up under the pubic bone.

Check the placement of the diaphragm by inserting one finger into the vagina and feeling for the firm cervix through the flexible rubber of the dome of the diaphragm.

The diaphragm may be inserted up to 2 hours before intercourse. Some women routinely insert the diaphragm every day or night so that they will not have to interrupt love-making.

The diaphragm should be left in place for 6 to 8 hours after inter-course because it takes that long for the spermicide to be completely effective. If you douche, do not do so until after you remove the diaphragm. You can urinate and defecate without dislodging the diaphragm, but it is a good idea to check the position of the diaphragm after having a bowel movement.

If you have intercourse again before the diaphragm is supposed to be removed, leave it in place and add a full applicator of the jelly or cream. Add a full applicator of spermicidal jelly or cream each time you have intercourse. Do not remove the diaphragm until from 6 to 8 hours after the last intercourse.

To remove the diaphragm, insert your finger in your vagina, hook your finger under the rim of the diaphragm, and bear down while pulling the diaphragm in a downward and outward direction.

The diaphragm can be left in place for 24 to 36 hours, but it should be removed to be washed after that time. It can then be reinserted.

Wash the diaphragm with a mild soap and warm water. Pat dry. If desired, cornstarch may be used to powder the diaphragm. Harsh soaps, perfumed powders, Vaseline, etc., should not be used on the diaphragm because they may be harmful to the rubber. Heat may also be harmful to the rubber, so store the diaphragm in a cool place.

Frequently check the diaphragm for holes by holding it up to a light and stretching the rubber. A diaphragm will usually last 2 years or more.

You will have the diaphragm fitted at your 4- to 6-week postpartum visit. At that visit, you will be given the opportunity to practice inserting, checking the placement of, and removing the diaphragm. You will be asked to practice with it for 1 to 2 weeks while using a backup method of contraception, and then to return for an evaluation of the fit. If the fit is good, and you are comfortable with using it, you will need to return for yearly visits.

You will need to have the fit of the diaphragm rechecked after a pregnancy (or an abortion), if you gain or lose 10 to 15 pounds, or if you have pelvic surgery.

SPERMICIDES

Definition

Spermicides are preparations that consist of an agent in an inert base that immobilizes and kills sperm.

Contraceptive action

The primary contraceptive action of spermicides is the immobilization and killing of sperm. Secondarily, the base may mechanically block the cervical os to prevent entry of sperm.

Types of spermicides

Because most spermicides use the same chemical, the types of spermicides depend primarily on their form. Forms include jelly, cream, foam, and vaginal suppositories. (Suppositories may foam, and there are sponges saturated with a substance that foams when moisture is added.) Spermicidal preparations may be quite similar in appearance and packaging to feminine hygiene products, and clients should be instructed to check products carefully to be sure of their intended use.

Effectiveness

Theoretical effectiveness for spermicidal preparations varies according to the preparation. The theoretical effectiveness for foam is about three pregnancies per 100 woman-years. Actual effectiveness is much less: about 30 pregnancies per 100 woman-years. The actual effectiveness is thought to be much lower than the theoretical effectiveness because of the numerous opportunities for error: not using the spermicide consistently, not using enough, not using more for each act of intercourse, inadequate supply, not timing insertion for adequate effectiveness, etc. The effectiveness of spermicides can be increased by using them in conjunction with condoms. The actual effectiveness of the concomitant use of foam and condoms approaches that of the pill: 5 to 10 pregnancies per 100 woman-years of use.

Contraindications

The only contraindication to the use of spermicidal preparations is allergy. Alternative forms or brands that contain different ingredients may alleviate this problem.

Side effects

The side effects of spermicides are limited. Rare allergic reactions are possible. Some women notice warmth and burning with use of foaming suppositories. Couples who enjoy oral sex may find that spermicides have an unpleasant taste.

Counseling

Instructions will depend on the specific spermicide used. Foam and condoms are a frequently used method of contraception (1) before the initiation of pills, insertion of an IUD, or fitting of a diaphragm, (2) until another method is well established, (3) when another method is terminated for any of a number of reasons, (4) midcycle for extra protection in conjunction with another method, or (5) as a couple's preferred method of contraception. Spermicides are used very frequently in the postpartum period before the initiation of another method. The discussion that follows is limited to the use of foam. The client should be instructed to consult package directions for other preparations because they may vary in some points, such as timing of insertion vis-a-vis timing of intercourse.

For maximum effectiveness, insert the foam no more than 30 minutes before intercourse, and insert it at the place where intercourse will occur, so the foam will not drip out as you walk around.

Shake the can 15 to 20 times, then fill the applicator. Insert the applicator deeply in your vagina, as far as it will go, withdraw ½ inch, and push in the plunger. For maximum effectiveness, use two full applicators.

If coitus does not occur within 30 minutes or if it is repeated, insert two more full applicators of foam each time.

Douching is not recommended, but if you do, wait until 6 to 8 hours after the last act of intercourse. You may want to insert a tampon to minimize messiness if you must get up soon after using the foam.

Keep an extra can of foam handy so that you will not run out. If the can freezes, the foam is not effective and must be discarded. The effectiveness of foam is greatly increased by using it in conjunction with condoms.

CONDOMS

Definition

The condom is a rubber or collagenous sheath that fits over the penis.

Contraceptive action

The condom acts as a mechanical barrier by keeping sperm within the sheath and away from the cervical os.

Types of condoms

Most condoms are made of rubber, but for those who are sensitive to rubber there are "natural skin" condoms, made of lamb cecum. Some condoms have reservoir tips at the end that collect the ejaculate.

Effectiveness

The theoretical effectiveness of the condom is three pregnancies per 100 woman-years. The actual effectiveness is much lower: approximately 15 to 20 pregnancies per 100 woman-years. Defects in condoms that are produced in the United States are rare because of high quality standards. Most failures with condoms result from inconsistent or improper use. Actual effectiveness is increased considerably by using condoms in conjunction with a spermicidal foam: 5 to 10 pregnancies per 100 woman-years.

Contraindications

The contraindications to condom use are minimal. Allergy to rubber is one contraindication to the use of rubber condoms, but "natural skin" condoms can be used instead.

Side effects

Some men complain of decreased sensation when using a condom. Some are unable to maintain an erection while using a condom, although others may maintain an erection longer because of the slight constriction from the rim of the condom at the base of the penis. Condoms may have the added benefit of preventing the spread of sexually transmitted diseases from one partner to the other.

Counseling

Condoms are frequently used in the postpartum period before another method is initiated. It is preferable in all contraceptive counseling to include the woman's partner, and this is especially true when the condom is to be used. Instructions for using the condom are provided below:

Use a new condom for each act of intercourse. Preferably, use a condom manufactured in the United States because you can be reasonably sure that it will be free from defects. Otherwise, check the condom for holes. Heat and time may deteriorate the rubber in condoms, so use only condoms that are less than 2 years old and that have been kept away from heat.

Put the condom on the penis before the penis comes near the vagina. To put it on, either partner can unroll it down over the erect penis. If the condom does not have a reservoir tip, pinch about ½ inch of the tip of the condom between two fingers before unrolling it on the penis. This will allow a space for the ejaculate to collect during intercourse.

If lubrication is needed, avoid using petroleum jelly because it causes rubber to deteriorate. Instead, use a spermicidal preparation, saliva, or a water-soluble lubricant jelly.

If the condom breaks or if any ejaculate leaks onto the woman's genitalia, some spermicidal preparation should be inserted into the vagina at once.

The effectiveness of condoms can be greatly increased by the concomitant use of a spermicide.

After intercourse, withdraw the penis from the vagina before it becomes flaccid, holding the condom securely in place at the base of the penis.

NATURAL METHODS OF FAMILY PLANNING

Definition

The natural methods of family planning are all based on abstinence from sexual intercourse during the time in a woman's menstrual cycle when she is potentially fertile. They are based on the following three assumptions:

1. Ovulation occurs 12 to 16 days before the beginning of the menstrual period.
2. The ovum is viable for up to 24 hours.
3. Sperm is viable for up to 48 hours.

Because there is no mechanical or medicinal interference with the body's normal functioning, this method is the most acceptable form of contraception for some couples.

Contraceptive action

The contraceptive action is based on preventing the release of sperm in the woman's genital tract when there is the possibility that a viable ovum may be present.

Types of natural family planning methods

There are three basic methods of natural family planning, which can be used singly or, more often and more effectively, in conjunction with each other.

The calendar method. The calendar method is based on the length of the woman's menstrual cycle, which is determined over a base-line period of 8 to 12 months. The shortest cycle during that period of time indicates the earliest likely time of ovulation, which usually occurs 14 days before menstruation. For example, if the woman's shortest cycle was 26 days, ovulation probably occurred on day 12 (14 days before her period began), but could have occurred as early as day 10 (16 days before her period). Because sperm may be viable for up to 48 hours, the woman must avoid intercourse for 2 days before the earliest possible time of ovulation. Her "unsafe" period begins on day 8. The end of her unsafe, or fertile, period is based on her longest menstrual cycle. For example, if her longest cycle was 28 days, ovulation probably occurred 14 days before, on day 14, but it could have occurred as late as 12 days before, on day 16. Because the ovum may be viable for 24 hours, she is potentially fertile until day 17. Therefore, her potentially fertile period, during which she must abstain from intercourse, is from day 8 to day 17.

The calendar method is more reliable in a woman with very regular cycles, but, even so, ovulation may occasionally occur outside the calculated time, thus making her fertile during what is normally a "safe" period. This method is particularly unreliable in women with irregular cycles (including women in the immediate postpartum period and lactating women). At least three cycles of similar length are required to establish a pattern before *resuming* this method if a woman has used it previously.

The basal body temperature method. The basal body temperature (BBT) method is based on the fact that the BBT drops slightly just before ovulation and then rises under the influence of progesterone during the luteal phase to approximately 0.5 °F above the base line established in the follicular phase. These temperature changes help to determine the time of ovulation. In general, the BBT method is combined with the calendar method: the earliest unsafe day is determined by the calendar method, and intercourse is resumed after the BBT has been elevated for 3 days, indicating that ovulation has already occurred.

This method requires consistency and motivation. The woman's temperature should be obtained every morning at about the same time of day, with a BBT thermometer, which is marked off in tenths of degrees. The BBT is obtained by the same route on awakening — before talking, eating, smoking, getting up, or moving about. It is plotted on a BBT graph that makes the rises and falls in temperature obvious. Of course, illness, stress, the use of electric blankets, irregular hours of sleep, and a host of other factors may influence the temperature reading. These should be noted on the graph to aid in interpretation.

The cervical changes method.   The cervical changes method is based on changes that occur in the cervix and cervical mucus near the time of ovulation. Immediately after menstruation, cervical secretions are scant and tacky. Before ovulation, secretions become noticeably present, opaque, and sticky. At about the time of ovulation, secretions become cloudy or clear, greater in amount, and slippery. A bit of mucus can be stretched between two fingers to a thin thread of 6 centimeters or more in length. A bit of this mucus dried on a slide and examined under a microscope would reveal a fernlike pattern. At the time of ovulation, the cervix becomes softer and the cervical os dilates slightly. After ovulation, the cervix becomes firm, the os closes, and the cervical mucus becomes opaque, tacky, and less in amount. "Safe" days are the days with opaque, tacky, and dry mucus. Unsafe days are those characterized by the preovulatory, or wet, ovulation mucus. Some women find that their secretions do not present clear changes, thus making interpretation difficult. Others use changes in cervical mucus as a useful adjunct to the other natural family planning methods and avoid intercourse on days that might be unsafe according to any one of the three methods.

Effectiveness

Effectiveness rates vary, depending on which method(s) are used, regularity of menstrual cycles, and education and motivation of clients. Constant users of natural family planning methods achieve a rate of about 15 pregnancies per 100 woman-years. However, all users of the method achieve a rate of 25 to 30 pregnancies per 100 woman-years. The principles of natural family planning methods may be used by women using other methods of contraception to increase their effectiveness. For example, couples relying on IUDs or diaphragms may abstain from intercourse or use an additional method (such as foam and/or condoms) during the fertile period.

Contraindications

Because there are no medicinal or mechanical components to this method, there are few contraindications: irregular menses, irregular temperature charts, anovulatory cycles, and lack of motivation to adhere to the method by either partner.

Counseling

In the immediate postpartum period, counseling on the natural methods will be limited to an explanation of the methods and how they work. The woman's partner should be included in the counseling because his participation is crucial to the success of the method. The woman can be encouraged to begin to keep records of her cycles: length, BBT, and changes in cervical mucus. However, even if she has used the method previously, she should not rely on it until she has reestablished regular menstrual cycles, which can be evidenced by three successive regular periods. This will take several months in all postpartum women and, perhaps, longer in lactating women. Women who have never used the method before will need a period of 6 to 12 months to establish their own base line and to become skilled at interpreting the signs of ovulation that are exhibited by their bodies. It will be most helpful for new users of the method to attend a clinic where an experienced clinician can help in the interpretation of the charts until the couple is comfortable with it.

STERILIZATION

Definition

Sterilization is a permanent method of contraception. Immunologic, hormonal, and other nonsurgical methods for sterilization are being studied for both men and women; however, at present, the regularly used methods are surgical: tubal ligation for women and vasectomy for men. Tubal ligation is the interruption of the patency of the fallopian tubes by cutting, tying, cauterizing, or sclerosing the tubes to prevent sperm from reaching the ovum to achieve fertilization. Vasectomy is a similar interruption of the patency of the vas deferens to prevent sperm from entering the man's ejaculate.

Effectiveness

The effectiveness of both male and female sterilization is quite high, with less than one pregnancy per 100 users.

Counseling

Counseling regarding sterilization is of utmost importance. Couples should be informed that sterilization should be considered irreversible. Although new techniques are being developed that may increase reversibility, it cannot be guaranteed in any individual case. Couples should be informed that the surgery involves all of the risks inherent in any surgery, and that, rarely, the surgery is not effective in preventing conception.

Many states, hospitals, and individual practitioners will have policies or procedures governing sterilization that are designed to protect the rights of clients. These may include eligibility criteria, content of counseling, method for obtaining informed consent, or a waiting period between signing the consent and performance of the procedure in order to give the couple sufficient time to consider the procedure and change their minds. It is important that the nurse counselor know the local policies governing sterilization so that accurate, complete information can be provided to the clients.

Tubal ligations are frequently performed in the postpartum period when the mother is already hospitalized. In general, tubal ligations are only performed on clients who have considered it thoroughly and signed consent forms during the antepartum period. Clients who first decide on sterilization during the postpartum period should be given complete counseling, perhaps sign the consent forms, and be scheduled for the procedure at a later date. An interim method of contraception should be provided to such a couple. It must be clear that a couple that desires sterilization in the postpartum period is doing so out of a sincere desire to prevent future childbearing and not out of labile reactions to a negative experience in pregnancy, labor, or delivery.

OTHER METHODS

There are a number of other methods of contraception that are under investigation in the United States and throughout the world. Although a few of these will be mentioned below, the list is by no means exhaustive.

One method currently receiving a great deal of attention in the United States is the cervical cap. The cervical cap looks much like a diaphragm, but it is smaller in diameter and the cup is deeper. The cervical cap is designed to fit snugly over the cervix, as a mechanical barrier, and it may be used with a spermicide to enhance effectiveness. Because it may be left in place several days, it is not intercourse related, as is the diaphragm. It can be used by some women who cannot use the diaphragm, such as those with lax vaginal muscles. The cervical cap is being used in other countries and is undergoing clinical trials in the United States (before Food and Drug Administration approval).

Progesterone injections ("the shot") are administered every 3 months to provide contraception. Contraindications are similar to those of other hormonal methods of contraception, although the risk of thromboembolic diseases is not clear. Women may experience intermenstrual bleeding, heavy menstrual bleeding, irregular bleeding, or amenorrhea while taking progesterone injections. It is currently not recommended for women who may desire pregnancies in the future.

Research is being conducted on other types of contraceptives: subdermal implants that provide slow release of hormones, immunologic methods, "plugs" for fallopian tubes that can be removed if pregnancy is desired. At present, these methods are available only as part of research protocol.

SUMMARY

Although many of the contraceptive methods cannot be initiated in the immediate postpartum period, clients do need to have some method readily available when they decide to resume sexual intercourse. Very often, resumption of intercourse will occur before the 4- to 6-week postpartum examination. Clients also need information on all of the available contraceptive options so that they can consider which method(s) to use until they are ready to plan another pregnancy.

REFERENCES

1. Siemens and Brandzel. 282-283.

2. Hatcher et al. 18-19.

3. Hatcher et al. 19-20.

4. Hatcher et al. 22-24.

5. Hatcher et al. 23-24.

6. Hatcher et al. 53.

7. Hatcher et al. 58-59.

8. Hatcher et al. 79.

CHAPTER 21

ASSESSMENT OF THE NEWBORN

Dorothy Allbritten

NURSING CARE AND EVALUATION IN THE DELIVERY ROOM

Apgar scoring

Nursing care must be administered with an awareness that maternal-infant attachment can be optimized during this period (*see* Chapter 14).

Once the delivery is complete, and the infant is received by the maternity nurse, Apgar scoring is performed and recorded at 1 and 5 minutes after birth (Table 21-1). Five categories are observed and scored from 0 to 2, with a maximum total score of 10.

1. *Heart rate* is auscultated for a minimum of 30 seconds before scoring.
2. *Respiratory rate* is inspected and counted for a full 60 seconds to obtain an accurate rate.
3. *Muscle tone* is scored on the basis of the degree of flexion and the amount of resistance that the infant offers when the examiner attempts to extend the extremities.
4. *Reflex irritability* is elicited in the infant by inserting a cotton-tipped swab into the nostril or flicking the sole of the foot. A vigorous cry and withdrawal response are expected.

TABLE 21-1
Apgar Scoring Chart

	Score*		
Sign	0	1	2
Heart rate	Absent	Slow (below 100)	Fast (over 100)
Respiratory rate	Absent	Slow, irregular	Good, crying
Muscle tone	Flaccid	Some extremity flexion	Active motion
Reflex irritability‡	No response	Grimace	Cry
Color	Blue, pale	Body pink, extremities blue	Completely pink

*The Apgar method is used for evaluating the immediate postnatal adjustment of the newborn baby. If the total score of the five signs is 8 to 10, the initial adjustment is good. Infants with lower scores require special attention. Scores under 4 indicate that the child is seriously depressed.
‡Tested by inserting the tip of a catheter into the nostril.
Courtesy of Virginia Apgar, MD, and Smith, Kline & French Laboratories, Philadelphia.

5. *Color* is scored simply by observing the degree and location of the infant's pinkness.

The scores in each of the five sections are totaled. A score below 7 is abnormal and indicates that the infant requires immediate attention. A score of 7 to 10 indicates a healthy infant, who needs only brief oral and nasal suctioning to clear the airway.

Maintaining body temperature

A prime nursing activity in the delivery room is maintaining the infant's temperature while initial identification and care are being performed. Radiant heaters, warmed blankets, and/or heated isolettes are used to retain infant body heat. An equally effective method of maintaining the infant's body temperature is to place him or her next to the mother, with both covered by a warm blanket. Axillary or cutaneous temperatures should be taken and recorded soon after birth and frequently thereafter until they are stable. Identification and eye and umbilical cord care procedures (*see below*) should be performed in a warm area, with an awareness of the need to maintain the infant's body heat.

Vital signs

During the first hour, the neonate's vital signs must be measured and recorded at least every 15 to 20 minutes. After the first hour, vital signs should be monitored hourly until they stabilize: pulse, 120 to 160 beats/min; respirations, 20 to 60 breaths/min.[1] If instability is noted, medical intervention and cardiac monitoring may be required.

Prophylactic medications

Eye drops of 1 percent silver nitrate solution are routinely instilled into both eyes of the newborn to prevent ophthalmia neonatorum — a gonococcal infection. An intramuscular injection of 1 milligram of vitamin K (AquaMephyton) is administered to supplement the neonate's normally low level of this vitamin and to prevent hemorrhage.[2]

Cord care

Once the umbilical cord is clamped and cut, it should be inspected to determine the presence of two arteries and one vein. The goals of cord care are to promote drying and to prevent infection. The umbilical cord may be treated with 70 percent alcohol or Triple Dye during the 5- to 10-day process of healing before it necroses and drops off.

Identification

Before leaving the delivery room and the mother, the infant must be properly identified. In general, the practice is to document the mother's name and hospital number, the baby's sex, and the date and time of birth on two wrist bands. These two bands should be verified against the record and by the mother before the nurse places both of them around the infant's ankle or wrist. At this time, the baby's footprints and the mother's fingerprint are recorded in the baby's hospital record.

Observation of physical status

An initial observational assessment of physical status (Table 21-2) should be performed between the 1- and 5-minute Apgar scoring tests. At this point in the birth recovery process, the infant is in stage 1: the alert and active phase (see Table 21-3). During the initial 30 minutes of life, there is usually an increase in motor activity, with respiratory and cardiac rate acceleration to accommodate for the lowered body temperature.[3]

The infant's chest is observed for equal expansion during respiration. The respirations are counted for a full minute, and the

TABLE 21-2

Checklist for Screening the Newborn in the Delivery Room

Criterion	No	Yes*
Respirations exceed 60 breaths/min?		
Chest expansion unequal?		
Intercostal retraction?		
Substernal retraction?		
Nasal flaring?		
Cardiac rate exceeds 160 beats/min?		
Circumoral cyanosis?		
Trunk cyanosis?		
Visible chest heave?		
Physical anomalies?		
Asymmetrical facial features?		
Missing facial features?		
Missing digits?		
Extra digits?		
Spinal deviations?		
Breaks or abrasions of skin?		
Misshaped head?		

*Any positive response requires further pediatric assessment.

regularity of the rate is noted. The normal range is 30 to 60 respirations/min. The presence of any respiratory distress, manifested by intercostal or substernal retractions accompanied by flaring of the nasal alae, must be noted.

The color of the infant's skin is an indicator of cardiac functioning. The nurse should identify the presence of cyanosis at the distal portion of the extremities — a condition called acrocyanosis, which is a normal finding in neonates. Acrocyanosis is self-limiting and resolves within 4 to 12 hours when cardiac perfusion is complete. The skin, the nail beds, and the mucous membranes normally have a rosy hue. Any findings that contradict these are significant and should be brought to the pediatrician's attention.

This initial observation period is also used to identify the presence of any obvious physical anomalies. Are all four extremities intact, each with its five digits? Are facial features present, intact, and symmetrical? Is the spine at the midline, without masses or a break in its continuity? Is the head round to ovoid with no masses or discoloration? Is the skin intact over the body without edema, markings, or abrasions? A negative response to any of these questions signifies the need for further pediatric assessment and possible medical intervention.

THE PHYSICAL EXAMINATION

Because the maternity nurse is the 24-hour caregiver for the infant's first few days of life, he or she must continually use assessment skills to monitor the newborn's state of health. Performing a complete physical assessment enables the maternity nurse to determine the health status of each newborn. From these base-line data, plans for health care may be formulated.

Triage and newborn physical assessment

Complete assessment of the newborn includes detailed evaluation of all body systems. However, the nurse should remember that there are certain broad indicators of well-being that unfailingly alert caregivers to the overall health of the newborn. These include skin color, temperature, gastrointestinal activity and feeding patterns, breathing patterns, and activity (Table 21-3).

Preparation

Before the examination of the newborn is begun, the examiner should prepare the needed supplies and equipment to facilitate inspection, percussion, palpation, and auscultation. The needed supplies include an ophthalmoscope or flashlight, a tongue blade, a stethoscope, a measuring tape, and behavioral assessment equipment.

The optimal time for performing a neonatal physical examination is when the infant's thermal, cardiac, and respiratory statuses are stabilized, after the birth recovery period is completed. Moreover, it is wise to perform the examination at least 1 hour after feeding in order to minimize interference with gastrointestinal functioning.

Once the appropriate time for the examination is chosen and the equipment is assembled near the infant, the examiner organizes the sequence of the examination to conserve body heat and energy. The infant should be disturbed as little as possible. Table 21-4 displays the sequence that facilitates an energy-efficient physical examination. The following descriptive narrative will proceed in a cephalocaudal manner after the preliminary inspection and auscultation stages have been discussed.

Inspection

By observing the newborn in the resting, untouched state, the

TABLE 21-3
Indicators of Newborn Well-Being

Parameter	Normal finding	Sign of disease
Color	Generally pink to light brown. Occasional cyanosis around mouth, hands, or feet. Variations include mottling when unclothed, harlequin color change, and/or ruddiness several hours after birth.	*Jaundice:* Before 24 hr: Erythroblastosis fetalis, cytomegalic inclusion disease, congenital rubella, toxoplasmosis. After 24 hr: Physiological, anemia, galactosemia, hepatitis, congenital atresia of bile duct. *Pallor:* Anemia, hemorrhage, hypoxia, hypoglycemia, sepsis, shock, adrenal failure. *Beefy redness:* Hypoglycemia. *Cyanosis:* Respiratory insufficiency, pulmonary anomaly secondary to intracranial hemorrhage, cyanotic heart disease, methemoglobinemia, hypoglycemia, bacteremia, meningitis.
Respiration	30-60 breaths/min within a range of 20-60 breaths/min. May be irregular and is influenced by activity.	*Apnea:* Metabolic as well as respiratory or CNS disturbance. *Grunting:* Pneumonia, RDS, left-sided heart failure. *Retraction, nasal flaring, or cyanosis:* On inspiration: Block in large bronchi. On expiration: Block in small bronchi.

Feeding and GI activity	Daily requirements: 150 ml and 120 cal/kg/day. Feeding: 60-120 ml of formula/feeding. Stooling: Varies with feeding method and individual baby. Voiding: 6-8 times/day.	*Poor sucking/feeding*: Seen in most sick newborns. *Vomiting*: 1st day of life: Obstruction in GI tract or increased intracranial pressure. Later: Still points to GI or CNS system, but may be sign of any disease. *Diarrhea*: Overfeeding, acute gastroenteritis, infection (parenteral diarrhea). *Abdominal distention*: Intestinal obstruction, intra-abdominal mass, enteritis, ileus, sepsis, or RDS.
Activity	Goes through three stages, then settles into individual pattern. *Stage 1*: Alert and active phase (first 30 min of life). *Stage 2*: Quiet phase (30 min-2 hr). *Stage 3*: Alert and active phase (2-10 hr).	*Floppiness/lethargy*: Hypoxia, sedation (maternal analgesia/anesthesia), cerebral defect, severe infection. *Irritability*: Discomfort. *Failure to move an extremity*: Fracture, dislocation, nerve injury. *Hyperactivity*: CNS damage, hypoxia, pneumothorax, emphysema, hypoglycemia, hypocalcemia. *Convulsions*: CNS damage, withdrawal, vitamin B6 dependency, intracranial pressure, tetany, severe infection, rapid electrolyte change.
Temperature	Axillary temperature of 36.5-37.0°C (97.7-98.6°F) within a range of 35.7-37.2°C (96.3-99.0°F).	*Fever (above 37.2°C [99°F])*: Environmental temperature too high, "dehydration fever," infection. *Subnormal*: Infection, metabolic disturbance.

CNS, central nervous system; GI, gastrointestinal; RDS, respiratory distress syndrome.

TABLE 21-4
Sequence of Newborn Examination

Assessment	Assessment factors
Inspection Untouched Observe	General appearance and posture, position of extremities, placement of features, respiratory rate and ease, color and condition of skin, body symmetry, and motor activity.
Listen	Cry (pattern, pitch, and tone), respirations, and heart sounds.
Unclothe chest, loosen diaper	Anomalies, contour of abdomen, and condition of umbilical cord.
Auscultation	Chest (heart and lungs), abdomen, and head.
Systematic examination	General appearance, skin, head, face, eyes, ears, nose, throat and mouth, neck, thorax, abdomen, genitalia, anus, spine, extremities, and neuromuscular.
Measurement of growth	*See* p. 524.
Gestational age	*See* p. 524.

nurse can ascertain many facts about his health. The newborn's general appearance may be described as "struggling," "alert and quiet," "crying," "sleeping," "contentedly moving extremities," etc. The respiratory rate is observable as chest movement, and respiratory effort should be noted (*see* Table 21-3). Skin color (e.g., mottled, cyanotic, or jaundiced) indicates the status of thermoregulation, cardiac perfusion, and liver functioning. The newborn position is characteristically one of symmetrical flexion: with elbows, knees, and hips bent. The infant's general appearance and respiratory rate will indicate his progress through the birth recovery period. In stage 2 (the quiet stage), which lasts from 30 minutes to 2 hours, the infant is asleep and has lowered heart and respiratory rates. After this quiet period comes stage 3, in which the neonate becomes as alert and active as in stage 1. Vital signs increase, and there may be increased mucus production or meconium passage.[3] The nurse should identify the neonate's stage of birth recovery (*see* Table 21-3).[4]

The newborn's facial features should be observed for position and placement, symmetry and balance. Body symmetry in the resting and active state indicates the absence of motor problems, fractures, and/or nerve injury.

While listening to the newborn without the stethoscope, the examiner may identify moist or impaired respirations; the bounding heart sound of an organic murmur; or the unique pattern, pitch, and tone of the cry of a child with congenital heart problems.

At this point, the examining nurse should approach the infant only to loosen the clothing to expose the chest, abdomen, and genitalia. Nursing observation should continue by assessing and describing the contour of the abdomen, the condition and contents of the umbilical cord, and the presence of any structural anomalies (*see* Table 21-8).

Auscultation

With the infant quietly resting with his anterior trunk exposed, the examiner should use the warmed diaphragm of a stethoscope to auscultate the infant's heart, lungs, abdomen, and head. The heart sounds should be auscultated at the base and apex of the heart for at least 1 minute each, and the nurse should identify the intensity, quality, duration, location, and radiation of any murmur. The clarity of respirations is identified by listening to the anterior and posterior chest and comparing the right and left sides from apex to base of both lungs. The nurse should listen in each of the four quadrants of the abdomen until bowel sounds occur (up to 3 minutes). The nurse should then auscultate the right and left temporoparietal and parietal frontal regions of the cranium for any bruits and, if present, note their location.

Systematic examination

Skin. The nurse should keep in mind that the skin gives clues to the health of the entire body. In general, normal skin color is pink to light brown. However, several normal variations may be noted (*see* Table 21-3), and these variations should be explained to parents for their information and reassurance that the findings are within normal limits. The newborn's skin should be smooth, soft, and of medium thickness. Subcutaneous fat will be present in the term newborn. Vernix — a creamy, protective coating of sebum, peridermal cells, and other skin debris — will be present.

The nurse should evaluate skin turgor, which is an indicator of hydration status. This is best accomplished by grasping a large amount of skin over the abdomen and gently lifting. Well-hydrated skin rises when pinched and falls back into place. Dehydrated skin remains in the pinched position.

Head.   The head should be symmetrical and in proportion to the rest of the body. Cranial sutures and fontanels should be open and palpable. Immediately after birth, sutures are normally felt as ridges. Within a day they become slightly depressed. A bulging fontanel is normal when the newborn is crying, coughing, or vomiting. However, it may also indicate increased intracranial pressure. An accurate evaluation of the fontanels can be made with the infant in a semi-Fowler's position.

Molding and caput succedaneum are normal findings at birth. Molding, the overlapping of the cranial bones as a result of head compression during descent through the pelvis, disappears within 2 days. Caput succedaneum, a diffuse, edematous swelling of the soft tissue of the scalp, also disappears within the first few days of life. Caput succedaneum should be carefully differentiated from cephalhematoma. Caput succedaneum is a discolored, soft tissue swelling resulting from superficial head trauma during birth. It is palpated as a soft, fluctuant mass on the head that may cross over or obliterate suture lines. Caput is a self-resolving condition. Cephalhematoma is a malformation of the head resulting from hemorrhage under the cranial bone, subperiosteal. It is palpated as a tense mass within the perimeter of a cranial bone. The swelling does not cross the suture line. Cephalhematoma requires medical supervision, and the pediatrician should be informed of this finding.

The nurse should measure the infant's head circumference. The average is 34 to 36 centimeters within a range of 32 to 38 centimeters.[5] The tape should be placed over the occipital, parietal, and frontal prominences in order to obtain the correct measurement. Most practitioners take three measurements and record the mean score as the actual circumference. Extremes in head size usually indicate pathology (e.g., microcephaly or hydrocephalus).

The nurse should also inspect the scalp for scaling, distribution and texture of hair, and location of the hairline. (One is able to feel individual hairs in a term newborn.) The hair should be smooth and fine. The color and amount should be evenly distributed throughout. Chopped, brittle hair may be a sign of hypothyroidism. A low-set hairline may be indicative of mental retardation.

Face.   The nurse should observe for symmetry and relative size of facial features and identify the presenting facial expression (e.g., bland, alert, fussing, crying, or frowning). The nurse should attempt to elicit Chvostek's sign by gently tapping over the parotid gland. The sign is negative if no facial twitch occurs. When the infant is hypocalcemic or hypoglycemic, a positive sign or twitch will be elicited. A gentle stroking motion at the side of the mouth will stimulate the rooting reflex. When positive, the infant turns his face toward the side being stroked and begins sucking. To test the masseter reflex, the examiner places the side of the index finger along the infant's chin and taps that finger briskly with the other hand. This motion will stimulate the masseter muscle to contract, and the chin will rise as a normal response. When the examiner taps one finger over the nasal bridge between the eyebrows, the infant should close both eyes tightly and quickly. If there is a facial nerve paresis, there will be an asymmetric response.

Eyes. The newborn's eyes are slate blue or dark. The infant should be able to focus briefly on the face. In most states, antibiotic or chemical prophylaxis to prevent gonococcal eye infection is required by law. This may produce reddened, edematous eyelids and a discharge, both of which disappear within 24 to 48 hours after birth. Conjunctival hemorrhage (bleeding into the sclera as a result of the trauma of the birth process) may be present. Infants usually do not produce tears until approximately 3 months of age. Excessive tearing in the newborn may indicate plugged lacrimal ducts.

The nurse should evaluate the symmetry, position, and placement of the eyes. Very wide-set eyes may indicate mental retardation. Very close-set eyes may indicate absence of the nasal bridge.

Nystagmus is normal unless excessive. The newborn's pupils should be symmetrical, round, and reactive to light. With the ophthalmoscope or a flashlight, in an area of subdued light, the examiner may stimulate pupillary constriction by shining the light beam on the pupil from a 45-degree lateral position. The examiner must elicit the red reflex, thus ascertaining the presence of retinas.

Ears. In the first 2 to 3 days of life, the ears are filled with debris from the birth process. Therefore, it is useless — as well as dangerous — to examine the ears with an otoscope. The nurse should inspect the position and palpate the consistency of the newborn's ears.

At least part of the external ear should be above a line extending from the outer canthus of the eye to the external occipital protuberance.[6] Low placement is associated with congenital defects, especially renal anomalies.

A term newborn's ears should have enough cartilage to make them stand out from the head. The amount of cartilage varies from baby to baby: preterm infants, for example, have less cartilage.

Nose. The nose should be at the midline and should seem flattened, with little nasal bridge. The nurse should be mindful of the fact that newborns breathe through their nose, and should test nasal patency by holding the infant's mouth closed and by occluding only one naris at a time. Absence of the nasal bridge (saddle nose) or excessive discharge (snuffles) may be indicative of congenital syphilis.

Mouth. The neonate's mouth should be edentulous and shallow. The tongue should be relatively large, and saliva scanty. The frenulum should allow the tongue to protrude beyond the lower dental ridge.

An otoscope (without aural speculum attached) or flashlight is used to inspect the oral mucosa, tongue, palate, gums, and throat. A tongue blade is used to depress the tongue to aid visualization of the soft and hard palates. The tongue blade may also stimulate the gag reflex, during which the nurse should observe the symmetrical rise of the uvula.

Natal teeth and/or Epstein's pearls (small gum cysts that resolve spontaneously) may be present.[7] The nurse may elicit the sucking reflex by placing a finger in the infant's mouth. During this procedure, it is a good practice to palpate the hard and soft palates to reconfirm their intactness.

Neck. The infant's neck should be short and straight. Full range of motion should be present. The nurse should palpate the neck and note the position and consistency of the trachea and thyroid gland. The nurse should perform a meticulous palpation of the clavicles in order to assess intactness. Broken clavicles may occur as a result of birth trauma — especially after shoulder dystocia.

Thorax. The nurse should add to the inspection and auscultation findings the following information: chest circumference (approximately 2 centimeters less than the head circumference), position and distance between nipples, size of breast tissue, presence of nipple discharge, symmetry of chest expansion, presence of xiphoid prominence, precordial activity, location of the point of maximal impulse, and femoral and peripheral pulses. An absence of femoral pulses is indicative of aortic coarctation.

Abdomen. Before performing light palpation, the size, shape, and movement of the abdomen should be observed to determine the tension of the abdominal wall and to identify the rectus muscle. Midline diastasis (separation) of the recti may be present. The nurse should palpate deeply (1 to 2 inches) to identify masses and any malformation of the liver, spleen, bladder, or kidneys. The nurse should also check the umbilical stump for redness, swelling, or purulent drainage.

Genitalia.

Male: The foreskin is adherent to the glans and covers it. It will not retract until 4 to 6 months of age.[8] The scrotum is fully rugated in the term newborn. The testes are palpable in the scrotum or inguinal canal. The examiner should take care to block off the inguinal canal when palpating in order to prevent the testis from ascending. The meatus should be at midposition at the tip of the glans penis.

Female: The labia minora appear prominent. The urethral orifice, hymen, and vaginal mucosa can be visualized. Mucoid or serosanguineous discharge may be present. This discharge is the result of maternal hormones, and will disappear spontaneously.

Anus. The anus should be patent, with good muscle tone, and a purse-string sphincter. Tags, fissures, and fistulas are abnormal findings. The anal reflex is elicited by stroking briskly at the side of the anus with a tongue depressor. A positive response is the tightening of the anal sphincter and closure of the purse string. Patency is evidence by the passage of the meconium plug.

Spine and extremities. Upper extremities usually move together, whereas lower extremities move alternately. The spine should be examined for its midline position and the presence of dimples, masses, hair tufts, discontinuity, or lateral curvature. The nurse can test Galant's reflex by briskly stroking along the lateral border of the spine while the infant is prone. A healthy response — an incurving of the spine toward the stroked side — indicates neural intactness.

It is most important to diagnose dislocation (luxation) of the hips. Failure to make a diagnosis at birth will delay treatment and may result in permanent disability. In luxation, the femoral head is completely dislocated above the acetabular rim. The following is a list of early signs and symptoms of luxation:

1. Asymmetrical skin folds of gluteal, adductor, and inguinal areas. Redundancy of skin on the affected side results in extra skin folds on the inner aspect of the thigh. This is seen in all three areas (Fig. 21-1).
2. Limitation of abduction (away from the median plane) of the hip.
3. Shortening of the affected leg.
4. Prominence and elevation of the greater trochanter on the affected side.
5. Broadening of the perineum on the affected side.
6. Ortolani's sign. To elicit this sign, the infant is placed on a firm mattress with hips and knees flexed. The examiner places both thumbs over the medial aspect of the infant's knees and spreads the fingers over the lateral aspect of the thighs and hips. As the thighs are gradually spread apart (abducted), a palpable jerk or click can be felt as the head of the femur slips over the acetabular rim (Fig. 21-2).

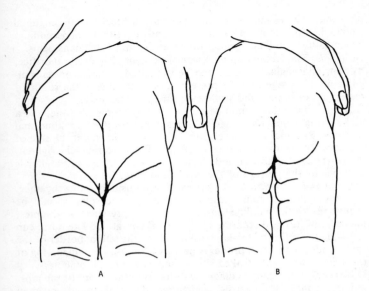

Figure 21-1. (A) Normal and (B) abnormal gluteal and popliteal skin creases. (*See* p. 521 for discussion.) Courtesy of Mead Johnson Laboratories, Evansville, Ind.

7. Telescoping of the affected side. The infant is placed on a firm mattress with hips and knees flexed. The examiner places one hand over the infant's pelvis while grasping the infant's knee and the distal end of the femur with the other hand. The examiner then applies alternate traction and compression (push and pull). Telescoping of the femoral head can be felt as it glides back and forth. This is demonstrable when the hip is dislocated.

Neuromuscular. In addition to those reflexes that were mentioned in the systematic examination, the following reflexes may be elicited to complete the neuromuscular assessment (Table 21-5 contains a list of the important reflexes of early infancy.):

1. Babinski's sign: A brisk stroke over the lateral plantar surface from the heel forward, across the metatarsal arch, stimulates great toe flexion, with the remainder of toes extending.
2. Biceps: Percussion on the flexed biceps tendon stimulates the biceps muscle to contract and flex the lower arm.
3. Grasp: Pressure on the palmar and plantar surfaces stimulates the flexion of the fingers and toes, as if they were grasping.

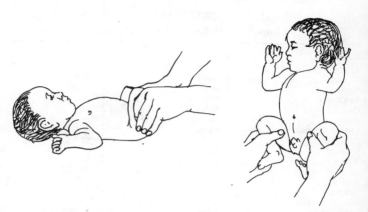

Figure 21-2. Elicitation of Ortolani's sign to determine dislocation of the hip. (*See* p. 521 for discussion.) *Adapted from* Bates, B. A. Guide to Physical Examination. J. B. Lippincott Co., Philadelphia. 1979. Second edition. 415-416.

4. Moro's: A sudden, rapid movement of the infant's head (e.g., when support is withdrawn as if the infant is about to fall or be dropped) stimulates quick flexion of the forearms at the elbow and extension of the fingers, followed by abduction of the upper extremities at the shoulders. This is frequently called the "startle reflex" or "tree-climber's reflex" because of the movements produced.
5. Patellar: Percussion on the stretched patellar tendon (between the patella and tibial head) stimulates the extension of that leg.
6. Placing: Holding the infant in vertical suspension with the dorsum of the foot touching an obstacle will stimulate the infant to raise the foot up and over the obstacle and place it on the surface.
7. Stepping: Holding the infant in vertical suspension with the feet touching a flat surface will stimulate the infant to alternate lifting of the feet as if walking or stepping. (The placing and stepping reflexes may be altered after breech delivery. Absence or alteration of the reflex should be verified with the pediatrician.)

Absence of any of these reflexes may be due to a physical problem with the infant or to improper technique by the examiner. Absence or alteration of a reflex response should be medically validated.

TABLE 21-5
Important Reflexes of Early Infancy

Reflex	Appears	Disappears
Rooting	At birth.	By 12 mo.
Sucking	At birth.	By 12 mo.
Swallowing	At birth.	Persists.
Gag	At birth.	Persists.
Grasp	At birth.	3 mo.
Lateral eye movement	At birth.	Persists.
Optic blink	At birth.	Persists.
Traction	At birth.	
Biceps	At birth.	Persists.
Masseter	At birth.	10 days.
Babinski's	At birth.	At ambulation.
Achilles	At birth.	Persists.
Chvostek's sign	At birth.	Persists.
Doll's eyes	At birth.	10-12 days.
Moro's	At birth.	3-4 mo.
Clonus	At birth.	
Patellar	At birth.	Persists.
Stepping	2nd-3rd day.	4-8 wk.
Placing	4th day.	By 24 mo.
Galant's	5th-6th day (optimal).	
Tonic neck	2nd-3rd mo (optimal).	By 6 mo.

Growth parameters

The nurse should measure each of the following parameters of the infant's growth: height, weight, head circumference, chest circumference, and the anterior and posterior fontanels. These measurements should be recorded and plotted on a growth grid (Fig. 21-3) in order to provide the beginning points for serial measurements. This record should be maintained with the infant's health record for subsequent growth measurements. In general, an infant's measurement percentiles will all fall into the same quartile when his body is proportional.

Gestational age assessment

The Dubowitz guide for the rating of external and neurological criteria elicited in the newborn is a tool that enables the examiner to make a gestational age assessment. Instructions for its use are provided below:

Using Table 21-6, rate the infant on each of the 11 listed criteria described. Add up the scores for each for a total external score.

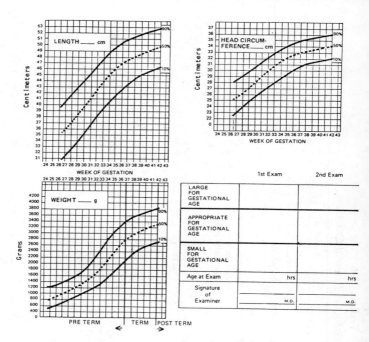

Figure 21-3. Classification of newborns based on maternity and intrauterine growth. *Adapted from* Dubowitz, L., V. Dubowitz, and C. Goldberg. Clinical assessment of gestational age in the newborn infant. *Journal of Pediatrics* (July 1970). 1-10.

Using Figure 21-4 in conjunction with Table 21-7 (which explains how to score each of the 10 items in the figure), rate the infant and total the neurological scores. Combine the external criteria with the neurological total for a combined total score, which will range between 0 and 70.

Using Figure 21-5, locate the point on the x axis (or total score axis) that indicates the infant's combined total score and draw a line perpendicular to that axis up to intersect the angled line. To determine the gestational age in weeks, draw a line (parallel to the x axis) to the y axis. To validate the assessment, use the formula as shown in the figure by inserting the total score in the "x" position and compute for "y." Both scores should match the point on the y axis, indicating the correct gestational age in weeks.

TABLE 21-6

Scoring System for External Criteria

External sign	Score*				
	0	1	2	3	4
Edema	Obvious edema of hands and feet; pitting over tibia.	No obvious edema of hands and feet; pitting over tibia.	No edema.		
Skin texture	Very thin, gelatinous.	Thin and smooth.	Smooth; medium thickness; rash or superficial peeling.	Slight thickening; superficial cracking and peeling, especially of hands and feet.	Thick and parchment-like; superficial or deep cracking.
Skin color	Dark red.	Uniformly pink.	Pale pink; variable over body.	Pale; only pink over ears, lips, palms, or soles.	
Skin opacity (trunk)	Numerous veins and venules clearly seen, especially over abdomen.	Veins and tributaries seen.	A few large vessels clearly seen over abdomen.	A few large vessels seen indistinctly over abdomen.	No blood vessels seen.
Lanugo (over back)	No lanugo.	Abundant; long and thick over whole back.	Hair thinning, especially over lower back.	Small amount of lanugo and bald areas.	At least one half of back devoid of lanugo.
Plantar creases	No skin creases.	Faint red marks over anterior half of sole.	Definite red marks over greater than anterior one half; indentations over less than anterior one third.	Indentations over anterior one third.	Definite deep indentations over greater than anterior one third.

Nipple formation	Nipple barely visible; no areola.	Nipple well defined; areola smooth and flat. Diameter <0.75 cm.	Areola stippled; edge not raised; diameter <0.75 cm.	Areola stippled; edge raised; diameter >0.75 cm.
Breast size	No breast tissue palpable.	Breast tissue on one or both sides; <0.5 cm diameter.	Breast tissue on both sides; one or both 0.5-1.0 cm.	Breast tissue on both sides; one or both >1 cm.
Ear form	Pinna flat and shapeless; little or no incurving of edge.	Incurving of part of edge of pinna.	Partial incurving of whole of upper pinna.	Well-defined incurving of whole of upper pinna.
Ear firmness	Pinna soft, easily folded; no recoil.	Pinna soft, easily folded; slow recoil.	Cartilage to edge of pinna, but soft in places; ready recoil.	Pinna firm, cartilage to edge; instant recoil.
Genitals Male	Neither testis in scrotum.	At least one testis high in scrotum.	At least one testis right down.	
Female (with hips one half abducted)	Labia majora widely separated; labia minora protruding.	Labia majora almost cover labia minora.	Labia majora completely cover labia minora.	

*If score differs on two sides of the body, take the mean.

Adapted from Dubowitz, L., V. Dubowitz, and C. Goldberg. Clinical assessment of gestation age in the newborn infant. *Journal of Pediatrics* (July 1970). 1-10.

Neurological sign	SCORE					
	0	1	2	3	4	5
Posture						
Square window	90°	60°	45°	30°	0°	
Ankle dorsiflexion	90°	75°	45°	20°	0°	
Arm recoil	180°	90-180°	<90°			
Leg recoil	180°	90-180°	<90°			
Popliteal angle	180°	160°	130°	110°	90°	<90°
Heel to ear						
Scarf sign						
Head lag						
Ventral suspension						

Figure 21-4. Scoring system for neurological signs of the newborn. *Adapted from* Dubowitz, L., V. Dubowitz, and C. Goldberg. Clinical assessment of gestational age in the newborn infant. *Journal of Pediatrics* (July 1970). 1-10.

TABLE 21-7
Techniques for Neurological Assessment

Assessment	Technique
Posture	Observed with infant quiet and in supine position. Score 0: arms and legs extended; 1: beginning of flexion of hips and knees, arms extended; 2: stronger flexion of legs, arms extended; 3: arms slightly flexed, legs flexed and abducted; 4: full flexion of arms and legs.
Square window	The infant's hand is flexed on the forearm between the thumb and index finger of the examiner. Enough pressure is applied to achieve as full a flexion as possible, and the angle between the hypothenar eminence and the ventral aspect of the forearm is measured and graded accordingly. (Care should be taken not to rotate the infant's wrist while performing this maneuver.)
Ankle dorsiflexion	The foot is dorsiflexed onto the anterior aspect of the leg, with the examiner's thumb on the sole of the foot and the other fingers behind the leg. Enough pressure is applied to achieve as full a flexion as possible, and the angle between the dorsum of the foot and the anterior aspect of the leg is measured.
Arm recoil	With the infant in the supine position, the forearms are first flexed for 5 sec, then fully extended by pulling on the hands, and then released. The sign is fully positive if the arms return briskly to full flexion (score 2). If the arms return to incomplete flexion or the response is sluggish, the score is 1. If they remain extended or are only followed by random movements, the score is 0.
Leg recoil	With the infant supine, the hips and knees are fully flexed for 5 sec, then extended by traction on the feet, and released. A maximal response achieves full flexion of the hips and knees (score 2). A partial flexion scores 1, and minimal or no movement scores 0.
Popliteal angle	With the infant supine and his pelvis flat on the examining couch, the thigh is held in the knee-chest position by the examiner's left index finger and thumb, which supports the knee. The leg is then extended by gentle pressure from the examiner's right index finger behind the ankle, and the popliteal angle is measured.
Heel-to-ear maneuver	With the infant supine, draw the foot as near to the head as it will go without forcing it. Observe the distance between the foot and the head as well as the degree of extension at the knee. Grade accordingly. (Note that the knee is left free and may draw down alongside the abdomen.)

Assessment	Technique
Scarf sign	With the infant supine, take the hand and try to put it around the neck and as far posteriorly as possible around the opposite shoulder. Assist this maneuver by lifting the elbow across the body. See how far the elbow will go across and grade accordingly. Score 0: elbow reaches opposite axillary line; 1: elbow reaches between the midline and opposite axillary line; 2: elbow reaches the midline; 3: elbow will not reach the midline.
Head lag	With the infant supine, grasp the hands (or the arms, if a very small infant) and pull slowly toward the sitting position. Observe the position of the head in relation to the trunk and grade accordingly. In a small infant, the head may initially be supported by one hand. Score 0: complete lag; 1: partial head control; 2: able to maintain head in line with body; 3: brings head anterior to body.
Ventral suspension	The infant is suspended in the prone position, with the examiner's hand under the infant's chest (one hand for a small infant, two for a large infant). Observe the degree of extension of the back and the amount of flexion of the arms and legs. Also note the relation of the head to the trunk. Grade accordingly.

Adapted from Dubowitz, L., V. Dubowitz, and C. Goldberg. Clinical assessment of gestational age in the newborn infant. *Journal of Pediatrics* (July 1970). 1-10.

The maternity nurse will find the physical assessment checklist (Table 21-8) to be a complete guide for the assessment of newborn health status. It provides a visual summary of the findings obtained during the examination process, and it includes space for a detailed description of abnormal findings. The use of this checklist will promote the completion of a thorough newborn health assessment.

SUMMARY

Nursing care of the newborn, which begins in the delivery room and continues in the nursery after the physical assessment, is the connecting link in the chain of continuity for parent-child attachment (Chapter 14) and preparation for home life (Chapter 23). Although periods of separation occur, the maternity nurse can provide the communication that promotes togetherness for the infant and his family while in the hospital. Reassuring information about the positive health status of the infant, identified during the assessment process, should be shared with the parents (e.g., growth parameters, vital signs, and endearing behaviors or expressions that

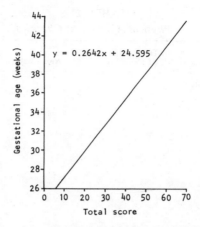

Figure 21-5. Graph for reading the gestational age from the total score obtained on the gestational age scale. The formula for obtaining the gestational age score is shown above, with *x* as the total score and *y* as the gestational age score. *Adapted from* Dubowitz, L., V. Dubowitz, and C. Goldberg. Clinical assessment of gestational age in the newborn infant. *Journal of Pediatrics* (July 1970). 1-10.

occurred during the exam). It is helpful, too, to demonstrate portions of the physical examination. Parents delight to see positive responses to reflex testing and frequently express their appreciation to the nurse who plans this type of parent education time into a busy work schedule. Questions from parents should be willingly addressed and therapeutically encouraged. Depending on administrative policy and local custom, the maternity nurse can sensitively deal with parents' concerns about any negative aspects of their newborn's health status and facilitate the resolution of problems — present and anticipated. It is the maternity nurse who can provide the coordination, collaboration, and communication within and between the health care team and the newborn's family.

REFERENCES

1. Vaughan et al. 358.
2. Vaughan et al. 1782.
3. Desmond.
4. Vaughan et al. 352.
5. Vaughan et al. 22.
6. Bates. 395.
7. Bates. 399.
8. Bates. 410.

TABLE 21-8
Physical Assessment Checklist

Feature	Description of abnormal	Abnormal	Normal
General appearance			
Activity level			
Posture and position			
Skin (color, turgor, and markings)			
Head			
Circumference			
Shape			
Scalp			
Hair			
Fontanels			
Face			
Symmetry			
Movement			
Eyes			
Symmetry			
Movement			
Pupillary reaction			
Corneal light reflex			
Cornea			
Corneal reflex			
Optic blink			
Conjunctiva			
Sclera			
Ears			
Placement			
Position			
Configuration			
Symmetry			
Acoustic blink			
Nose			
Placement			
Patency			
Septum			
Throat and mouth			
Cry			
Placement			
Movement			
Mucosa			
Structures			
Suck			
Gag			
Neck			
Structures			
Movement			

Feature	Description of abnormal	Abnormal	Normal
Thorax			
Circumference			
Symmetry			
Movement			
Breasts			
Heart			
Rate and rhythm			
Point of maximal impulse			
Pulses			
Lungs			
Rate and rhythm			
Respirations			
Abdomen			
Umbilicus			
Shape			
Bowel sounds			
Musculature			
Organs			
Genitalia			
Male			
Testicles			
Scrotum			
Meatal opening			
Female			
Labia			
Clitoris			
Drainage			
Anus			
Patency			
Reflex			
Spine			
Continuity			
Mobility			
Extremities			
Symmetry			
Length			
Range-of-motion, hips			
Digits			
Palmar creases			
Neuromuscular			
Spontaneous activity			
Symmetry			
Reflexes			
Babinski's sign			
Biceps			
Clonus			

Feature	Description of abnormal	Abnormal	Normal
Grasp			
Traction			
Patellar			
Placing			
Stepping			
Moro's			
Growth parameters			
Blood pressure			
Temperature			
Height (length)			
Weight			
Gestational age			

Adapted from Dubowitz, L., V. Dubowitz, and C. Goldberg. Clinical assessment of gestational age in the newborn infant. *Journal of Pediatrics* (July 1970). 1-10.

CHAPTER 22

INFANT FEEDING

Nancy Kulb

Whether a new mother chooses to breast-feed or bottle-feed her infant, she will undoubtedly be very concerned about feeding her infant properly. A study of mothers in the early postpartum period revealed that they had more questions and concerns about infant feeding than about any other aspect of infant care.[1] Because feeding is viewed as a primary part of the maternal role, the client may assess her success as a mother by how expertly she feeds her baby. She may believe that the baby naturally knows how to eat and is hungry from birth, and she may, therefore, feel frustrated or rejected if the baby does not feed easily in the first few attempts. Nursing support is important, regardless of the method of feeding the client has chosen. The nurse must help the client to understand her infant's needs and to feel competent and confident in her new maternal role.

NUTRITIONAL NEEDS OF THE INFANT

Normal infants are born with sufficient nutrient stores to sustain them until they have mastered eating.

There are several newborn reflexes that are important in feeding: rooting, sucking, swallowing, and gag reflexes. Although all normal babies are born with these reflexes, each baby is an individual: some eat quickly and energetically; some suck quickly but are unable to

535

swallow as quickly; some suck initially but get "excited," lose the nipple, and are unable to find it again; some eat well initially, but fall asleep before they are full; and others just lick the nipple and take their time in feeding. The mother and her infant must both adapt to the needs and expectations of the other, which is normally a time-consuming process. The mother must also be aware that the infant may take a few days to establish eating patterns, especially if she received sedatives, analgesics, or anesthetics during labor.

The newborn's stomach is small, with a capacity of 50 to 60 milli-liters (approximately 2 ounces) when empty. During feedings, the newborn's stomach is able to stretch in order to hold more milk in addition to the air that frequently enters the stomach from gulping or crying. Gastric emptying time is slow in the newborn. Often, milk from a feeding will still be in the infant's stomach 3 or 4 hours later.[2]

The Recommended Dietary Allowances for infants from birth to 6 months of age are listed in Table 22-1. Table 22-2 lists the percentage of calories derived from the fat, protein, and carbohydrates in milk.

The protein in the milk that is fed to infants must contain all of the essential amino acids. The carbohydrates should consist primarily of monosaccharides and disaccharides because they are more easily digested and absorbed by the newborn than are polysaccharides. The fats should contain the essential fatty acids and be readily digestible. In general, unsaturated fats of medium-chain length are absorbed best. Breast milk and prepared formulas meet these requirements and provide most of the vitamins and minerals required by the newborn.[3] (The need for vitamin and mineral supplementation is discussed in the sections on breast- and bottle-feeding.)

It is common for a mother to wonder whether her infant is receiving enough to eat, especially if she is breast-feeding and cannot measure the amount of milk the infant is ingesting. The mother can be reassured that her baby is ingesting enough milk if (1) the baby urinates at least six to eight times each day, (2) the urine is pale in color, (3) he has bowel movements at least every 2 days, (4) he is satisfied for 2 to 3 hours between feedings, and (5) he gains about 113 grams (4 ounces) or more each week after the first week. Babies are expected to double their birth weight by 6 months, and triple it by 1 year of age; however, immediately after birth the baby may lose a few ounces as a result of the passage of urine and meconium. Consequently, a small weight loss should not be cause for alarm.

Many mothers ask when to start feeding solids to their infants. Often, the mother's family will encourage her to begin feeding solids to the baby in the first few weeks of life, or at least to add cereal to the baby's bottle, to help him sleep through the night. This practice is

TABLE 22-1

Recommended Dietary Allowances for Infants from Birth to 6 Months

Parameter	Value
Weight	6 kg (13 lb)
Height	24 in (61 cm)
Energy	117 × weight (in kg) = calories
Protein	2.2 × weight (in kg) = grams of protein
Vitamin A	420 μg RE
Vitamin D	10 μg CE
Vitamin E	3 mg α-TE
Vitamin C	35 mg
Thiamine	0.3 mg
Riboflavin	0.4 mg
Niacin	6 mg NE
Vitamin B6	0.3 mg
Folacin	30 μg
Vitamin B12	0.5 μg
Calcium	360 mg
Phosphorus	240 mg
Magnesium	50 mg
Iron	10 mg
Zinc	3 mg
Iodine	40 μg

CE, cholecalciferol equivalents; NE, niacin equivalents; RE, retinol equivalents; α-TE, tocopherol equivalents.
Adapted from the Food and Nutrition Board, National Academy of Sciences-National Research Council, Washington, D. C.

TABLE 22-2

Nutrient Composition of Calories in Milk

Nutrient	Percentage of calories needed by infant	Percentage in breast milk	Percentage in cow's milk
Fat	30-55	55	50
Carbohydrate	35-65	38	30
Protein	7-16	7	20

Adapted from Bender, K. J., M. W. McKenzie, and A. J. Seals. Infant formulas. *Journal of the American Pharmaceutical Association* (May 1975). 230.

to be discouraged beause (1) solids may take the place in the baby's diet of the milk or formula, which is generally higher in nutritional value and which ensures an adequate fluid intake, (2) the milk or formula has adequate nutrients for the young infant, (3) ingesting solids apparently does *not* help the baby to sleep through the night, (4) food allergies are more likely to develop with early introduction of solids, and (5) solids are more expensive and take more of the mother's time in preparation and feeding. Current recommendations call for solid foods to be initiated between 4 and 6 months of age.[4] The mother should be advised to consult her pediatrician or pediatric nurse practitioner before beginning to feed solids to her baby.

BREAST-FEEDING

Advantages

There are a number of reasons why women choose to breast-feed their infants, not the least important of which is the logical rationale that human milk is meant for human babies. The types of proteins, fats, carbohydrates, vitamins, and minerals in breast milk are appropriate for the needs of the newborn, are absorbable, and are present in adequate amounts. Breast-feeding may have psychological benefits, which are difficult to determine, for both the mother and her baby as they establish their relationship with each other.

There are specific advantages of breast-feeding for the mother. Postpartum blood loss is minimized and involution is hastened by the intermittent release of oxytocin, a hormone released during the let-down reflex (*see* Chapter 19). The incidence of breast cancer is lower in women who have breast-fed than in women who have not. Although lactation is not to be relied on as a method of contraception, the resumption of ovulation and menstruation is often delayed in breast-feeding mothers. Many mothers find that breast-feeding is more convenient than bottle-feeding because there is minimal preparation for feeding. Many also view the time spent in breast-feeding as a guaranteed time for rest.

In addition to the appropriate nutrients, breast-fed babies also receive other benefits from breast-feeding. Unlike formula, breast milk is not subject to contamination. Breast milk also provides antibodies and macrophages to the immunologically immature newborn. The result is that breast-fed babies have fewer gastrointestinal and respiratory infections than do bottle-fed babies. There is some evidence (although controversial) that breast-fed babies are less likely to develop obesity. Finally, because of the technique of sucking required for breast-feeding, the sucking needs of the infant may be met more adequately during feeding in breast-fed than in bottle-fed infants.

Disadvantages

The disadvantages of breast-feeding are few. No one else can help the mother by feeding the baby for her. It is time-consuming for her, and it is always her responsibility — even in the middle of the night.

In recent years, there has been increased concern over the presence of environmental pollutants in breast milk — particularly polychlorinated biphenyl (PCB). PCBs have been shown to cause cancer, skin disorders, hyperactivity, learning disorders, and even death in laboratory animals. Unfortunately, PCBs are widespread in the environment, and they become concentrated in humans because humans are at the top of the food chain. There are no inexpensive, reliable tests for determining the levels of PCBs in one's milk, and there is no easy way to rid the body of the contaminant. In general, it is recommended that women not be discouraged from breast-feeding because of PCBs unless it is known that they work and/or live in an area with unusually high levels of PCBs.[5]

Prenatal preparation for breast-feeding

Clients who plan to breast-feed may be encouraged to begin breast preparation in the last month of pregnancy. Because of the theoretical possibility of premature labor resulting from oxytocin release stimulated by breast manipulation, it is recommended that breast preparation not begin before the 36th week of gestation. Preparation of the breasts is intended to decrease sensitivity of the nipples, to "draw out" and strengthen the erection of the nipples, to clear the lactiferous sinuses and ducts of viscid early colostrum in order to facilitate the postpartum flow of colostrum and milk, and to increase the client's comfort and skills in caring for her breasts. The same techniques may prove invaluable during the postpartum period.

Breast massage.   Breast massage increases the blood circulation to the breasts and aids in the passage of milk through the ducts to the lactiferous sinuses. The client should remove her bra and wash her hands. She should lubricate her hands with a cream, lotion, or oil. The massage begins with both hands placed palmar surface down on the upper part of the breasts. While firm, even pressure is exerted, the hands separate, moving down the sides of the breast. The thumbs meet on the upper part of the breast, and the fingers meet at the lower margin of the breast. While even pressure is maintained all around, the breast is drawn out. When the areola is reached, the breast is allowed to slip between the hands. This procedure is repeated 10 to 15 times on each breast (Fig. 22-1).

Manual expression.   Manual expression of milk out of the lactiferous sinuses should be performed after breast massage. The client should support the breast with one hand. With the other, she places the thumb on one side of the areola, and the index finger on the

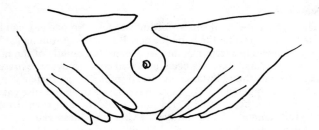

Figure 22-1. Breast massage. Used to increase blood circulation to the breasts and aid in the passage of milk through the ducts of the lactiferous sinuses. (*See* text for specific procedure.)

other. The finger and thumb are drawn back (not slid over the skin); gentle, but firm, pressure is applied, and the finger and thumb are drawn toward the nipple; then the pressure is released. Any colostrum or milk that is expressed should be gently wiped off. This should be repeated at various locations around the areola to ensure emptying of all the lactiferous sinuses. Initially, this procedure should not be repeated more than two or three times in the same place in order to avoid traumatizing the tissue. Later, it may be repeated until all the colostrum or milk is expressed (Fig. 22-2).

Nipple rolling. The nipple is gently held on the sides between the thumb and index finger of one hand while the other hand supports the breast. The nipple is gently rolled as far as it will go in one direction without letting it slip through the fingers. It is then rolled in the other direction as far as it will go. This procedure is repeated for about 30 seconds on each side (Fig. 22-3).

Nipple toughening. There are several techniques for toughening the nipples. The nipples can be rubbed briskly with a towel after a

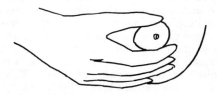

Figure 22-2. Manual expression. Used to express milk out of the lactiferous sinuses. (*See* text for specific procedure.)

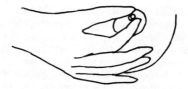

Figure 22-3. Nipple rolling. Used to draw out, and strengthen the erection of, the nipples. (*See* text for specific procedures.)

bath or shower; or instead of being protected by a bra, they can be exposed to the friction of clothes rubbing over them. Support of the breasts may be maintained by wearing a bra with holes cut in the cups to allow the nipples to be exposed. The use of soap on the nipples and areolae should be discouraged in the last month of pregnancy in order to avoid washing away protective secretions.

Inverted nipples.   Inverted nipples are a problem for breast-feeding mothers because the baby cannot get a good grasp on the nipple and areola. To check for inverted nipples, the mother should place the areola between her thumb and forefinger and apply pressure. An everted nipple will project out, but an inverted nipple will be drawn in. The best time to deal with inverted nipples is during the antepartum period, when nipple-rolling exercises and the use of Woolwich breast shields are usually sufficient to draw out the nipples before the initiation of breast-feeding. (A Woolwich breast shield is a hard plastic shield with a hole cut out for the nipple. Worn inside the bra, it pushes back on the areola, thus everting the nipple.) During the postpartum period, nipple shields can be used while breast-feeding in order to draw out the nipple, and Woolwich breast shields can be worn for a few days or weeks until the nipple is drawn out.

Initiation of breast-feeding

A significant alteration in maternal hormones occurs at delivery. One of the results of this change is the initiation of lactation (*see* Chapter 19).

The first secretion from the breasts in the first 2 or 3 days postpartum is colostrum, a yellowish fluid that provides nutrients and antibodies to the newborn. Colostrum contains twice as much protein as milk, and it has fat globules, which make it slightly thick and sticky. Colostrum contains antibodies to a number of bacteria and viruses, and it also has a laxative effect that aids in the passage of meconium. Gradually, during the second or third postpartum day, colostrum is replaced by milk, which is thinner and bluish white. Breast milk will replace the colostrum more quickly if the mother has performed prenatal breast preparation, if she has breast-fed previously, or if she was able to breast-feed within the first hour postpartum and regularly and frequently thereafter.

During the first hour after birth, most babies are in a quiet but alert state. This is an ideal time for breast-feeding to begin. Although many babies just lick their mother's nipples, most, with encouragement, will latch on and suck. The baby should be allowed to feed only 5 minutes on each side at first, until the nipples get used to it. The feeding time can be extended by 2 to 4 minutes each day over the first week or so until the baby empties one breast (usually about 20 minutes) before beginning to feed on the other side. The baby should be allowed to feed about every 2 to 3 hours, starting on one breast at one feeding, and on the other breast at the next feeding. It may help the mother to remember which side to start on at the next feeding by placing a safety pin on that side of her bra.

Breast-feeding technique

Preparation.   The mother should wash her hands before breast-feeding. It is not necessary to wash her breasts, but she may wipe off the nipples with plain water. The mother should be comfortable — her bladder should be empty, and any comfort measures for episiotomy or afterbirth pains should have been completed. She may wish to have something to drink while she nurses. The baby should be clean and dry. A baby that is crying loudly should be calmed before breast-feeding. The mother and her baby should be allowed uninterrupted time for feeding. They should be given privacy from other patients and unnecessary staff. However, a supportive nurse and/or significant others who are in attendance or nearby can help the mother while she and her baby are learning to breast-feed.

Positions.   The mother and her baby should both be in a position of comfort. The baby's mouth should be in alignment with his mother's breast, and his head and body should be supported. When sitting, the mother may find it comfortable to have the arm holding the baby resting on a chair arm or on a pillow placed on her lap. When lying down, she may lie on her side with her lower arm around the baby or extended toward the head of the bed. She should place the baby parallel to her body, either with the baby's feet toward her feet, or with the baby's feet near her head. The mother should learn to use various positions while in the hospital. The side-lying position may prove particularly useful for night feedings or for feedings when the mother needs to rest.

Feeding. The baby's cheek should be stroked with the breast to help him root to it. Initially, the mother may need to grasp her breast between her thumb and forefinger and guide it into the baby's mouth. If her breasts are large, she may use a finger to depress the breast in order to keep it from pressing tightly against the baby's nares.

The entire nipple and most of the areola should be in the baby's mouth when he sucks. The areola should be drawn farther into the baby's mouth with sucking. If the baby's grasp on the nipple is not correct, sucking may cause nipple soreness.

A baby who is uninterested in feeding may be enticed by having the mother express a few drops of colostrum or milk onto the surface of her nipple. A baby that drifts off to sleep after only a few minutes of feeding should be encouraged to stay awake longer in order to eat enough to satisfy him for 2 to 3 hours. Otherwise, he may want to feed again in 1 to 2 hours. Loosening his clothing, rubbing his feet, and/or changing his position will usually help to keep him awake during the entire feeding.

Before the baby is taken off the breast, the suction of the baby's mouth must be broken. Pulling the baby off the breast can be very uncomfortable for the mother, and may cause sore nipples. Suction can be broken by inserting a finger into the corner of the baby's mouth, by squeezing the cheeks together, or by applying downward pressure on the baby's chin, thereby causing the mouth to open.

Care of the breasts after feeding. After feeding, the nipples should be exposed to air for 15 to 30 minutes, preferably to sunshine or to the warmth of a 25-watt light bulb. A nipple cream (e.g., Masse or A and D Ointment) should then be applied. A well-fitting bra that does *not* have plastic liners should be worn. The client should continue to wash her nipples only with water — not soap or alcohol.

Burping. Although babies usually do not swallow as much air during breast-feeding as they do during bottle-feeding, they still may get air into the stomach and need to be burped or "bubbled." The most convenient times for burping the baby are after feeding on one breast but before going on to the other, and at the end of the feeding. The baby can be placed over the mother's shoulders or can be sat up on her lap. The baby's back should be gently rubbed or patted until he burps. It is wise to have a cloth under the baby because a little milk may come up with the air.

Maternal nutritional needs. The additional Recommended Dietary Allowances for lactating mothers are listed in Table 22-3. Because she is still eating for two, the lactating mother's caloric requirements are much greater (500 cal/day more) than those of the nonlactating, nonpregnant woman. Because she needs more calcium

TABLE 22-3
Additional Recommended Dietary Allowances for the Lactating Mother*

Parameter	Value
Energy	+ 500 cal/day (More if lactation continues >3 mo.)
Protein	+ 20 g
Vitamin A	+ 400 μg RE
Vitamin D	+ 5 μg CE
Vitamin E	+ 3 mg α-TE
Vitamin C	+ 40 mg
Thiamine	+ 0.5 mg
Riboflavin	+ 0.5 mg
Niacin	+ 5 mg NE
Vitamin B6	+ 0.5 mg
Folacin	+ 100 μg
Vitamin B12	+ 1 μg
Calcium	+ 400 mg
Phosphorus	+ 400 mg
Magnesium	+ 150 mg
Iron	+ 0‡
Zinc	+ 10 mg
Iodine	+ 50 μg

CE, cholecalciferol equivalents; NE, niacin equivalents; RE, retinol equivalents; α-TE, tocopherol equivalents.
*Basic requirements vary according to the age, size, and specific needs of the mother.
‡Despite the lack of an increased need of iron, supplementation is advised in order to replenish stores that were depleted during pregnancy.
Adapted from the Food and Nutrition Board, National Academy of Sciences-National Research Council, Washington, D. C.

(400 mg/day more), milk is recommended in her diet. The nursing mother also needs plenty of fluids — at least 3,000 ml/day.

Many nursing mothers are concerned about avoiding spices, chocolate, or other foods that might affect the baby. Occasionally, a baby may react to something the mother has consumed by experiencing diarrhea or gastrointestinal distress. If one food consistently affects the baby, it should be eliminated from the mother's diet. In general, however, the mother does not need to restrict her diet. She should be encouraged to eat a well-balanced diet and to consume a variety of foods.

Supplements.   In general, the totally breast-fed infant does not need other foods or supplements during the first few months of life. The mother may occasionally wish to give the baby a bottle if she will be separated from him at feeding time. Some working mothers are able to successfully combine breast-feeding and bottle-feeding on a routine basis. The mother may choose to give the baby formula while she is away, or she may manually express milk in advance to leave for the baby. She may manually express milk while she is away to relieve uncomfortable fullness and to stimulate her breasts to maintain her milk supply. Expressed milk should be kept in a clean bottle in the refrigerator for no longer than 24 hours.

The use of vitamin and mineral supplements in totally breast-fed infants is generally not necessary. If the baby is not exposed to sunlight at all, or if the mother is deficient in vitamin D, a daily vitamin D supplement (10 micrograms cholecalciferol equivalents) may be indicated. Infants of vegan mothers may need vitamin B12 supplementation. Although breast milk contains a relatively small amount of iron, it is readily absorbed and in sufficient quantity until the baby is 6 months of age, at which point iron-fortified cereals or iron supplements should be initiated. Although the content of fluoride in breast milk is minimal, the use of fluoride supplements is controversial. There is insufficient evidence to suggest that the administration of fluoride supplements in the first 6 months prevents dental caries. The mother should be encouraged to discuss fluoride supplementation with her pediatrician.

Management of problems and concerns

Engorgement.   Engorgement is a short-lived problem that many mothers, both breast-feeding and non-breast-feeding encounter. (*See* Chapter 19 for the physiological basis of engorgement and the appropriate nursing relief measures.)

Sore, cracked nipples.   Many mothers, especially if they are fair-skinned, experience sore nipples. The cause may be an improper breast-feeding technique, such as failure of the infant to grasp most of the areola in his mouth, or failure of the mother to break suction before removing the infant from the breast; or it may occur as a transient discomfort while the mother is becoming accustomed to breast-feeding. Prenatal breast preparation, proper breast-feeding technique, and proper breast care will help to prevent sore, cracked nipples.

Once sore nipples have developed, the nurse should encourage the mother to breast-feed more frequently for shorter periods of time. Before feeding, the mother should be encouraged to perform breast massage on the affected side so the milk will be in the lactiferous sinuses when the baby begins feeding. She should be encouraged to alternate positions for breast-feeding in order to change the points of pressure on the nipples. She might begin the feeding on the less sore side in order to initiate the let-down reflex, switch to the other side in order to empty that breast, then return to the less sore side. If the baby has a need to suck after feeding, he should be given a pacifier instead of being allowed to suck unnecessarily on an empty breast. Attention to proper breast-feeding technique, exposure of the nipples to air and warmth after feeding, and application of a nipple cream will also help sore nipples.

Tension.   The let-down reflex may be inhibited if the mother is tense or in pain. She should be given time in the hospital (and she should be encouraged to take time at home) to nurse when she will not be interrupted. A supportive family is invaluable in initiating and maintaining lactation. The nurse should be very supportive of her efforts in the first few days, so the mother can relax and be assured that she is a competent mother.

Maternal medications.   Many medications are secreted in breast milk. Appendix A lists commonly used medications, and what effect they may have on the breast-fed neonate. The mother should be encouraged to check with her pediatrician before taking medications if she is unsure of their effect on the baby.

Twins.   The mother who wants to breast-feed twins will be able to do so, but will need extra support and organization. For example, when one twin is awake and ready to eat, she will probably need to wake up the other so that her day is not totally taken up with feeding them. She will need to experiment with, or be shown the technique for, holding them both at the same time. She might choose to breast-feed one at one feeding and bottle-feed the other, then switch at the next feeding.

Mastitis.   Mastitis usually occurs as a result of stasis of milk, and appears as a firm, reddened area of the breast. The mother may feel feverish or sick. If such symptoms occur, she should report them to her physician, who may wish to prescribe antibiotics. She should take measures to restore the free flow of milk from that area (e.g., apply warm compresses for 5 to 10 mintues each hour, massage that area before breast-feeding, and increase the frequency of nursing on that side). It is rarely necessary to stop breast-feeding as a result of mastitis. If it becomes necessary, however, the mother should be encouraged to manually empty her breast often, until she can resume breast-feeding. The problem usually resolves itself in 2 or 3 days.

Follow-up care

The nurse can help the new mother to establish breast-feeding in the hospital through teaching and encouragement. The nurse can also prepare the mother for the problems or concerns she may experience at home. A follow-up visit or telephone call during the first few days or weeks at home is often of great help to the new mother. It allows her to ask questions or express concerns for which she would not call her physician. In addition, the nurse can suggest literature on breast-feeding or referral to La Leche League for continued help with nursing.

BOTTLE-FEEDING

Advantages

Bottle-feeding provides an adequate supply of nutrients for the neonate. It also provides time for closeness and interaction between the mother and her baby. Mothers should not be made to feel that they are making a wrong or inferior choice when they choose to bottle-feed. It allows other members of the family to participate in the feeding of the baby, which may be something that (1) they enjoy immensely, (2) facilitates family attachment, and (3) the mother may welcome, especially in the middle of the night or when she must be away from home. Although working mothers who desire to breast-feed can do so, many working mothers choose to bottle-feed their infants.

Disadvantages

Bottle-feeding requires time for preparation of the formula. In addition, it may be more expensive than breast-feeding because of the cost of the formula, the bottles, and the other equipment needed to prepare the formula.

Preparation of formula

There are many commercial formula preparations available. Table 22-4 lists several, and shows their nutrient content in comparison with breast milk.

Commercial formulas are generally available in three forms: ready-to-feed, concentrated, and powdered. The ready-to-feed formula is the most expensive, and the powdered is the least expensive. The powdered formulas may be difficult to dissolve in water; the use of warm water and, perhaps, a beater will help.

Noncommercial formula may also be prepared at home according

TABLE 22-4

Nutrient Content of Milk and Infant Formulas*

Parameter	Infant requirements	Human milk	Cow's milk (whole, fortified)	Enfamil (Mead Johnson)	Similac (Ross)	SMA (Wyeth)
Calories	117 × weight (in kg) = calories	75	69	66	66	66
Protein, g	2.2 × weight (in kg) = protein	1.1	3.5	1.5	1.8	1.5
Fat, g	ND	4.5	3.5	3.7	3.6	3.5
Carbohydrate, g	ND	6.8	4.9	7	7	6.8
Vitamin A, μg RE	420	240	185	160	250	250
Vitamin D, μg CE	10	0.5	40	40	40	40
Thiamine, mg	0.3	0.016	0.029	0.04	0.065	0.055
Vitamin E, mg α-TE	3	0.2	0.04	0.8-1.3	0.85-1.30	0.95
Vitamin C, mg	35	4.3	1.1	5.5	5.5	5.8
Niacin, mg NE	6	0.35	0.1	0.70-0.85	0.70-0.85	0.7
Riboflavin, mg	0.4	0.04	0.17	0.06-0.10	0.06-0.10	0.1
Vitamin B6, mg	0.30	0.01	0.06	0.03-0.04	0.03-0.04	0.04
Vitamin B12, μg	0.50	0.03	0.4	0.15-0.20	0.25	0.11
Folacin, μg	30	5.2	5.5	5-10	5-10	3.2
Calcium, mg	360	34	117	55-60	55-60	44.5
Iron, mg	10	0.5	0.5	Trace-0.15	Trace-0.15	1.3
Iodine, μg	40	3	4.7	4.0-6.9	4.0-6.9	6.9
Magnesium, mg	50	4	12	4.0-4.8	4.0-4.8	5.3
Phosphorus, mg	240	14	92	44-45	44.8	33
Sodium, mEq	ND	0.7	2.2	1.1-1.7	1.1-1.7	0.7

CE, cholecalciferol equivalents; ND, not determined; NE, niacin equivalents; RE, retinol equivalents; α-TE, tocopherol equivalents.

*Values shown are per 100 milliliters.

Adapted from Bender, K. J., M. W. McKenzie, and A. J. Seals. Infant formulas. Journal of the American Pharmaceutical Association (May 1975). 230; and Slattery, J. S., G. A. Pearson, and C. T. Torre. Maternal and Child Nutrition: Assessment and Counseling. Appleton-Century-Crofts, East Norwalk, Conn. 1979. p. 66-69.

to the following guidelines. An infant will usually take 3 ounces more than his age in months at each feeding. For example, a 3-month-old infant would take 3 ounces plus his age in months (3) — or 6 ounces at each feeding. He would probably take five feedings each day, or 30 ounces of formula. The 3-month-old baby needs the following requirements each day:

1.5 ounces of cow's milk per pound of body weight.
1.0 ounce of carbohydrate per 10 ounces of milk required.
1.5 to 2.5 ounces of water (part of which is supplied by the milk) per pound of body weight. That is, enough water is needed to make up the fluid requirement determined above.

The above requirements could be supplied by either whole milk, sugar, and water; or by evaporated milk (1 ounce per pound of body weight), corn syrup, and water. It should be noted that casein, the protein in cow's milk, is a "tough" curd that may slow gastric emptying time and cause gastrointestinal distress.

Clean technique. In the past, great emphasis was placed on the sterilization of bottles and formula to prevent infection. Today, the trend is toward using commercial formulas, preparing each bottle immediately before use, and using clean, rather than sterile, technique. Commercial formula preparations are much more convenient to use than formulas that must be prepared at home. The availability of clean tap water and refrigeration has improved sanitary conditions in most homes. It has been shown that bottles prepared immediately before use, by means of clean technique, have acceptably low bacterial counts. Bottles may be considered clean if they have been washed in hot, soapy water, or in a dishwasher. If the formula is prepared in advance, it should be kept in the refrigerator for no longer than 24 hours before use.

Sterilization. Aseptic and terminal methods of sterilization will be briefly discussed so that the nurse can properly instruct the mother who chooses to use a sterile technique.

Aseptic: In this method, all equipment is cleaned and sterilized before the formula is made. A glass pitcher for mixing the formula, a measuring cup, measuring spoons, a funnel (if needed), tongs, bottles, nipples, and caps are boiled vigorously for 10 mintues in a large pan of water. The tongs are used as forceps to manipulate the other equipment. They should be boiled with the other equipment with the handles up so the mother's hand does not have to enter the water to retrieve them. After the equipment is sterilized, the formula is prepared and poured into the bottles, which are then nippled, capped, and placed in the refrigerator for storage (for up to 24 hours). Care should be taken during this entire procedure in order to avoid touching any surface that will come in contact with the formula.

Terminal: In this method of sterilization, the prepared formula is poured into clean bottles, and the nipples and caps are loosely applied. The bottles are then placed in a sterilizer or a large pan with water in the bottom, and the pan is covered with a tight lid. The water is boiled vigorously for 25 minutes. The bottles are allowed to cool, the caps are tightened, and the bottles are placed in the refrigerator (for up to 24 hours).

Bottle-feeding technique

The mother should assume a comfortable position for feeding the infant: e.g., sitting up with the infant's head cradled in one arm. Once again, her arm may be more comfortable if it is resting on the arm of a chair or on a pillow on her lap. The baby's head and body should be straight and supported. The mother should be relaxed and free from pain or tension.

The milk should be warmed to body temperature before feeding. To check that the holes in the nipple are the appropriate size (i.e., large enough to allow the milk to run out easily as the baby sucks, but not large enough to cause the baby to choke as the milk quickly runs out), the mother should hold the bottle upside down. The milk should drop out, rather than flow out.

Like the breast-fed baby, the bottle-fed baby may drift off to sleep before getting a sufficient amount to satisfy him. He should be encouraged to stay awake to complete the feeding. Bottle-fed babies that are receiving enough formula at each feeding usually do not demand to be fed again for 3 to 4 hours.

The baby will need to be burped in the middle of the feeding and again at the end. The same techniques for burping may be used for the bottle-fed baby as for the breast-fed baby. After the baby is fed and burped, he should be placed on his side, rather than on his back, to minimize the chances of aspiration if he should regurgitate.

The mother should be discouraged from propping the bottle for a feeding. The baby needs the warmth and security of being held, as well as someone to burp him and to help him if he chokes or loses the nipple.

Infants receiving commercially prepared formulas generally do not require supplementation in the first 6 months of life. After 4 months of age, iron-fortified formula or cereal may be recommended. Commercial formulas are low in fluoride, but the fluoride content of concentrated and powdered preparations depends on the fluoride content of the water with which it is mixed. Fluoride supplementation is controversial, but may be prescribed in communities where the water contains less than 0.3 parts per million of fluoride.

Infants receiving home-prepared formulas may require supplementation of vitamins C and D. By 4 months of age, they will need supplemental iron (1 mg/kg/day) or iron-fortified formula or cereal.

SUMMARY

Feeding is a time of special closeness between a mother and her baby. Both breast-feeding and bottle-feeding are nutritionally adequate for the newborn, and both require skills that must be learned by the mother in the first few days postpartum. The nurse is in a unique position to teach the mother the skills she will need to care for her infant, and to support the mother in her early efforts at mothering.

REFERENCES

1. Adams.

2. Fitzpatrick et al. 377.

3. Bender et al.

4. American Academy of Pediatrics. (June 1980)

5. Mosher and Meyer.

CHAPTER 23

THE NEWBORN: DISCHARGE PLANNING

Dorothy Allbritten

Discharge planning is a process by which families prepare for the forthcoming transition from hospital care to home care. The process begins on admission to the hospital and continues through discharge. Although the primary people involved are nurses and their clients, other health care professionals (e.g., the physician, social worker, or psychologist) may be active participants in the process. The purpose of discharge planning is to provide a smooth transition from hospital to home without interrupting the therapeutic regimen that the client is following.

PREDISCHARGE ASSESSMENT OF NEEDS

A complete assessment of the client's needs includes all components of the client's health status. To identify all of these components, the involved parties must collaborate and identify the needs from each of their perspectives. In general, there are three perspectives in hospital-related parent-child issues: that of the family, that of the nurse, and that of the physician or nurse-midwife.

The family's concerns frequently center on the mother's need for rest, emotional support, "catch-up" time, support with routine household maintenance, and adaptation to the 24-hour demands of the new family member. The mother's assessment of her own discharge needs may be as stated above, or she may focus on infant care or be concerned that the sibling(s) accept and adapt to their new family member without disruptive behaviors. Whatever the perceived need, it is imperative that the family's perspective be identified for accurate and sensitive discharge planning.

The nursing perspective may focus on issues of child health, maternal recuperation, family adaptation, and education regarding continued health-maintenance care. The specifics for each client will usually include components from the above issues. Nursing assessment ensures the integration and coordination of the various components of the discharge planning process.

The medical perspective in the assessment of discharge needs focuses on the healing process occurring in the mother and her new infant. Medical concerns focus on compliance with prescriptions and therapies, closure of wounds, and the return of laboratory values and body functions to a normal range.

The three perspectives, when combined, provide a complete assessment of the discharge needs of the family. The forum that facilitates the combining of the three perspectives is that of the predischarge planning conference.

Predischarge planning conference

The scope of predischarge planning conferences varies with the needs of individual families. For healthy mothers and infants who have experienced an uncomplicated birth, the planning will be brief and less involved than for a mother or baby with complications. There are, nevertheless, several basic considerations to review with each client before the maternity nurse completes the discharge process (Table 23-1).

Activity and life-style. Part of the conference discussion should include exploration of the roles of various family members in the household and projections about how these roles may vary when the new family member joins the group. The nurse should assist the mother to begin considering the possible changes she may face when reentering the world of "home." The mother's initial feelings of elation, relief, and creativity that follow delivery may change into feelings of fatigue and overwhelming responsibility at homecoming. Care of her infant will be a 24-hour job, as the mother leaves the hospital nursing staff behind. Keeping the baby clean and dry, attempting to feed the baby in some synchrony with the family routine, and keeping up with the increased laundry load on less-than-usual sleep frequently leads to discouragement and the onset of postpartum blues. If the nurse and mother identify the need for

TABLE 23-1

Checklist for Discharge Planning Conference

Basic consideration	Specific topic
Topics for discussion	Activities and life-style: a. Role changes in family members. b. Activities of daily living: Rest. Exercise, stimulation, and sex. Nutrition (*see* Chapter 22). Elimination. Interaction. Education and anticipatory guidance: a. Supplies and equipment for parenting. b. Primary health care and health maintenance. c. Growth and development. Follow-up appointments (*see* Fig. 23-1): a. Continuity of care. b. Referral to special services.
Discharge activities	Give verbal and written instructions: a. Educational pamphlets. b. Discharge plan (*see* Fig. 23-2). Notify involved specialist or service.

assistance in this coping process, they may decide to use the services of the social worker and to include that person in their planning.

Once at home, the family begins to reorganize. There are new needs apparent, and there are new ways to meet the needs. There are family values that need reorienting as the family pair becomes a threesome. There are new roles to assign: the husband now becomes husband and father, and the wife becomes wife and mother. This reorganization stage of family development is facilitated by maturity in the parents.

As the nurse and new mother review the activities of daily living (ADL) required to return to home living, they may identify some limitations to ADL that require the services of an extended family member or a community service. When considering the components of ADL — rest, exercise, stimulation, nutrition, elimination, and interaction — the mother should be assisted by the nurse to plan for the known limitations and to anticipate some unknown problems. Together they may assess the need for public health nursing services, homemaker visits, or occasional home health aide service to smooth the transition to normalcy.

Education and anticipatory guidance.   Education of the family is an ongoing nursing responsibility. The predischarge planning conference will focus on the client's educational needs and provide the setting to begin anticipatory guidance for discharge. Supplies and equipment for caring for the infant are major topics for discussion. The nurse should help the mother differentiate between the "need-to-have" and the "nice-to-have" items (Table 23-2). The primary focus of the nurse is on the short-term needs assessed, but guidance should be offered regarding long-term needs as the infant grows and develops. Table 23-3 provides a list of the infant activities that change as the infant develops from birth to 1 month of age. The maternity nurse who teaches parents about these activities bridges the information gap between hospital discharge and the first pediatric visit.

The mother should be assisted in decision-making about selecting a single source of primary health care for both herself and the infant. She should have access to information about a variety of health care providers that are available in her area (if she has not already chosen one). The nurse should stress the need for health-maintenance visits for the baby from infancy through adolescence (Fig. 23-1). The mother should also be informed that immunizations are one means of preventing disease (Table 23-4).

Follow-up appointments.   It is a good idea to schedule a return appointment in 2 weeks in order to validate parenting techniques and to evaluate the infant's well-being. Parenting crises occur early and are frequently resolved without professional assistance during the usual 6-week gap between hospital discharge and the first office visit. When a 2-week visit is planned, seemingly "silly or trivial" questions and concerns can be resolved before they turn into problems or result

TABLE 23-2

Infant Supplies and Equipment*

Need-to-have items	Nice-to-have items
Bath towel	
Blanket, heavyweight — one	Baby bed with infant rail pads
Blanket, lightweight — four	Bathinette
Bottles	Changing table
Bottle-feeding	Gowns or sleepers
Two 4-oz. bottles	Socks or booties
Eight 8-oz. bottles	Vaporizer (cool mist)
Breast-feeding	
One 4-oz. bottle	
Two 8-oz. bottles	
Bottle brush	
Bulb syringe	
Diapers (preferably cloth) — 4 dozen	
Infant car seat	
Mild soap	
Protected sleeping area (e.g., basket, crib, or bassinet)	
Shirts — six	
Sweater and cap	
Terry washcloth	
Thermometer (axillary)	
Tub or basin for bathing	

*Numbers provided are suggestions only. Individual families may need to alter these suggested quantities.

in unhealthy coping patterns. The nurse can promote continuity of care by arranging the first pediatric appointment for the mother. Subsequent preventive health care visits are recommended every other month for the first 6 months (*see* Fig. 23-1).

If mutually validated needs have been identified and a special service is required, the nurse should assist the family to obtain that service. Consideration of each of the above-mentioned topics will provide a complete assessment for each family, whether the individual situation is uncomplicated or complicated with medical, health, and/or psychosocial problems.

Discharge activities.   At the actual time of discharge from the hospital, the greater part of the maternity nurse's discharge work has been accomplished. The final activities include providing last-minute

TABLE 23-3

Developmental Signs of Early Infancy

From birth	From 1 month
Cries, yawns, sneezes, hiccups, sucks, swallows.	Coos, gurgles.
Makes spontaneous crawling movements.	Smiles responsively.
Responds to loud noise or bright light with a startle.	Quiets to vocalization.
	Cries for hunger or discomfort.
Makes fist and flexes elbows.	Lifts head while lying on stomach.
Turns head to side when prone.	Turns head toward sound.
Regards human face.	Holds head up momentarily while sitting.
Smiles fleetingly.	
Moves extremities vigorously during crying.	Visually follows movement to midline.
Urinates, stools.	
Sleeps 18-22 hr daily.	

answers to questions, notifying involved specialists or services, and providing the mother with a written copy of the discharge plan (Fig. 23-2). The plan provides a visual summary of the outcomes of the nurse-client conference(s), with a display of the information required to resume life at home.

SUMMARY

The importance of discharge planning cannot be overemphasized. The discharge plan for the maternity nurse is as important as the blueprint is to the architect, the gameplan is to the coach, and the script is to the director. It provides the coordination, direction, and continuity needed for a successful outcome. The maternity nurse is the prime factor in providing a smooth transition for the mother and her infant from hospital to home.

AGE	2-4 wk	2-3 mo	4-5 mo	6-7 mo	9-10 mo	12-15 mo	16-19 mo	23-25 mo	36-37 mo	5-6 yr	8-9 yr	11-12 yr	13-15 yr	16-21 yr
HISTORY														
Initial	–					← At first visit →								–
Interval	–					← At each visit →								–
MEASUREMENTS														
Height and weight	–					← At each visit →								–
Head circumference	✓	✓	✓	✓		✓		✓						
Blood pressure									✓	✓	✓	✓	✓	✓
SENSORY SCREENING														
Sight	✓	✓		✓					✓	✓ OR		✓	✓	
Hearing	✓	✓		✓					✓	✓ OR		✓	✓	
DEVELOPMENTAL APPRAISAL	–					← At each visit →								–
PHYSICAL EXAMINATION	–					← At each visit →								–
PROCEDURES														
Immunization		✓	✓	✓		✓	✓		✓	✓			✓	
Tuberculin test			✓	✓					✓	✓	✓	✓		
Hematocrit or hemoglobin				✓					✓ OR	✓	✓		✓	
Urinalysis								✓		✓		✓		
Urine culture (girls only)														
DISCUSSION AND COUNSELING	–					← At each visit →								–
DENTAL SCREENING	–					← At each visit →								–
INITIAL DENTIST'S EXAMINATION									✓					

Figure 23-1. Recommendations for preventive health care. A guide for the care of well children who exhibit no untoward psychosocial or physical manifestations, who receive competent parenting, and who demonstrate progressive growth and development.

TABLE 23-4

Recommended Schedule for Immunization of Healthy Infants and Children

Time period	Vaccine
2 mo	DTP and TOPV
4 mo	DTP and TOPV
6 mo	DTP*
12 mo	Tuberculin test
15 mo	Measles, rubella, mumps
18 mo	DTP and TOPV
4-6 yr	DTP and TOPV
14-16 yr	Td‡

DTP, diphtheria and tetanus toxoids combined with pertussis vaccine; Td, combined tetanus and diphtheria toxoids (in contrast to diphtheria and tetanus — DT — toxoids, which contain a larger amount of diphtheria antigen); TOPV, trivalent oral polovirus vaccine.

*A third dose of TOPV is optional at this time.

‡Repeat every 10 yr.

Adapted from Committee on Infectious Diseases. Report of the Committee on Infectious Diseases. American Academy of Pediatricians, Evanston, Ill. 1977. Eighteenth edition.

DISCHARGE PLAN

Mother's name: _____ Date of plan: _____

Baby's name: _____ Date of birth: _____

Primary health care provider: _____

                    Telephone: _____

Obstetrician/midwife: _____

           Telephone: _____

Pediatrician/PNP: _____

       Telephone: _____

MOTHER

    Activity:

    Treatments:

    Medication:

    Return visit:

INFANT

    Activity:

       Feeding:

       Bathing:

    Treatments:

       Cord care:

       Circumcision care:

    Medications:

    Return visit:

Referral:

Literature given:

Signatures: _____   _____
                   (mother)   (nurse)

Figure 23-2.   Example of a discharge plan sheet. A copy should be given to the mother on discharge. PNP, pediatric nurse practitioner.

APPENDIX A: MEDICATIONS

MEDICATIONS

Pregnancy is a time of rapid and complex changes for the client and the fetus. Caregivers must pay special attention to the fact that agents that affect one will probably affect the other. Medications must be prescribed with particular attention to the risk:benefit ratio (i.e., Is the risk to the client and/or the fetus/newborn outweighed by the anticipated benefits of the drug?). Because safety during human pregnancy is so difficult to prove, many drug companies include a statement in their product information to the effect that safety during pregnancy has not been established. Clients should be fully informed of the potential risk of the medications prescribed, but also of the potential harm from the condition that is being treated by medication. In general, medications should be avoided during pregnancy whenever possible, but treatment for pathological conditions should not be withheld. In some cases, a medication may be changed during pregnancy to one that has minimal fetal, neonatal, and/or maternal side effects. There is still much to be learned about the effects of specific drugs on the client and the fetus during pregnancy.

Many factors influence how a drug may affect the fetus. The effect may be indirect, via the effect of the drug on the client. For example, hydralazine hydrochloride (Apresoline), which may be administered to control moderate to severe hypertension in a preeclamptic client, has not been shown to have direct effects on the fetus. However, the maternal hypotension that may result from the administration of hydralazine may result in fetal hypoxia.

On the other hand, the drug may have a direct effect on the fetus. In order to do so, it must cross the placental barrier from the maternal to the fetal circulation. There are a number of factors that determine whether, and how readily, a medication may pass from the maternal to the fetal circulation:

1. *Size of the molecule.* Small molecules pass the placental barrier more readily than large ones.

2. *Lipid solubility*. Medications that are lipid soluble cross the membrane more readily than those that are not.

3. *Ionization*. Drugs that are ionized pass through the barrier more slowly than those that are not.

4. *Acid-base balance*. Differences in maternal-fetal pH will facilitate or hinder the passage of certain drugs.

5. *Concentration gradient*. The greater the difference in concentration of medication on the two sides of the placental barrier, the more rapidly will the medication cross the barrier.

6. *Characteristics of the placental membrane*. During pregnancy, the surface area of the placental membrane progressively increases while the thickness of the membrane decreases. A large surface area and a thin membrane tend to promote rapid crossing of a medication. This effect, however, is not as great as might be expected.

7. *Characteristics of circulation*. Fetal absorption of medication will be diminished whenever placental circulation is impaired on either the maternal or fetal side of the membrane.

Once the medication has reached the fetal circulation, it passes through the umbilical vein to the fetus. Some of the drug goes to the liver, where it may be metabolized, and most passes through the inferior vena cava to the heart. The concentration of medication will be diluted by blood returning from the systemic circulation to the heart. From the heart, it will be distributed to the tissues of the fetus.

Early in gestation, during the time of organogenesis, medications may exert a teratogenic effect on the fetus. Teratogenic effects usually occur during the first 8 to 10 weeks after fertilization. The effects may be so profound as to cause spontaneous abortion, or defects that are incompatible with extrauterine life. Teratogenicity depends on the particular drug, the gestational time at which it is taken, the dose, and a host of other factors that are unique to the individual (e.g., susceptibility, nutritional status, presence of medical disease, presence of other medications, etc.).

Later in pregnancy, medications may alter fetal growth and development on a less obvious scale — in the growth or functioning of particular organs, in behavioral functioning, or in a predisposition to cancer. Some of these effects may not be obvious at birth or in every individual, but they may be discovered only after long-range studies of large numbers of individuals.

At the end of pregnancy, some drugs must be used with caution because of their effect on the neonate. Many of the analgesic and sedative drugs are in this group. When delivery is imminent, administration may cause sedation or respiratory depression of the neonate at the time of crucial adjustment to extrauterine life. These and other drugs, which are easily metabolized by the client, must now be metabolized by the neonate, with an immature and not fully functioning liver. It may require days or weeks for the infant to rid his system of medications that were in his circulation at birth.

It is important, therefore, that medications and other chemical agents be taken only when necessary during pregnancy. Many clients may not be aware that over-the-counter drugs (e.g., Tums, Dristan, Dramamine, Pepto Bismol) are medications and should be taken with the same caution that applies to prescription drugs. The nurse should encourage the client to call her physician or clinic before taking any medication.

Other chemicals not usually considered to be drugs have also been shown to affect the fetus. Caffeine (found in coffee, tea, cola beverages, and cocoa) may cause increased fetal activity and fetal tachycardia. In very high amounts, it may cause chromosome breakage. Cigarette smoking has been shown to cause low birth weight, and to increase the risk of fetal wastage. The nurse should encourage the client to eliminate these substances, if possible; or, if it is not possible, to decrease their use.

There are other drugs that are not used therapeutically during pregnancy, but may be abused by some clients. Examples include marijuana, heroin, cocaine, and phencyclidine (PCP). Table 15-7 lists some commonly abused drugs with their effect on both the mother and fetus. Clients using "street drugs" should be referred to a drug treatment center for follow-up care.

Medications should be administered only when necessary. The specific effects of the drug on the fetus and on the client's altered physiology during pregnancy must be considered. The client must be fully informed about the known risks and benefits of the medication and about what is as yet unknown. Following is a list of medications used during pregnancy and the postpartum and neonatal periods. The list is not exhaustive, but it includes a representative group of medications that may be used during pregnancy. Representative dosage regimens, indications, contraindications, and side effects are included. Readers are encouraged to check up-to-date references before administering medications because knowledge in the area of pharmacology is constantly increasing. It is the responsibility of the nurse, before administering any medication, to be certain that the correct medication is administered to the right person, in the correct dose, by the correct route, at the correct time. The nurse must also observe the client for the expected therapeutic effects and side effects of the medication. The client has the right to know what the medication is, why it is being administered, how to take it (if she is expected to take it herself), the expected therapeutic effects, the possible side effects, and the danger signs that require consultation with the physician.

LACTATION

There are many medications that are excreted in breast milk. Frequently, the concentration in breast milk is much less than that in the maternal circulation, although alkaline drugs may be more highly concentrated in breast milk than in maternal plasma. Small-molecule, water-soluble drugs will easily pass into breast milk. Other factors influencing passage of drugs into breast milk include lipid solubility, ionization, plasma protein binding, pH and fat content of the milk, drug concentration in maternal circulation, and adequacy of maternal hepatic and renal functioning.

Medications with minimal side effects should be used in order to minimize the effects of maternal drugs on breast-feeding infants. When possible, the initiation of drug therapy should be delayed until the infant is several days or weeks old and his enzyme functioning has been established. When possible, administer the medication immediately after a feeding, and consider delaying the next feeding or substituting a bottle for one feeding with manual expression of the breasts (see p. 539).

This appendix has two sections:

1. Medications used during pregnancy and the postpartum and neonatal periods. Included is an alphabetical list of medications and their classification, dose/route, indications, contraindications, maternal and fetal side effects, and, where appropriate, specific comments regarding drug usage.

2. Excretion of drugs in breast milk. Included are (a) an alphabetical list of drugs that are excreted in breast milk and their effects on the infant, and (b) a list of drugs that are known not to be excreted in breast milk.

For further information on medications, the reader is referred to the following texts:

Berkowitz, R. L., D. R. Coustan, and T. K. Mochizuki. Handbook for Prescribing Medications During Pregnancy. Little, Brown & Co., Boston. 1981.

Dickason, E. J., M. O. Schult, and E. M. Morris. Maternal and Infant Drugs and Nursing Intervention. McGraw-Hill Book Co., New York. 1978.

Lawrence, R. A. Breast-feeding: A Guide for the Medical Profession. C. V. Mosby Co., St. Louis. 1980.

Physicians' Desk Reference. Medical Economics Co., Oradell, N. J. 1981. Thirty-fifth edition.

MEDICATIONS USED DURING PREGNANCY AND THE POSTPARTUM AND NEONATAL PERIODS*

acetaminophen (Tylenol, Datril). *Classification:* Analgesic, antipyretic. Elevates pain threshold. Acts on hypothalamic heat-regulating center. *Dose/route:* 325-650 mg PO q 4 hr prn. Maximum daily dose: 2.6 g/day. *Indications:* Analgesic and antipyretic of choice during pregnancy. *Contraindications:* Hypersensitivity to acetaminophen. May be contraindicated in G6PD deficiency. *Maternal side effects:* Central nervous system symptoms: drowsiness, stimulation, euphoria, lightheadedness, dizziness, detachment. Skin rash with fever, hemolytic anemia, and other blood dyscrasias. Nephrotoxicity, myocardial damage, hypoglycemia, coma, hepatic necrosis with prolonged, excessive use. *Fetal side effects:* In large doses, renal damage.

acetylsalicylic acid (aspirin). *Classification:* Salicylate analgesic, antipyretic, anti-inflammatory drug. Inhibits prostaglandin synthesis in inflamed tissue. Inhibits histamine release. *Dose/route:* 325-650 mg PO q 4 hr prn. Higher doses may be required for treatment of severe arthritis. *Indications:* Use during pregnancy limited to anti-inflammatory effect in treating arthritis. *Contraindications:* Sensitivity to salicylates, peptic ulcer, bleeding disorders. *Maternal side effects:* Prolonged bleeding time, prolonged gestation, longer labor. Gastrointestinal irritation and bleeding, pyloric spasm, vomiting, tinnitus, sweating, drowsiness, thirst, headache. Toxic doses may cause renal damage or central nervous system disturbances. *Fetal side effects:* Prolonged bleeding time with possible gastrointestinal bleeding or hemorrhage at birth. Teratogenicity is suspected, but not proven. *Comments:* Administer with milk or on a full stomach to help reduce gastrointestinal irritation. Do not administer during organogenesis in the first trimester or near the expected date of delivery.

alcohol, ethyl. *Classification:* Tocolytic agent. Inhibits release of oxytocin from posterior pituitary. *Dose/route:* Loading dose of 7.5-15.0 mg/kg/hr IV for 2 hr, followed by 1.5 mg/kg/hr for 10 hr.

Abbreviations used in this section: bid, twice a day; D5W, 5% dextrose water; G6PD, glucose-6-phosphate dehydrogenase; IM, intramuscular(ly); IV, intravenous(ly); NPO, nothing by mouth; PO, oral(ly); prn, as necessary; qd, every day; q ___ hr, every ___ hours; qhs, every night at the hour of sleep; qid, four times each day; SC, subcutaneous(ly); SGOT, serum glutamic oxaloacetic transaminase; SGPT, serum glutamic pyruvic transaminase; tid, three times each day; tsp, teaspoon(s).

Also used socially. *Indications:* Treatment of premature labor. *Contraindications:* Conditions requiring prompt delivery (e.g., abruptio placentae, ruptured membranes). Chronic use is contraindicated. Data are insufficient to determine whether occasional social drinking is harmful to the fetus. *Maternal side effects:* Slurred speech, headache, nausea and vomiting, hypoglycemia, tachycardia, central nervous system depression, mood swings, mild hypotension. Chronic excessive intake can cause alcoholic hepatitis and cirrhosis, hyperlipemia, and fatty liver. Other effects include diuresis, vasodilation, and stimulation of gastric secretions. *Fetal side effects:* Fetal anomalies with chronic use, including growth retardation, craniofacial abnormalities, microcephaly, and maxillary hypoplasia. *Comments:* Observe client closely because her control will be inhibited. Place client on bed rest with side rails up. Keep client NPO, with emesis basin available. Offer bedpan frequently because incontinence may occur. Monitor maternal vital signs and fetal heart tones. Monitor contraction pattern, and stop infusion if labor continues and delivery is inevitable. Offer comfort measures for hangover after infusion is stopped, such as an ice pack for her head.

alphaprodine hydrochloride (Nisentil). *Classification:* Narcotic analgesic. *Dose/route:* 40-50 mg SC. 30-40 mg IM. 15-20 mg IV slowly. *Indications:* Moderate to severe pain of active labor in client at term. More rapid onset of action and shorter duration than other narcotics. *Contraindications:* Hypersensitivity. Latent phase of labor, labor before term, or fetal distress. *Maternal side effects:* Allergic reactions, drowsiness, respiratory depression, orthostatic hypotension, urinary retention, delayed gastric emptying, constipation. Less nausea and vomiting than with other narcotics. *Fetal side effects:* Decreased fetal heart rate variability, neonatal respiratory depression. Effects on fetus from use in early pregnancy are unknown. Neonate of addicted mother will have narcotic withdrawal. *Comments:* Have naloxone hydrochloride ready at delivery for possible narcotic-induced respiratory depression.

aluminum hydroxide (*see* **Gelusil, Maalox**).

aminophylline. *Classification:* Bronchodilator. Relaxes smooth muscles while stimulating cardiac muscle. Increases rate and depth of respirations, stimulates the central nervous system, increases renal blood flow. *Dose/route:* Loading dose: 6 mg/kg IV over 20 min. Maintenance dose: 0.9 mg/kg/hr. Dose may be increased if bronchospasm continues and signs of toxicity are not present. Long-term treatment with theophylline may be initiated. Usual dose is 100-200 mg PO tid or 125-500 mg rectally qd. *Indications:* Treatment of choice for asthma in pregnant clients. Adjunctive therapy for acute pulmonary edema. *Contraindications:* Hypersensitivity to aminophylline or theophylline. *Maternal side effects:* Anorexia, nausea and vomiting, fever, diuresis, abdominal distention, palpitations, tachycardia, excitation, anxiety, insomnia, tremor. Convulsions may occur secondary to toxic level of drug. Adverse effects usually occur when normal therapeutic dose is exceeded. *Fetal side effects:* Vomiting, jitteriness, tachycardia, cardiac arrhythmias, transient hyperglycemia. Teratogenesis is not proven. Toxicity for breast-fed neonate may vary from infant to infant. *Comments:* Administer aminophylline at a rate of no more than 1 ml/min. Faster administration may cause hypotension. Monitor vital signs and relief of bronchospasm.

ampicillin (Omnipen, Polycillin). *Classification:* Broad-spectrum antibiotic. Interferes with bacterial cell wall production. *Dose/route:* 250-500 mg q 6 hr PO, IM, or IV. *Indications:* Infection with susceptible organisms. Particularly effective for treatment of urinary tract infection because ampicillin is excreted primarily unchanged in the urine. *Contraindications:* Allergy. Infection with resistant organisms. *Maternal side effects:* Allergic reactions, rash, diarrhea, nausea and vomiting, epigastric distress, black hairy tongue, vaginitis flare-up. Hypersensitivity may cause hemolytic anemia, thrombocytopenia, leukopenia, nephritis, or anaphylactic reactions. *Fetal side effects:* None known. *Comments:* Always check for allergy before administration.

Anusol suppository (contains bismuth subgallate, bismuth resorcin compound, benzyl benzoate, Peruvian balsam, and zinc oxide). *Classification:* Rectal analgesic. *Dose/route:* Insert one suppository rectally bid (may also be used after each stool). *Indications:* Symptomatic relief of pain and itching of internal and external hemorrhoids, of anal fissures, or after rectal/anal surgery. Frequently used during the postpartum period. *Contraindications:* Hypersensitivity to any of the components. *Maternal side effects:* Burning, irritation, sensitivity reactions. *Fetal side effects:* None known.

Apresoline (*see* **hydralazine hydrochloride**).

AquaMephyton (*see* **vitamin K**).

Aspirin (*see* **acetylsalicylic acid**).

AVC cream (contains sulfanilamide, aminacrine hydrochloride, and allantoin). *Classification:* Antibiotic. Interferes with growth and enzyme system of susceptible organisms. *Dose/route:* 1 applicator or 1 suppository inserted vaginally qd or bid for 14 days. *Indications:* Vaginal infection when specific cause cannot be determined and treated specifically. *Contraindications:* Hypersensitivity to sulfonamides. *Maternal side effects:* Skin rashes, local burning or itching of vagina. *Fetal side effects:* Systemic absorption thought to be minimal. Theoretical possibility of sulfonamide side effects: kernicterus, hemolytic anemia in G6PD-deficient neonates.

Bendectin (*see* **doxylamine succinate**).

Benemid (*see* **probenecid**).

betamethasone (Celestone). *Classification:* Corticosteroid. Has numerous effects throughout the body. Mechanism for inducing fetal lung maturation is unknown. *Dose/route:* 12 mg IM q 24 hr for 2 doses for inducing fetal lung maturation. Otherwise, dose depends on condition being treated. *Indications:* Chronic adrenal insufficiency, anti-inflammatory agent for a large number of diseases. Also for prevention of respiratory distress syndrome when premature delivery (before 34 wk) is anticipated, but will not occur until 24 hr after treatment is initiated. *Contraindications:* Systemic fungal infections. *Maternal side effects:* Fluid and electrolyte imbalance, hypertension, hyperglycemia, peptic ulcer, vertigo, headache, skin reactions, sterile abscess at injection site. Rarely, anaphylactic reactions have occurred. *Fetal side effects:* Transient adrenocortical insufficiency.

bisacodyl (Dulcolax). *Classification:* Laxative. Acts directly on intestinal mucosa to stimulate peristalsis. *Dose/route:* 2 tablets PO, or 1 rectal suppository, when immediate effects are desired. *Indications:* Constipation during prenatal or postpartum course. Sometimes used in place of enemas during the first stage of labor. *Contraindications:* Any acute abdominal situation necessitating prompt operation (acute surgical abdomen). *Maternal side effects:* Abdominal cramps.

Brethine (*see* **terbutaline sulfate**).

Bricanyl (*see* **terbutaline sulfate**).

bromocriptine mesylate (Parlodel). *Classification:* Lactation inhibitor. *Dose/route:* 2.5 mg PO bid for 5-14 days. *Indications:* Maternal desire for lactation suppression. *Contraindications:* Pregnancy. Hypersensitivity to ergot alkaloids. *Maternal side effects:* Hypotension, dizziness, weakness, nausea, headache, abdominal cramps, diarrhea, constipation.

calcium gluconate. *Classification:* Mineral. *Dose/route:* 500 mg PO bid. *Indications:* Calcium deficiency. Used especially in clients with milk intolerance to meet the calcium needs of the fetus. *Contraindications:* Digitalis therapy, hypercalcemia, predisposition to renal stones.

Celestone (*see* **betamethasone**).

cephalexin (Keflex). *Classification:* Antibiotic (cephalosporin). *Dose/route:* 250-1,000 mg PO q 6 hr for 10 days. *Indications:* Infection with susceptible organisms. *Contraindications:* Allergy to cephalexin or penicillin. (There is a possibility of cross-sensitivity to penicillin.)

Maternal side effects: Allergic reactions: fever, rash, pruritus. Nausea and vomiting, diarrhea, vaginal flare-up, dizziness, headache. *Fetal side effects:* No known side effects for fetus. Neonate of a woman who took it during pregnancy may have a positive Coombs's test.

chlorotrianisene (TACE). *Classification:* Lactation suppressant. Estrogen. *Dose/route:* 12 mg PO qid for 7 days, 25-50 mg PO q 6 hr for 6 doses, or 72 mg PO bid for 2 days. *Indications:* Maternal desire for lactation suppression. *Contraindications:* Estrogen-dependent cancer; hepatic, cardiac, or renal disease; pregnancy; undiagnosed abnormal genital bleeding; thrombophlebitis or thromboembolic disorders. May be contraindicated if postpartum surgery is anticipated. *Maternal side effects:* Adverse effects similar to those of oral contraceptives: skin rash, nausea, vomiting, edema. Rarely, increased postpartum bleeding, postpartum thromboembolism. Estrogen therapy increases risk of endometrial cancer, although short-term effect is probably minimal. *Fetal side effects:* None known. *Comments:* Begin administration immediately postpartum.

Cleocin (*see* **clindamycin**).

clindamycin (Cleocin). *Classification:* Antibiotic. *Dose/route:* 150-450 mg PO q 6 hr, up to 600 mg IM or IV q 6 hr. *Indications:* Serious infection suspected or known to be a result of *Bacteroides fragilis* or other susceptible organisms, when less toxic agents will not suffice. *Contraindications:* Hypersensitivity to drugs containing clindamycin or lincomycin. History of colitis and severe renal disease are relative contraindications. *Maternal side effects:* Abdominal cramps, diarrhea, colitis, allergic reactions, leukocytosis, leukopenia, jaundice, altered liver functioning, pain or abscess at injection site. *Fetal side effects:* None known. *Comments:* Observe for signs of abdominal cramps, diarrhea, or colitis, which may require discontinuation of the drug.

clotrimazole (Gyne-Lotrimin, Mycelex, Mycelex-G). *Classification:* Antibiotic (antifungal). *Dose/route:* 1 tablet or 1 applicator of cream inserted vaginally qhs for 7 days. Alternatively, for nonpregnant women, 2 tablets or applicators for 3 days. *Indications:* Treatment of vaginal candidiasis. (Also treatment of fungal infections of the skin.) *Contraindications:* Hypersensitivity. *Maternal side effects:* Redness, burning, itching, urticaria, irritation, lower abdominal cramps, urinary frequency. *Fetal side effects:* None known.

Colace (*see* **dioctyl sodium sulfosuccinate**).

Darvon (*see* **propoxyphene hydrochloride**).

Datril (*see* **acetaminophen**).

Deladumone OB (*see* **testosterone enanthate and estradiol valerate**).

Demerol (*see* **meperidine hydrochloride**).

diazepam (Valium). *Classification:* Antianxiety agent. *Dose/route:* ≤ 30 mg IV for status epilepticus. 2-20 mg PO qd up to tid for other uses (e.g., mild anxiety, alcohol withdrawal). *Indications:* Treatment of status epilepticus and acute anxiety states. Otherwise, not warranted during pregnancy because there are other agents available. *Contraindications:* Hypersensitivity, acute narrow-angle glaucoma. Long-term use in pregnancy is contraindicated. *Maternal side effects:* Drowsiness, lethargy, ataxia, skin rashes, nausea, paradoxical anxiety. Prolonged use can lead to addiction. *Fetal side effects:* Fetal tachycardia, decreased fetal heart rate variability, neonatal respiratory depression, increased serum bilirubin. Associated with cleft lip, but causation is not proved. Breast-feeding neonate may experience lethargy, sedation, weight loss, poor sucking.

Dilantin (*see* **phenytoin sodium**).

dioctyl sodium sulfosuccinate (Colace). *Classification:* Stool softener. *Dose/route:* 50-200 mg PO qd. *Indications:* Constipation as a result of hard stools and painful anorectal conditions. Does not stimulate peristalsis. *Contraindications:* None known. *Maternal side effects:* Nausea and vomiting, mild abdominal cramps, rash.

dioctyl sodium sulfosuccinate with casanthranol (Peri-Colace). *Classification:* Laxative with stool softener and peristalsis stimulant. *Dose/route:* 1-2 capsules PO qhs or 1-3 tablets PO qd. *Indications:* Constipation, where peristalsis stimulation is needed. Frequently used during the postpartum period. *Contraindications:* Diarrhea, intestinal obstruction, nausea and vomiting, abdominal pain. *Maternal side effects:* Nausea, loose stools, rebound constipation, abdominal cramps, rash. Dependence may occur after prolonged use.

doxylamine succinate with pyridoxine (Bendectin). (Each tablet contains 10 mg doxylamine and 10 mg pyridoxine.) *Classification:* Antinauseant and antihistamine. Also corrects possible vitamin B6 deficiency, which is common during pregnancy. *Dose/route:* Usual dose: 2 tablets PO at bedtime. For severe nausea and vomiting, an additional tablet may be taken in the morning. *Indications:* Nausea and vomiting of pregnancy. *Contraindications:* Some clinicians consider pregnancy a contraindication, especially in the first trimester because of the potential for teratogenicity. Certainly, it should not be used unless clearly needed. *Maternal side effects:* Dizziness, drowsiness, dry mouth, thirst, nervousness, headache, palpitations, dysuria, epigastric pain, disorientation, irritability, diarrhea, constipation, anorexia. *Fetal side effects:* Teratogenicity suspected but not proved. *Comments:* Encourage clients to use dietary measures to try to relieve nausea and vomiting when possible (*see* Chapter 6). Warn that drowsiness may occur; therefore, driving or operating machinery should be avoided while under the effects of Bendectin.

Dulcolax (*see* **bisacodyl**).

Empirin (*see* **phenacetin**).

ergonovine maleate (Ergotrate). *Classification:* Oxytoxic (uterine stimulant). *Dose/route:* 0.2 mg IM or PO q 6 hr. *Indications:* Prevention and treatment of postpartum or postabortion hemorrhage. Also used to treat subinvolution. *Contraindications:* Hypersensitivity, pregnancy, hypertension, breast-feeding. *Maternal side effects:* Nausea and vomiting, hypertension, diaphoresis, dizziness, headache, palpitations, tinnitus, dyspnea, delayed or inhibited lactation, allergic reactions. *Fetal side effects:* Ergotrate is secreted in breast milk. Breast-feeding infant may experience vomiting, diarrhea, or cardiovascular abnormalities. *Comments:* Do not administer if client is hypertensive. Check blood pressure before and after administration. Observe for excessive uterine cramping. Offer analgesic or other relief measures with PO doses.

Ergotrate (*see* **ergonovine maleate**).

Ferro-Sequels (*see* **iron preparations**).

ferrous sulfate (*see* **iron preparations**).

Filibon (*see* **vitamins, prenatal**).

Flagyl (*see* **metronidazole**).

folic acid (folacin). *Classification:* Vitamin. A member of B-complex vitamins. Required for normoblastic bone marrow. *Dose/route:* 1.5-1.0 mg PO qd. *Indications:* Prevention or treatment of folate-deficiency anemia. *Contraindications:* Hypersensitivity. *Maternal side effects:* Allergic reactions. May lower phenytoin sodium levels in woman on this anticonvulsant, thus allowing more seizures. *Fetal side effects:* No known effects from folate supplementation. *Deficiency* may cause congenital malformation.

furosemide (Lasix). *Classification:* Diuretic. *Dose/route:* 40 mg PO qd up to qid or 20-40 mg/dose IV. *Indications:* Congestive heart failure or some cases of chronic renal disease. Not indicated for the treatment of physiological edema of pregnancy or for routine treatment of preeclampsia. *Contraindications:* Allergy to furosemide or sulfonamides (which are similar in chemical structure), anuria. *Maternal side effects:* Weakness, dizziness, nausea and vomiting, leg cramps, anorexia, confusion, hypovolemia, hyponatremia, hypokalemia, hypochloremia, uricemia, nephritis, paresthesias, alkalosis. *Fetal side effects:* Maternal hypovolemia, decreasing placental perfusion, causes fetal distress. Increased fetal urine output. Congenital anomalies have been observed in animals. *Comments:*

Monitor vital signs and intake and output closely. Observe for side effects and for fetal distress.

Garamycin (*see* **gentamicin sulfate**).

Gelusil, Mylanta (contain aluminum hydroxide, magnesium hydroxide, and simethicone). *Classification:* Antacid and antiflatulent. *Dose/route:* 2 tsp PO or 2 tablets PO 1 hour after meals and at bedtime. Maximum of 12 tablets or tsp in 24 hr. *Indications:* Relief of heartburn, acid indigestion, and flatulence. *Contraindications:* Renal disease. Hypersensitivity to any of the ingredients. Do not administer with concurrent tetracycline therapy. *Comments:* (*See* Chapter 6.)

gentamicin sulfate (Garamycin). *Classification:* Antibiotic of aminoglycoside group. Inhibits protein synthesis in susceptible bacteria. *Dose/route:* 3-5 mg/kg/day IM or IV. *Indications:* Treatment of serious infections of susceptible aerobic, gram-negative organisms. *Contraindications:* Impaired renal functioning, hypersensitivity. *Maternal side effects:* Damage to 8th cranial nerve, auditory damage, rash, renal impairment, lethargy, neuromuscular blockade, apnea, overgrowth of nonsusceptible organisms, nausea and vomiting, weight loss, hypotension, hypertension. *Fetal side effects:* Safety to fetus not established. *Comments:* Do not mix with other drugs. IV infusion must be slow, intermittent infusion.

guaifenesin (Robitussin). *Classification:* Expectorant. *Dose/route:* 2 tsp PO q 4 hr, not to exceed 12 tsp in 24 hr. *Indications:* Cough of common cold, bronchitis, laryngitis, influenza, etc. *Contraindications:* Hypersensitivity. *Maternal side effects:* No serious side effects reported.

Gyne-Lotrimin (*see* **clotrimazole**).

Heparin. *Classification:* Anticoagulant. *Dose/route:* Varies, depending on client's condition and laboratory reports. On average, may be 20,000-40,000 U/day. May be administered SC, by intermittent IV, or by continuous IV infusion. *Indications:* Treatment and prevention of pulmonary embolism and thromboembolic disease, prevention of clotting with arterial or cardiac surgery, or with prosthetic implants. *Contraindications:* Any condition that increases bleeding tendency, suspected intracranial bleeding, threatened abortion, pericarditis, or subacute bacterial endocarditis. Should not be used with drugs that tend to increase bleeding, such as aspirin and indomethacin. Hypersensitivity to heparin and inability to perform coagulation studies at indicated intervals are also contraindications. *Maternal side effects:* Hypersensitivity reactions: urticaria, fever, chills, conjunctival itching, alopecia. Osteoporosis and renal dysfunction with long-term use. Thrombocytopenia. Overdose may cause bleeding from body orifices, petechiae, bruises, vasospasm. *Fetal side effects:* Large molecule that does not cross the placenta and does not affect breast-feeding infants. *Comments:* When administering heparin, have antidote available. Protamine sulfate is the antidote for overdosage, and it is administered at 1 mg/1 mg (100 U) of heparin by slow IV push. Check for bleeding and subinvolution if administered postpartum. Always check clotting time before administration.

hydralazine hydrochloride (Apresoline). *Classification:* Antihypertensive. Relaxes smooth muscles of arterioles, especially in the coronary, cerebral, splanchnic, renal, and uterine circulation. *Dose/route:* 10-50 mg PO qid or 5-20 mg IM or IV, which may be repeated. The daily dose should not exceed 300 mg. *Indications:* Drug of choice for control of the moderate to severe hypertension of preeclampsia. May be used in concert with other drugs to control chronic hypertension in the pregnant client, but is not the drug of choice for this purpose. *Contraindications:* Hypersensitivity, coronary artery disease, rheumatic heart disease. It is not the drug of choice for chronic hypertension because the other drugs used with it (diuretics and propranolol) are not recommended during pregnancy. *Maternal side effects:* Chills, fever, depression, headaches, dizziness, palpitations, nausea and vomiting, tachycardia, flushing, anxiety, dry mouth, perspiration, nasal congestion, angina. Chronic use may cause peripheral neuropathy, blood dyscrasias, rheumatoid arthritis, symptoms of systemic lupus erythematosus, and sodium and water retention. *Fetal side effects:* Fetal side effects not proved, although animal studies indicate teratogenicity. *Comments:* Administer 5-mg test dose to evaluate chance of precipitous hypotension in client with vascular depletion. Monitor vital signs frequently. Notify physician of precipitous fall in blood pressure because it can cause fetal hypoxia. Observe for fetal distress. Check list of interacting drugs before introducing a new medication.

hydroxyzine pamoate (Vistaril). *Classification:* Ataractic, antihistamine, antiemetic. *Dose/route:* 25-100 mg IM only. *Indications:* Relief of anxiety, prevention of nausea and vomiting. Used alone or with narcotic analgesic. Potentiates analgesic effect of narcotics. *Contraindications:* Hypersensitivity. *Maternal side effects:* Drowsiness, dry mouth, pain and irritation at injection site, tremor, convulsions. *Fetal side effects:* Sedation of neonate. Animal studies indicate teratogenicity.

Insulin. *Classification:* Hormone. *Dose/route:* Varies according to individual needs. Generally decreases in the first third to one half of pregnancy, then increases to two to three times the prepregnant dose. Generally decreases dramatically in the postpartum period. *Indica-*

tions: Diabetes mellitus when the diabetes cannot be controlled by diet and exercise alone. *Contraindications:* Allergy to the animal component. This may be alleviated by switching to insulin from another animal. *Maternal side effects:* Hypertrophy or atrophy at injection site. Allergy to the animal component. Overdose may cause hypoglycemia. *Fetal side effects:* Insulin does not cross the placenta to any great extent. Maternal hyperglycemia of diabetes stimulates fetal insulin secretion, possibly causing the macrosomia and neontal hypoglycemia seen in infants of diabetic mothers. *Comments:* Provide full education about diabetes control, including diet, exercise, and medications, and about the interactions between pregnancy and diabetes (*see* p. 363). Be alert to changing insulin needs during pregnancy, labor and delivery, and the postpartum period.

iron preparations (ferrous sulfate, Ferro-Sequels, Mol-Iron). *Classification:* Mineral. *Dose/route:* 180 mg elemental iron PO qd in 3 divided doses. *Indications:* Iron-deficiency states. Because the average American diet does not contain enough iron for the pregnancy, preventive supplementation is common. *Contraindications:* Thalassemia or chronic hemolytic anemia. *Maternal side effects:* Nausea, vomiting, constipation, diarrhea, black stools. *Fetal side effects:* None. Generally, the fetus will get the iron it needs at the mother's expense. *Comments:* Advise taking iron 30 min after meals in order to minimize gastrointestinal upset; take with vitamin C source to enhance absorption. Warn that black stools may occur. Advise dietary measures to prevent/relieve constipation.

isoxsuprine hydrochloride (Vasodilan). *Classification:* Tocolytic agent (beta-receptor stimulant). *Dose/route:* A number of treatment regimens are currently being used. Usually 0.25-0.50 mg/min by continuous IV infusion pump for 8-12 hr, followed by 5-20 mg IM or PO q 3-6 hr. (Some sources recommend an IV loading dose of up to 20 mg in the first 30 min.) *Indications:* Treatment of premature labor, when delivery is not indicated for maternal or fetal reasons (such as hemorrhage or fetal distress). *Contraindications:* Immediate postpartum period. Administer with care to clients with hypotension or tachycardia. *Maternal side effects:* Hypotension, tachycardia, hyperglycemia, allergic skin reactions, tremors, palpitations, restlessness, nausea and vomiting. *Fetal side effects:* Accelerated fetal lung maturity. May cause neonatal hypotension, hypoglycemia, and ileus. *Comments:* Keep client in left lateral position to maintain optimal uterine perfusion. Monitor vital signs, including blood pressure, frequently. Monitor contraction status and fetal response.

Keflex (*see* **cephalexin).**
Konakion (*see* **vitamin K).**

Lasix (*see* **furosemide**).

lidocaine hydrochloride (Xylocaine). *Classification:* Local anesthetic. Stabilizes the membrane of each nerve with which it comes in contact. *Dose/route:* Dosage depends on route, which may include local infiltration, or paracervical, pudendal, spinal, caudal, or epidural block. *Indications:* Local anesthesia by infiltration or regional nerve block. *Contraindications:* Hypersensitivity to amide local anesthetics. Shock, heart block, inflammation at site intended for injection. *Maternal side effects:* Allergic reactions. Excess dose, IV injection, or low tolerance may cause nervousness, dizziness, tremors, that progress to drowsiness, convulsions, respiratory arrest, hypotension, bradycardia, cardiac arrest. *Fetal side effects:* Teratogenic potential unknown. Fetal bradycardia when administered by paracervical route. *Comments:* Have emergency equipment available when local anesthetics are administered.

Maalox (aluminum hydroxide and magnesium hydroxide). *Classification:* Antacid. *Dose/route:* 2-4 tsp or 2-4 No. 1 tablets PO qid (20 min after meals and at bedtime). *Indications:* Heartburn, gastric acidity. *Contraindications:* Hypersensitivity to any of the components, concurrent tetracycline therapy, renal disease.

magnesium hydroxide (*see* **Gelusil, Maalox, Milk of Magnesia, and Mylanta**).

magnesium sulfate. *Classification:* Central nervous system depressant. (May also be used as a tocolytic agent.) *Dose/route:* 4 g in 250 ml D5W IV over 20 min, followed by 1-3 g/hr in IV fluids; or 10 g IM (5 g in each buttock) followed by 5 g IM q 4 hr. *Indications:* Prevention of seizures in patients with preeclampsia. Has been used as a tocolytic to stop premature labor. *Contraindications:* Respiratory depression or inability to elicit deep tendon reflexes. *Maternal side effects:* Decreased frequency and intensity of contractions, modest drop in blood pressure, flushing, nausea and vomiting, pain at injection site, diminished reflexes, respiratory and cardiac arrest. *Fetal side effects:* Decreased fetal heart rate variability, neonatal hypotonia, lethargy, low Apgar scores, hypermagnesemia. *Comments:* Check deep tendon reflexes, respirations, and urine output hourly and before administration of next dose of magnesium sulfate. Have calcium gluconate, 10 g IV, available as an antidote to magnesium sulfate.

meperidine hydrochloride (Demerol). *Classification:* Narcotic analgesic. *Dose/route:* 50-100 mg IM q 3-4 hr prn or 25-50 mg IV q 3-4 hr prn. *Indications:* Moderate to severe pain of active labor at term. *Contraindications:* Hypersensitivity, premature labor. *Maternal side effects:* Nausea and vomiting, dizziness, urinary retention, constipation, euphoria, dry mouth, flushing. *Fetal side effects:* Decreased heart rate variability, neonatal respiratory depression. *Comments:* Observe for untoward effects. Have naloxone hydrochloride available for treatment of narcotic-induced respiratory depression.

Metamucil (*see* **psyllium hydrophilic mucilloid**).

Methadone hydrochloride. *Classification.* Narcotic analgesic. *Dose/route:* Usually administered PO with dose titrated to client need. In the hospital, IM may be used for maintenance when PO medication cannot be administered. Dose is usually 10-100 mg. *Indications:* Detoxification and maintenance of narcotic addiction. *Contraindications:* Hypersensitivity to methadone. Should not be used in pregnancy unless physician believes benefits outweigh risks. *Maternal side effects:* Allergic reactions, analgesia, sedation, respiratory depression, shock, circulatory depression, cardiac arrest, nausea and vomiting, lightheadedness, dysphoria, constipation, urinary retention. *Fetal side effects:* Safe use during pregnancy not established. Neonate undergoes withdrawal.

Methergine (*see* **methylergonovine maleate**).

methylergonovine maleate (Methergine). *Classification:* Oxytoxic. *Dose/route:* 0.2 mg IM or PO q 4 hr for 6 doses. *Indications:* Postpartum atony, hemorrhage, or subinvolution. *Contraindications:* Pregnancy. *Maternal side effects:* Possible inhibition of lactation. Mild hypertension when administered PO. If administered IV, can cause acute hypertensive and cardiac crises, nausea and vomiting, dizziness, headache, tinnitus, dyspnea, diaphoresis, palpitations. Pain from uterine cramps. *Fetal side effects:* None. Administered after delivery. *Comments:* Obtain blood pressure before administration. Monitor vital signs after administration. May administer analgesic at same time to decrease pain from uterine cramps.

metronidazole (Flagyl). *Classification:* Antibiotic. *Dose/route:* 250 mg PO tid for 7 days, or 2 g PO (1 dose). *Indications:* Trichomoniasis or amebiasis. Used during pregnancy only if other agents do not prove effective. *Contraindications:* Pregnancy, especially during the first trimester. Hypersensitivity, active organic central nervous system disease, history of blood dyscrasias. *Maternal side effects:* Nausea and vomiting, flushing if used with alcohol. Animal studies indicate carcinogenicity. Abdominal cramps, nausea, diarrhea, metallic taste, rebound candidiasis, dizziness, vertigo, seizures, depression, weakness, insomnia, allergic reactions. *Fetal side effects:* None proven. Animal studies indicate genetic mutations secondary to metronidazole. Secreted in breast milk.

miconazole nitrate (Monistat). *Classification:* Antifungal agent. *Dose/route:* 1 applicator of cream inserted into the vagina at bedtime for 7 days. *Indications:* Vaginal candidiasis. *Contraindications:* Hypersensitivity to miconazole. *Maternal side effects:* Vaginal burning, itching, pruritus. Abdominal cramps, headache, hives, skin rash. *Fetal side effects:* None known.

Milk of Magnesia (magnesium hydroxide). *Classification:* Laxative and antacid. *Dose/route:* Laxative dose: 2-4 tsp PO followed by a glass of water. Antacid dose: 1-3 tsp PO up to qid. *Indications:* Constipation, heartburn, gastric acidity. *Contraindications:* Impaired renal functioning or cardiac disease, abdominal pain, nausea and vomiting, symptoms of appendicitis. *Maternal side effects:* Dehydration.

Mol-Iron (*see* **iron preparations**).

Monistat (*see* **miconazole nitrate**).

morphine sulfate. *Classification:* Narcotic analgesic. *Dose/route:* 5-15 mg SC q 3-4 hr or 2.5-15.0 mg IV diluted and injected slowly. *Indications:* Severe pain in labor. May be used for analgesia and sedation in hypertonic uterine dysfunction during early labor. *Contraindications:* Hypersensitivity, premature fetus, premature labor, preeclampsia. *Maternal side effects:* Respiratory depression, central nervous system depression, euphoria, dizziness, nausea and vomiting, itching, urticaria, urinary retention, orthostatic hypotension, decreased secretion of gastric acid, constipation, allergic reactions. *Fetal side effects:* Decreased fetal heart rate variability, neonatal respiratory depression. *Comments:* Have naloxone hydrochloride ready for treatment of narcotic-induced respiratory depression.

Mycelex, Mycelex-G (*see* **clotrimazole**).

Mycostatin (*see* **nystatin**).

Mylanta (*see* **Gelusil**).

naloxone hydrochloride (Narcan). *Classification:* Narcotic antagonist. *Dose/route:* Neonatal dose: 0.01 mg/kg IV, IM, or SC. Dose may be repeated up to 2 times if there is no response in 2-3 min. Maternal dose: 0.4 mg IM, IV, or SC. Dose may be repeated up to 2 times if there is no response in 2-3 min. *Indications:* Narcotic-induced respiratory depression. In the case where the client has no respiratory depression, but depression of the neonate is anticipated, it is generally preferable to administer naloxone to the neonate when the need for, and the response to, the drug can be monitored. The alternative is to administer the naloxone to the client 10-15 min before delivery. *Contraindications:* Hypersensitivity to naloxone. Must be administered with caution to women or neonates known to be addicted to narcotics because it will precipitate withdrawal. Should not be administered for respiratory depression attributable to other causes. *Maternal side effects:* Withdrawal symptoms in narcotic-addicted patient. Nausea and vomiting, sweating, tachycardia, hypertension, tremors resulting from rapid narcotic reversal. *Fetal side effects:* Withdrawal symptoms in neonate of addicted mother. *Comments:* Have naloxone ready if narcotic depression is anticipated. Continue other resuscitative measures while awaiting the effects of naloxone. Continue to observe the client after successful resuscitation because the effects of naloxone may wear off before the effects of the narcotic, thus causing a second narcotic-induced respiratory depression several hours after delivery.

Narcan (*see* **naloxone hydrochloride**).

Natalins (*see* **vitamins, prenatal**).

Neo-Synephrine Hydrochloride (*see* **phenylephrine hydrochloride**).

Nilstat (*see* **nystatin**).

Nisentil (*see* **alphaprodine hydrochloride**).

nitrous oxide. *Classification:* General anesthetic, analgesic. *Dose/route:* Administered by face mask, mixed with oxygen, for inhalation. Concentration varies, depending on degree of pain relief required. 80% concentration is maximum. *Indications:* Analgesia when used alone for difficult delivery or painful procedures immediately after delivery. Anesthesia when combined with other agents for cesarean sections. *Maternal side effects:* Nausea and vomiting. *Comments:* Ensure that only trained anesthesia personnel administer nitrous oxide.

nystatin (Nilstat, Mycostatin). *Classification:* Antifungal agent. *Dose/route:* Vaginal infection: 1 suppository or 1 applicator of cream inserted vaginally qd-bid for 14 days. Gastrointestinal infection: 500,000-1,000,000 U PO tid. Thrush: 400,000-600,000 U PO qid (retain in mouth as long as possible). Skin infection: apply cream liberally bid. *Indications:* Monilial infections of skin, mucous membranes, and gastrointestinal tract. *Contraindications:* Hypersensitivity. Vaginal medication is contraindicated after membranes have ruptured. *Maternal side effects:* Hypersensitivity reactions. Rarely, nausea and vomiting, diarrhea, irritation. *Fetal side effects:* None known.

Omnipen (*see* **ampicillin**).

Ornade Spansule capsules (contains chlorpheniramine maleate, phenylpropanolamine hydrochloride, isopropamide). *Classification:* Nasal decongestant, antihistamine. *Dose/route:* 1 capsule PO q 12 hr. *Indications:* Relief of sneezing, runny nose, and upper respiratory tract congestion. *Contraindications:* Hypersensitivity to any of the ingredients, concurrent use of monoamine oxidase inhibitors, hypertension, bronchial asthma, coronary artery disease, peptic ulcer. *Maternal side effects:* Drowsiness, excessive dryness of the mouth, nervousness, insomnia, nausea and vomiting, diarrhea, weakness, angina, abdominal pain, headache, palpitations, dysuria, visual disturbances, signs of iodine toxicity. *Fetal side effects:* Safety in pregnancy not established, but no known ill effects.

oxytocin (Pitocin, Syntocinon). *Classification:* Oxytoxic. *Dose/ route:* For induction or stimulation of labor: administered by continuous IV infusion pump, titrated to uterine and fetal response. Postpartum: 10-20 U IM or in 1,000 ml IV fluid to be infused at 125 ml/hr. *Indications:* Induction or stimulation of labor for a viable infant for any of a number of reasons, including premature rupture of membranes, prolonged labor, and diabetes. The physician must decide when induction is indicated, based on the risks and benefits to both the client and the fetus/baby. Also used to prevent or treat postpartum hemorrhage. Used antepartally to stimulate uterine contractions to test fetal well-being. *Contraindications:* Contraindications to induction or stimulation are relative and based on total assessment of the client. Possible contraindications: cephalopelvic disproportion, grand multiparity, previous cesarean section or other uterine scar, abnormal presentation or position, fetal distress. *Maternal side effects:* Intense labor. Hyperstimulation may cause uterine rupture, amniotic fluid embolism, cervical or perineal tears. Anaphylactic reactions rarely occur. Increased blood pressure is common, but, in large doses, a transient decrease in blood pressure may be followed by a slow increase. Nausea and vomiting may occur. Abdominal cramps after postpartum administration. Water intoxication, convulsions, coma. *Fetal side effects:* Fetal distress secondary to poor placental perfusion caused by hyperstimulation. *Comments:* Ensure that a physician or fully trained nurse stays with a laboring client on oxytocin to monitor progress, titrate the dose to client response, and observe for complications or rapid progress to delivery. Oxytocin infusion must be stopped if hyperstimulation or fetal distress occurs. A fetal monitor is a useful tool to help in monitoring maternal and fetal response.

Parlodel (*see* bromocriptine mesylate).

penicillins. *Classification:* Antibiotic. *Dose/route:* Varies, depending on the particular drug and the infection being treated. *Indications:* Treatment of infection with susceptible organisms. Drug of choice for treatment of gonorrhea and syphilis. *Contraindications:* Allergy. *Maternal side effects:* Allergic reactions, rash to anaphylactic shock. Nausea and vomiting, diarrhea, black hairy tongue, nephritis, vaginal candidiasis after treatment. Electrolyte imbalance may occur after IV administration. *Fetal side effects:* No fetal side effects known except decreased urinary estriol after ampicillin administration. In breast-feeding infant, may cause diarrhea or candidiasis. *Comments:* Administer probenecid before administration of penicillin for treatment of gonorrhea in order to slow excretion, thus increasing serum level and duration of penicillin.

Pentothal (*see* **thiopental sodium**).

Peri-Colace (*see* **dioctyl sodium sulfosuccinate with casanthranol**).

phenacetin (Empirin compound). *Classification:* Analgesic, antipyretic. *Dose/route:* 1-2 tablets PO q 3-4 hr prn for pain. *Indications:* Mild to moderate pain in postpartum period. *Contraindications:* Hypersensitivity. Phenacetin is generally contraindicated in pregnancy because it is always used in combination with other medications, such as caffeine and aspirin, which are not recommended during pregnancy.

Phenergan (*see* **promethazine hydrochloride**).

phenylephrine hydrochloride (Neo-Synephrine Hydrochloride). *Classification:* Nasal decongestant. *Dose/route:* 0.25% solution nose drops q 3-4 hr prn. *Indications:* Nasal congestion of common cold, allergies, or sinusitis. *Maternal side effects:* Tremors, insomnia, palpitations. Rebound congestion may occur with frequent or excessive use.

phenytoin sodium (Dilantin). *Classification:* Anticonvulsant. Acts at motor cortex to inhibit spread of seizure activity. *Dose/route:* Titrated to serum levels, but usually 100-600 mg PO qd. *Indications:* Prevention of epileptic seizures. *Contraindications:* Hypersensitivity to hydantoin products. *Maternal side effects:* Confusion, ataxia, drowsiness, irritability, gingival hyperplasia, nausea and vomiting, constipation, nystagmus, rash, lymphadenopathy, hematopoietic abnormalities, fever, hirsutism, hyperglycemia, osteomalacia, megaloblastic anemia. *Fetal side effects:* Increased risk of congenital heart disease and cleft palate, but it is unknown whether this is due to phenytoin or epilepsy. A syndrome thought to be associated with phenytoin includes intrauterine growth retardation, mental retardation, craniofacial abnormalities, and digital hypoplasia. *Comments:* Administer slowly if given IV ($\leq$ 50 mg/min).

Pitocin (*see* **oxytocin**).

Polycillin (*see* **ampicillin**).

probenecid (Benemid). *Classification:* Uricosuric and renal tubular blocking agent. *Dose/route:* 1 g PO 30 min before administration of penicillin. *Indications:* In treatment of gonorrhea, administered 30 min before penicillin in order to prolong duration and raise serum level of penicillin. Also used to treat gout and hyperuricemia. *Contraindications:* Hypersensitivity to probenecid, blood dyscrasias, uric acid, kidney stones, concurrent use of salicylates. *Maternal side effects:* Nausea and vomiting, anorexia, headache, dizziness, flushing, urinary frequency, anemia, sore gums, hypersensitivity reactions. *Fetal side effects:* None known.

promethazine hydrochloride (Phenergan). *Classification:* Phenothiazine. Antihistamine, antiemetic, anticholinergic, and sedative effects. *Dose/route:* 25-50 mg IM or IV. *Indications:* Potentiation of analgesic and sedative effect of narcotics by relieving anxiety. Used primarily during labor. May also be used during pregnancy to treat severe nausea and vomiting. *Contraindications:* Hypersensitivity, patients who are comatose or who have received large amounts of central nervous system depressants. Relative contraindications include glaucoma, asthma, peptic ulcer, pyloroduodenal obstruction, bladder-neck obstruction. *Maternal side effects:* Transient hypotension, drowsiness, dizziness, tinnitus, incoordination, blurred vision, nervousness, insomnia, convulsions, hysteria, tachycardia, bradycardia, nausea and vomiting, allergic reactions, leukopenia, agranulocytosis. *Fetal side effects:* Rarely, platelet aggregation is impaired in the neonate. Effect on fetal development is unknown.

propoxyphene hydrochloride (Darvon). *Classification:* Analgesic. *Dose/route:* 65 mg PO q 4 hr prn. *Indications:* Mild to moderate pain during the postpartum period. *Contraindications:* Hypersensitivity to propoxyphene hydrochloride. Late pregnancy, because it may have additive depressant effects with central nervous system depressants, such as narcotics. *Maternal side effects:* Nausea and vomiting, drowsiness, dizziness, rash, constipation, abdominal pain, headache, weakness, euphoria. Chronic excessive use may cause psychosis, convulsions, or dependence. *Fetal side effects:* Possible adverse effect on development. Neonates have exhibited withdrawal after use during pregnancy. *Comments:* Observe client for untoward effects, especially dizziness and drowsiness upon ambulation.

psyllium hydrophilic mucilloid (Metamucil). *Classification:* Laxative. Provides bland bulk. *Dose/route:* 1 tsp stirred into a glass of liquid PO qd-tid. *Indications:* Constipation, hemorrhoids. *Contraindications:* Intestinal obstruction, fecal impaction.

RhO(D) immune globulin (RhoGAM). *Classification:* Immunoglobulin. *Dose/route:* Must be titrated to the amount of Rh-positive blood that entered the circulation. 1 vial (300 μg) is usually sufficient after a normal term delivery. It must be administered within 72 hr of delivery. *Indications:* Prevention of active maternal formation of RhO(D) antibodies. To be administered to RhO(D)-negative D^u-positive or negative client after abortion, amniocentesis, ectopic pregnancy, or the birth of an RhO(D)-positive infant. May be administered to RhO(D)-negative client prophylactically between the 28th and 32nd wk of gestation. *Contraindications:* RhO(D)-positive blood or previous immunization to RhO(D) factor. *Maternal side effects:* Fever, myalgia, lethargy. *Fetal side effects:* None known. *Comments:* RhoGAM is cross-matched in the laboratory before administration. Verify lot number on RhoGAM and cross-match form with that on the vial. Administer IM. Return empty vial with its identification form to the lab.

ritodrine hydrochloride (Yutopar). *Classification:* Tocolytic agent. *Dose/route:* Administered IV by constant infusion pump with dose titrated to response. Starting dose is 100 μg/min increased by 50 μg/min every 10 min until response has been achieved. Maximum dose is 350 μg/min. *Indications:* Treatment of premature labor that has no obvious cause. (Used in other countries to treat intrapartum fetal distress.) *Contraindications:* Premature labor that should be allowed to continue (e.g., with 3rd trimester bleeding, severe pre-eclampsia, fetal death, chorioamnionitis). Relative contraindications include cardiac disease and diabetes mellitus. *Maternal side effects:* Tachycardia, premature ventricular contractions, increased systolic blood pressure and decreased diastolic blood pressure, hyperglycemia. Pulmonary edema may occur if used with glucocorticoids. *Fetal side effects:* Tachycardia, neonatal hypoglycemia. *Comments:* Observe client constantly for assessment of labor status and titration of dose. Monitor maternal vital signs and fetal heart rate frequently.

Robitussin (*see* guaifenesin).

silver nitrate. *Classification:* Anti-infective. *Dose/route:* 2 drops of 1% silver nitrate solution in each eye. *Indications:* Prevention of ophthalmia neonatorum. May be used routinely. *Fetal side effects:* Chemical conjunctivitis in neonatal period. *Comments:* Wash eyelids clean of blood, mucus, meconium, etc., before administration. Irrigation of eyes after instillation is not recommended.

simethicone (*see* Gelusil).

Stuart Prenatal tablets (*see* vitamins, prenatal).

succinylcholine chloride. *Classification:* Muscle relaxant. Causes paralysis by blocking nerve transmission at the myoneural junction. *Dose/route:* Dose varies according to individual and type of procedure. May be administered by IV push or constant IV infusion. *Indications:* Adjunct to general anesthesia. Should be used only when there is adequate anesthesia and when resuscitation equipment and personnel trained in resuscitation are present. *Contraindications:* Hypersensitivity. *Maternal side effects:* Respiratory depression, apnea, increase or decrease in heart rate and blood pressure, arrhythmias, cardiac arrest, hyperthermia, muscle fasciculation, postoperative muscle pain. *Fetal side effects:* No known effect from use in early pregnancy. Does not cross placental barrier so paralysis from anesthesia for cesarean section does not occur. *Comments:* Ensure that it is administered only by physician or anesthetist who is prepared to artificially assist respiration. Emergency equipment for cardiac and respiratory support should be available.

sulfonamides. *Classification:* Antibiotics. *Dose/route:* Depends on particular drug. In general 0.5-1.0 g q 4-8 hr PO. *Indications:* Treatment of urinary tract infections with susceptible organisms. *Contraindications:* 3rd trimester of pregnancy because of possibility of neonatal kernicterus. Allergy. *Maternal side effects:* Allergic reactions: rash, photosensitivity, drug fever. Gastrointestinal: nausea and vomiting, stomatitis. Blood dyscrasias, headache, depression, confusion, hepatic damage, hemolytic anemia (especially in clients with G6PD deficiency), vasculitis, renal damage from crystalluria if high urine volume is not maintained. *Fetal side effects:* Kernicterus in the neonate as a result of competition with bilirubin for binding. Hemolytic anemia in G6PD-deficient infants who are breast-feeding. *Comments:* Encourage large fluid intake to prevent formation of crystals.

Sultrin (contains sulfathiazole, sulfacetamide, sulfabenzamide). *Classification:* Antibiotic (sulfonamide). *Dose/route:* 1 applicator of cream or 1 suppository vaginally bid for 4-6 days. *Indications:* Treatment of *Hemophilus vaginalis* vaginitis. *Contraindications:* Kidney disease. Sensitivity to sulfonamides.

Syntocinon (*see* oxytocin).

TACE (*see* chlorotrianisene).

terbutaline sulfate (Bricanyl, Brethine). *Classification:* Tocolytic agent, bronchodilator. *Dose/route:* For tocolysis, administered by constant IV infusion at the rate necessary to inhibit uterine contractions. *Indications:* Preterm labor that has no obvious cause. Other medications (e.g., aminophylline) should be used for relief of bronchospasm. *Contraindications:* Gestation of less than 20 wk, premature labor that should be allowed to continue (e.g., with 3rd trimester bleeding, severe preeclampsia, etc.), hypersensitivity. Should be used with caution in clients with hypertension, diabetes, hyperthyroidism, cardiac arrhythmias. *Maternal side effects:* Nervousness, tremors, headaches, drowsiness, tachycardia, palpitations, sweating, nausea and vomiting. *Fetal side effects:* None known, but safe usage in pregnancy has not been established.

testosterone enanthate and estradiol valerate (Deladumone OB). *Classification:* Lactation suppressant (contains estrogen). *Dose/route:* 2 ml IM at onset of 2nd stage of labor or immediately after delivery. *Indications:* Lactation suppression for non-breast-feeding mothers. *Contraindications:* Thromboembolic disorders. May be contraindicated if postpartum surgery is anticipated. *Maternal side effects:* Pain at injection site, virilization. Potential for estrogen side effects, such as increased postpartum bleeding or embolism.

tetracycline. *Classification:* Antibiotic. Inhibits protein synthesis in susceptible bacteria. *Dose/route:* Varies, depending on specific drug and infection. Frequently is 1-2 g/day in 2 or 4 divided doses for at least 24-48 hr after fever has subsided. *Indications:* Infection with susceptible organisms. *Contraindications:* Pregnancy, because of fetal side effects and possibility of maternal hepatotoxicity. Allergy. *Maternal side effects:* Gastrointestinal: nausea and vomiting, diarrhea, glossitis, black hairy tongue. Hypersensitivity: rash, urticaria, anaphylactic reactions, pericarditis, photosensitivity. Other: vaginitis; hoarseness; fever; elevation of SGOT, SGPT, alkaline phosphatase, and bilirubin; hepatotoxicity. *Fetal side effects:* Brown discoloration of teeth (permanent) and decreased skeletal growth. *Comments:* Do not administer with antacids, milk, or iron because they interfere with absorption.

thiopental sodium (Pentothal). *Classification:* Barbiturate (very short-acting), central nervous system depressant that causes hypnosis and anesthesia. *Dose/route:* Individual response is so varied that there is no fixed dosage. *Indications:* Induction of general anesthesia, such as for cesarean section. *Contraindications:* Hypersensitivity to barbiturates, status asthmaticus, porphyria. Relative contraindications: shock, cardiovascular disease, hepatic or renal disease, severe anemia, asthma. *Maternal side effects:* Laryngospasm, bronchospasm, respiratory depression, decreased cardiac output. Restlessness and shivering may occur during recovery. Allergic reactions. *Fetal side effects:* Respiratory and cardiac depression in large doses. *Comments:* Ensure that it is administered only by persons qualified in the use of IV anesthesia. Resuscitation equipment should be ready for use.

Tucks pads (contains witch hazel and glycerin). *Classification:* Astringent cleansing agent. *Dose/route:* Apply to perineum prn. *Indications:* Compress for discomfort of hemorrhoids or episiotomy, or as a wipe after stooling in order to prevent irritation. *Contraindications:* Sensitivity. *Maternal side effects:* Irritation.

Tylenol (*see* **acetaminophen**).

Valium (*see* **diazepam**).

Vasodilan (*see* **isoxsuprine hydrochloride**).

Vistaril (*see* **hydroxyzine**).

vitamin K (AquaMephyton, Konakion). *Classification:* Vitamin. *Dose/route:* 0.5-2.0 mg IM immediately after birth. *Indications:* Prevention and treatment of neonatal hemorrhage secondary to hypoprothrombinemia. (Prothrombin levels reach normal at about 5 days of life when milk and intestinal bacteria are present in the gut.) *Contraindications:* None. *Fetal side effects:* Neonatal hyperbilirubinemia with high doses, inflammation of injection site.

vitamins, prenatal (Filibon, Natalins, Stuart Prenatal). *Classification:* Multivitamin preparations. *Dose/route:* 1 tablet or capsule PO qd. *Indications:* Because nutritional requirements are increased during pregnancy and lactation, and because vitamin and mineral deficiency may adversely affect the fetus, some clinicians routinely prescribe prenatal vitamins. Others prefer to assess nutritional intake and to supplement only if intake is low. *Contraindications:* None. *Maternal side effects:* Nausea and vomiting as a result of having to swallow the large vitamin capsule. Folic acid may mask symptoms of pernicious anemia. *Fetal side effects:* Fetal anomalies secondary to overdosage of vitamins A and D. Withdrawal from excessive vitamin B6 can cause neonatal convulsions. *Comments:* Instruct client that other supplements, particularly fat-soluble vitamins, should not be taken with prenatal vitamins because of the possibility of overdosage of fat-soluble vitamins.

Xylocaine (*see* **lidocaine hydrochloride**).

Yutopar (*see* **ritodrine hydrochloride**).

EXCRETION OF DRUGS IN BREAST MILK

The following is a list of medications that are excreted in breast milk. Their effects on the infant are also included.

acetaminophen (Tylenol, Datril). Detoxified in the immature neonatal liver. Avoid immediately after delivery. Later, there is no known problem with the therapeutic dose.

acetylsalicylic acid (aspirin). Can cause interference with blood clotting, although problems are rare. If mother requires high dose, observe infant for petechiae, bruises, and bleeding disorders.

alcohol, ethyl. Usually no problem. Excessive drinking may cause obesity, drowsiness, and depression of maternal milk-ejection reflex.

ampicillin (Omnipen, Polycillin). May cause diarrhea or secondary candidiasis. Sensitivity from repeated exposure.

caffeine. May cause jitteriness, sleep disorders, and irritability. May accumulate with moderate or continued use.

chloramphenicol (Chloromycetin). Contraindicated in mother of breast-feeding neonate because infant does not excrete drug well and the dose may accumulate.

coumarin. May cause bleeding disorders. Administer vitamin K to the infant and check prothrombin time periodically.

diazepam (Valium). May cause jaundice in the young infant. May also cause hypoventilation, drowsiness, lethargy, and weight loss.

epinephrine (Adrenalin). Broken down in gastrointestinal tract of the infant before absorption. Consequently, there is no effect on the infant.

ergonovine maleate (Ergotrate). May cause nausea and vomiting or cardiovascular abnormalities.

erythromycin. May cause an infant under 1 month old to develop jaundice.

hydralazine hydrochloride (Apresoline). May cause jaundice, electrolyte imbalance, or thrombocytopenia.

indomethacin (Indocin). May cause convulsions and may be nephrotoxic. Indocin is used therapeutically to close patent ductus arteriosus.

marijuana. May impair RNA and DNA formation. The infant may also inhale smoke if he is held while the mother is smoking.

methadone. May show depression or failure to thrive.

methyldopa (Aldomet). May cause galactorrhea.

metronidazole (Flagyl). Concentration in milk is high. Should not be administered if the infant is less than 6 months old because it may cause neurological disorders and blood dyscrasias and because it has been implicated in cancer.

narcotics. Single dose is usually not a problem, but narcotics can accumulate with repetitive doses, causing addiction, depression, drowsiness, and poor feeding.

nicotine. May interfere with milk production and the maternal let-down reflex. The infant may inhale smoke while feeding.

nitrofurantoin (Furadantin). No known problems except hemolysis in the glucose-6-phosphate dehydrogenase-deficient infant.

oral contraceptives. May decrease maternal milk production and alter the composition of milk. The long-range implications of the infant's receiving hormones are unknown.

penicillin. The infant may have an allergic response.

pentobarbital (Nembutal). No problem for the older infant. For the first week of life, however, while the liver is immature, the dose may accumulate, causing drowsiness and feeding disorders.

phenytoin sodium (Dilantin). May cause hemolysis, but usually causes no problem.

propoxyphene hydrochloride (Darvon). May cause failure to feed and drowsiness.

RhO(D) immune globulin (RhoGAM). Broken down in the infant's gastrointestinal tract before absorption.

streptomycin sulfate. May cause auditory and renal damage with prolonged use.

sulfonamides. May cause rash or hemolytic anemia. Should be avoided during the first month of life because of the risk of jaundice.

tetracycline. May cause discoloration of teeth. Should not be administered long-term or repeatedly.

theophylline. May cause irritability and fretfulness.

The following drugs are not excreted in breast milk:

cephalexin (Keflex).

cephalothin sodium (Keflin).

heparin.

magnesium hydroxide (Gelusil, Maalox, Milk of Magnesia, Mylanta).

nystatin (Mycostatin, Nilstat).

stool softeners and bulk-forming laxatives.

It is unknown whether **gentamicin sulfate (Garamycin)** or **insulin** is excreted in breast milk. However, if insulin is excreted in breast milk, it is broken down in the infant's gastrointestinal tract before absorption.

APPENDIX B: LABORATORY TESTS

Evaluation of Laboratory Data for the Maternity Client

Laboratory test/procedure	Normal values	Abnormal values and significance	Comments
Pap smear	Negative (Class I).	Class II: cellular atypia, not suggestive of malignancy. Class III: cellular atypia suggestive of, but not diagnostic of malignancy. Class IV: malignant cells. Class V: malignant cells more bizarre than Class IV.	Vaginal infections, such as *Trichomonas vaginalis*, may cause a Pap smear to be Class II. The procedure is usually repeated after treatment of the vaginal infection.
Gonorrhea culture	Negative.	Positive: treatment of client and all contacts is indicated (*see* Chapter 18).	
Tuberculin test	Negative.	Positive.	BCG vaccine, which is administered in many countries, will cause subsequent tine tests and PPD tests to be positive. Clients who have been administered BCG vaccine may be sent for a chest x-ray.
Rubella titer	Immune is at least 1:8 or 1:10, depending on the laboratory.	Susceptible is less than 1:8 or 1:10. Very high titers indicate current or recent infection.	Rubella-susceptible clients should be evaluated for rubella vaccination postpartum. After suspected exposure, an initial titer should be taken. A fourfold increase in a titer taken 3 weeks later indicates infection. A high

Laboratory test/procedure	Normal values	Abnormal values and significance	Comments
			initial titer followed by a lower titer on a repeat test indicates that the client initially had the infection.
Serologic test for syphilis or VDRL	Negative or nonreactive.	Positive or reactive. Does not become positive until 7-10 days after appearance of chancre (see Chapter 18).	A positive VDRL test should be confirmed with an FTA-ABS test — a more specific test for syphilis.
Blood type	All types are normal.	All Rh-negative women should be screened for Rh incompatibility by an evaluation of the Rh-antibody titers. All antibodies except anti-Lewis cross the placenta.	Rh-negative mothers should be evaluated for RhO (D antigen) immune globulin postpartum (see Appendix A).
Urinalysis Color	Yellow.		
Clarity	Clear.	Cloudy: infection or contaminated specimen.	
pH	5-7.		
Specific gravity	1.010-1.020.	<1.010: diluted urine, overhydrated client. >1.020: concentrated urine, dehydrated client.	
Protein	Negative.	+ to ++++: vaginal or urinary infection, preeclampsia, contaminated specimen, or renal disease.	
Glucose	Negative.	+ to ++++: high carbohydrate intake before specimen was obtained, or symptom of diabetes.	

Test	Normal Value	Interpretation	Comments
Ketones	Negative.	+ to + + + +: breakdown of fat secondary to insufficient dietary intake or utilization.	
WBC	Negative.	Few to many: contaminated specimen, or urinary or vaginal infection.	
RBC	Negative.	Few to many: vaginal infection, trauma, or renal disease.	
Bacteria	Negative.	Few to many: vaginal or urinary tract infection (not trauma).	
Epithelial cells	Negative.	Few to many: usually, specimen obtained was not a clean-catch.	
Casts	Negative.	Few to many: may state content, usually secondary to dietary intake.	
Urine culture and sensitivity	<100,000 colonies.	>100,000 colonies.	Specific infecting organism and its sensitivity to antibiotics will also be reported.
Complete blood count			
WBC	5,000-10,000.	Increased: may be secondary to infection.	During labor, an elevated WBC level may be normal.
RBC	$3.8-4.8 \times 10^6$.	Decreased: may be secondary to increased blood volume during pregnancy or anemia.	
Reticulocytes	0.5-1.5%.	Decreased: may be secondary to folic acid or vitamin B12 deficiency. Increased: may be secondary to bleeding.	
Hemoglobin	≥10 g.	Decreased: may be secondary to increased blood volume during pregnancy or anemia.	
Hematocrit	≥30%.	Decreased: may be secondary to increased blood volume during pregnancy or anemia.	

Laboratory test/procedure	Normal values	Abnormal values and significance	Comments
MCV	$87 \pm 5 \ \mu g^3$.	Increased: may indicate folic acid deficiency.	
Mean corpuscular hemoglobin	29 ± 2 pg.	Decreased: along with decreased MCV, may indicate iron deficiency.	
Mean corpuscular hemoglobin concentration	$34 \pm 2\%$.	Reduced: may indicate iron deficiency.	
Serum iron	50-180 μg/100 ml.	Reduced: may indicate iron deficiency and/or iron-deficiency anemia.	
TIBC	248-422 μg/100 ml.	Increased: may indicate iron-deficiency anemia or bleeding.	The TIBC level is elevated when the body is trying to capture more iron.
Sickle prep (note: this test is a screen for sickle cell disease only; a negative test does not rule out the presence of other hemoglobin-opathies)	Negative.	Positive: may indicate sickling trait or sickle cell disease.	A positive sickle prep should be followed up with a hemoglobin electrophoresis in order to determine whether the trait or the disease is present.
Hemoglobin electrophoresis	Negative or AA (normal adult hemoglobin).	AS: sickling trait. SS: sickle cell disease. AA_2: thalassemia minor. AF: thalassemia major.	

Test	Value	Notes
Oral glucose tolerance test (fasting and 2-hr postprandial values)	Whole blood: Fasting: 90 mg/100 ml. 1 hr: 165 mg/100 ml. 2 hr: 145 mg/100 ml. 3 hr: 125 mg/100 ml.	Oral glucose tolerance test: diagnostic for diabetes if two or more of the values are exceeded.	If plasma (rather than whole blood) is analyzed, all values are 15% higher.

Test	Value		Notes
Screening coagulation tests*			
Bleeding time	1-5 min.	Decreased.	Measures platelet and vascular integrity.
Platelet count	140,000-440,000/mm³.	Decreased.	Measures number of platelets.
Partial thromboplastin time	24-36 sec.	Decreased.	Measures factors II, V, VII, IX, X, and XI.
Prothombin time	11-12 sec.	Decreased.	Measures factors II, V, VII, and X.
Thrombin time	16-20 sec.	Decreased.	Measures factors I and II, and circulating split products.

Test	Value	Notes
Blood electrolytes		
Sodium	136-145 mEq/liter.	For all electrolytes, increased and decreased values are abnormal.
Potassium	3.5-4.5 mEq/liter.	
Chloride	100-106 mEq/liter.	
Calcium	8.5-10.5 mg/100 ml.	
Phosphorus	2.0-4.5 mg/100 ml.	
Magnesium	1.5-2.5 mEq/liter.	

Test	Value	Notes
Blood chemistries		
Uric acid	3.0-7.5 mg/100 ml.	Increased: may indicate kidney disease or preeclampsia.	Kidney perfusion is increased during pregnancy. Therefore, uric acid, BUN, and creatinine may be normally slightly decreased.
BUN	10-20 mg/100 ml.	Increased: may indicate kidney disease or preeclampsia.	
Creatinine	0.7-1.5 mg/100 ml.	Increased: may indicate kidney disease or preeclampsia.	

Laboratory test/procedure	Normal values	Abnormal values and significance	Comments

Protein
  Total
  Albumin
  Globulin
	6.0-8.9 g/100 mg.
	3.5-5.5 g/100 mg.
	2.5-3.5 g/100 mg.
		Decreased: may indicate kidney disease and preeclampsia as well as in malnutrition.	

G6PD	<40 IU/gram (confirm with laboratory).	>40 IU/gram.	Certain drugs or foods may cause a hemolytic reaction in clients with G6PD deficiency. (See Table 15-1). Some infections or diabetic acidosis may also cause a reaction.

BCG, bacille Calmette-Guerin; BUN, blood urea nitrogen; FTA-ABS, fluorescent treponemal antibody absorption (test); G6PD, glucose-6-phosphate dehydrogenase; MCV, mean corpuscular volume; Pap, Papanicolaou; PPD, purified protein derivative (of tuberculin); RBC, red blood cell(s); TIBC, total iron-binding capacity; VDRL, Venereal Disease Research Laboratories; WBC, white blood cell(s).
*Findings of coagulation tests are decreased or abnormal in these acquired conditions: disseminated intravascular coagulation, liver disease, and idiopathic thrombocytopenic purpura.

APPENDIX C: GLOSSARY

VITAL STATISTICS

Abortus. A fetus or embryo removed or expelled from the uterus during the first half of gestation (20 weeks or less), weighing less than 500 grams, or measuring less than 25 centimeters.

Birth. The complete expulsion or extraction of a fetus from a woman, regardless of whether the umbilical cord has been cut or the placenta is attached. Fetuses that weigh less than 500 grams are usually considered as abortions rather than births (for purposes of perinatal statistics). If the birth weight is unobtainable, a body length of 25 centimeters (crown to heel) is usually equated with 500 grams.

Birth rate. The number of births per 1,000 population.

Direct maternal death. Death of the mother resulting from obstetric complications of the pregnancy, labor, or puerperium; from interventions, omissions, or incorrect treatment; or from a chain of events resulting from any of the above. (Example: exsanguination from rupture of uterus.)

Fertility rate. The number of live births per 1,000 female population of 15 to 44 years of age.

Indirect maternal death. An obstetric death not directly resulting from obstetric causes. A death resulting from a previously existing disease or a disease that develops during pregnancy, labor, or the puerperium that is aggravated by the maternal physiological adaptation to pregnancy. (Example: mitral stenosis.)

Live birth. Whenever the infant at birth, or sometime thereafter, breathes spontaneously or shows any other sign of life (such as a heartbeat or definite spontaneous movement of voluntary muscles), a live birth is recorded.

Low birth weight. Birth weight of less than 2,500 grams.

Maternal mortality rate. The number of maternal deaths that occur as the result of the reproductive process per 100,000 live births. (Note: this rate is calculated per *100,000* live births, *not* per 1,000.)

Neonatal death. Early neonatal death refers to the death of a live-born infant during the first 7 days of life. Late neonatal death refers to a death occurring between 8 and 29 days of life.

Neonatal mortality rate. The number of neonatal deaths per 1,000 live births.

Nonmaternal death. Death of the mother resulting from accidental or incidental causes that are in no way related to the pregnancy. (Example: death from an airplane crash.)

Perinatal mortality rate. The number of stillbirths and neonatal deaths per 1,000 total births.

Postterm infant. An infant born after 42 weeks (294 days) of gestation.

Preterm or premature infant. An infant born before 37 completed weeks of gestation.

Stillbirth. A stillbirth is recorded if the infant shows no sign of life (e.g., heartbeat or spontaneous breaths and/or movements.)

Stillbirth rate. The number of stillborn infants per 1,000 births. Synonymous with the fetal death rate.

Term infant. An infant who is born no earlier than 38 completed weeks, but no later than 42 completed weeks, of gestation.

OTHER RELEVANT TERMS

Abruptio placentae. Separation of the placenta from its site of implantation before the birth of the fetus. Although the cause is unknown, maternal hypertension has a strongly positive correlation.

Amniocentesis. Withdrawal of a small amount of amniotic fluid from the uterine cavity. Most commonly performed for genetic studies or other analysis of fetal well-being.

Amnioscopy. Visualization of the amniotic fluid through the membranes when the cervix is sufficiently dilated. Used to diagnose the presence of meconium staining.

Android pelvis. Pelvic shape called "wedge" or "funnel," characterized by a progressive, downward narrowing of all pelvic diameters. Occurs in approximately 25 percent of women.

Anemia. A condition in which there is a reduction in the number of circulating red blood cells, hemoglobin, or both. It exists when the hemoglobin content is less than 13 to 14 grams for males and 11 to 12 grams for females.

Anthropoid pelvis. Pelvic shape characterized by a narrow and pointed subpubic arch, and a hollow, deep posterior segment. Occurs in approximately 25 percent of women.

Apgar score. Tool used to evaluate the newborn's cardiopulmonary status during the first 5 minutes of life.

Attitude. Relationship of the fetal parts to each other. The basic attitudes are flexion and extension.

Bacilluria. The presence of a significant number of bacteria in the urine (bacteriemia).

Ballottement. Near midpregnancy, when the volume of the fetus is much smaller than that of the amniotic fluid, sudden pressure exerted on the uterus may cause the fetus to sink into the fluid and then rise. This motion produces a tap felt by the examining hand.

Bilirubin. A reddish yellow pigment produced by the breakdown of hemoglobin. Found in bile, blood, urine, and gallstones.

Bimanual examination. Examination with two hands. Part of the pelvic examination. The examiner assesses the size, shape, and consistency of the uterus and the ovaries with the fingers of one hand in the vagina and the other hand on the abdomen.

Bishop score. Tool used to evaluate readiness for induction of labor.

Breast engorgement. A condition occurring in the first 24 to 48 hours after delivery in which the breasts become distended, firm, and nodular as a result of the normal venous and lymphatic stasis preceding lactation.

Candida albicans. A type of fungus or yeast that causes vaginal pruritus and thick, white, cheesy discharge.

Caput succedaneum. A diffuse swelling of the fetal scalp as a result of the forces of labor. Usually disappears within 24 to 48 hours.

Cephalhematoma. A subperiosteal hemorrhage of the newborn that is caused by trauma to the fetal skull during birth.

Chadwick's sign. A presumptive sign of pregnancy. The vaginal mucosa becomes dark blue or reddish purple and appears congested.

Chloasma. Irregular brownish patches on the face and neck that occur during pregnancy. Chloasma is thought to be the result of increased levels of estrogen and progesterone, which have a melanocyte-stimulating effect. Also called the "mask of pregnancy."

Colostrum. The precursor of breast milk. Colostrum is rich in nutritive value and immunoglobins. This thick, yellow substance may be manually expressed from the breast from the first few months of pregnancy until the breast milk supply starts on about the third postpartum day.

Congenital. Existing at, or dating from, birth. Acquired during development in the uterus and not through heredity.

Coombs's test. An antiglobulin test used in the diagnosis of various hemolytic anemias, including fetal Rh-sensitization anemia.

Couvade syndrome. A custom among some primitive peoples in accordance with which the father takes to bed when a child is born as if he is bearing the child. He cares for it and submits himself to fasting, purification, and taboos.

Crowning. Encirclement of the largest (biparietal) diameter of the fetal head by the vulvar ring during birth.

Curve of Carus. The J-shaped curve of the birth canal.

Cystocele. Prolapse of the bladder into the vagina. Caused by weakened muscle support.

Denominator. An arbitrarily chosen point on the presenting part that is used in describing position. Common denominators include the occiput and the sacrum.

Diaphoresis. Profuse perspiration.

Diastasis recti. Midline separation of the abdominal rectus muscles.

Diuresis. Increased excretion of urine.

Doppler effect. A change in the frequency with which waves (light, sound, or radio) from a given source reach an observer when the source and the observer are in rapid motion in respect to each other so that the frequency increases or decreases according to the speed at which the distance is decreasing or increasing.

Dyspareunia. Painful sexual intercourse.

Dystocia. Abnormal labor or childbirth.

Eclampsia. The occurrence of convulsions in a woman who has pre-eclampsia.

En face. A characteristic position assumed by the new mother in which she is face-to-face with the newborn and engages in eye-to-eye contact.

Engagement. The point at which the widest diameter of the presenting part has passed through the pelvic inlet.

Estimated date of confinement. Anticipated birth date. This is 280 days from the first day of the last normal menstrual period or 267 days from conception.

Ferning. A characteristic pattern of midcycle cervical mucus and/or amniotic fluid. When either of these is allowed to air-dry on a slide and then examined microscopically, a typical "palm leaf" pattern is seen.

Fetoscope. An instrument used to auscultate the fetal heart antenatally. Different types of fetoscopes are available: from a modified stethoscope to a device that uses ultrasound to elicit fetal heart valve movement.

Fibroid. Uterine myoma or benign tumor consisting of connective and muscular tissue.

Fontanels. Membrane-covered spaces where fetal or newborn skull sutures intersect. The anterior fontanel is a diamond-shaped space bordered by the sagittal and coronal sutures. The posterior fontanel is a triangular space bordered by the sagittal and lambdoidal sutures.

Glycosuria. The presence of glucose in the urine.

Goodell's sign. A presumptive sign of pregnancy. At 6 to 8 weeks of gestation, the cervix, which usually feels firm, becomes soft.

Gynecoid pelvis. Normal pelvic shape. Characterized by wide, deep diameters. Occurs in approximately 50 percent of women.

Heartburn. Reflux of gastric contents into the lower esophagus. A common occurrence in the third trimester of pregnancy.

Hegar's sign. A presumptive sign of pregnancy. At 6 to 8 weeks of gestation, the uterine body becomes doughy or elastic and the lower uterine segment becomes soft.

Hemorrhoids. Varicosities of the hemorrhoidal veins.

Hydatidiform mole. A disease of the trophoblast characterized by degeneration of the chorionic villi into a mass of fluid-filled vesicles. This condition is associated with the development of chorio-carcinoma.

Hydramnios. An excessive amount of amniotic fluid that leads to overdistension of the uterus and the possibility of cord prolapse, fetal malpresentation, and postpartum hemorrhage. A normal amount of amniotic fluid is from 800 to 1,200 milliliters. Hydramnios refers to greater than 2,000 milliliters of fluid.

Hypertension during pregnancy. A diastolic blood pressure of at least 90 mmHg or a systolic pressure of at least 140 mmHg; or a rise of 15 mmHg in the diastolic and/or a rise of 30 mmHg in the systolic blood pressure over base-line blood pressures.

Icterus neonatorum. Physiological jaundice of the newborn. Occurs in approximately one third of newborns between the second and fifth day of life. Thought to be a result of the immaturity of the newborn's hepatic system.

Interspinous diameter. Distance between the ischial spines. Usually 12 centimeters or less.

Interstitial. Related to, or situated in, a space that intervenes between things, especially body tissues.

Involution. Return of the reproductive organs to the nonpregnant state.

Kernicterus. A condition of the newborn in which severe neural damage is associated with high levels of bilirubin (18 to 20 mg/dl).

Ketoacidosis. A disturbance in the acid-base balance of the body in which there is an accumulation of acids as a result of excessive pro-duction of ketone bodies (seen in starvation or diabetes mellitus).

Ketosis. Accumulation of ketone bodies in blood and urine as a result of the breakdown of body fat stores for energy. Usually associ-ated with pathology, such as diabetes, nausea and vomiting, or starvation.

Lanugo. Downy hair covering the fetus from the 20th to 38th week of gestation.

Leopold's maneuvers. Four specific techniques of abdominal palpation used in conjunction to diagnose the presentation and position of the fetus.

Leukorrhea. Increased vaginal secretions.

Lie. The relationship between the long axis of the fetus and that of the uterus.

Lightening. A decrease in fundal height that occurs a few weeks before delivery as a result of the descent of the fetal head through the pelvic inlet and of a small decrease in amniotic fluid. This sensation may be reported by the client as "the baby dropped." It is most common in the first pregnancy.

Linea nigra. Pigmentation of the abdominal midline during pregnancy from the symphysis pubis to the umbilicus. It resembles a brownish black line, and is thought to be the result of the increased levels of estrogen and progesterone, which exert a melanocyte-stimulating effect.

Malpresentation. Abnormal fetal entry into the birth canal. Entry of any part other than the vertex.

Mechanisms of labor. A description of the ways that the fetus passively adapts itself to, and descends through, the maternal pelvis. Eight cardinal movements are descent, flexion, internal rotation, extension, restitution, external rotation, birth of the shoulders, and birth of the trunk (expulsion).

Meconium. The contents of the fetal and/or newborn colon. Comprised of epithelial cells from the intestinal tract, mucus, skin cells, and hair (lanugo) that the fetus had swallowed with the amniotic fluid. Passage of meconium in utero may indicate fetal distress.

Megaloblastic anemia. Anemia in which large, pale red blood cells (megaloblasts) are found in the blood. In pregnancy, a common cause of megaloblastic anemia is folic acid deficiency.

Montgomery's tubercles. Hypertrophic sebaceous glands that are scattered throughout the areola of the breast.

Nagele's rule. A method of estimating the estimated date of confinement. The rule is as follows: add 7 days to the first day of the last normal menstrual period; subtract 3 months; the date arrived at will be the estimated date of confinement.

Oligohydramnios. An abnormally small amount of amniotic fluid that may be symptomatic of a variety of problems, including fetal renal agenesis and intrauterine growth retardation.

Ophthalmia neonatorum. Gonorrheal infection of the newborn's eyes during birth if the mother has gonorrhea. May result in newborn blindness. Most states require prophylaxis, e.g., silver nitrate solution or antibiotic ointment applied to both eyes within the first hour of life.

Papanicolaou test. Pap smear. Microscopic examination of a slide that contains cells from the cervix and/or vagina in order to screen for the presence of cancer.

Paroxysm. A fit, attack, or sudden increase or recurrence of symptoms.

Pica. A craving for unusual substances like ice, refrigerator frost, laundry starch, or soil.

Placenta previa. The location of the placenta over, or very near, the cervical os. May result in hemorrhage and/or fetal death.

Platypelloid pelvis. Pelvic shape characterized by a wide transverse diameter and a short anterior-posterior diameter. Occurs in approximately 3 percent of women.

Position. The relationship of the denominator to the front, back, and sides of the maternal pelvis.

Postpartum hemorrhage (early). Loss of over 500 milliliters of blood during the first 24 hours after the birth of the infant.

Postpartum hemorrhage (late). Loss of at least 500 milliliters of blood after the first 24 hours after the birth of the infant, but within 6 weeks after the birth. Most often seen on postpartum days 4 through 9.

Postpartum morbidity. A temperature of 38 °C (100.4 °F) or higher occurring on any 2 of the first 10 days postpartum, exclusive of the first 24 hours. The temperature is taken orally at least four times a day.

Postprandial. After a meal.

Preeclampsia. The development of hypertension (with proteinuria, edema, or both) after the 20th week of gesation.

Premature rupture of the membranes. Rupture at least 1 hour before the onset of labor, regardless of the duration of gestation.

Presentation. The part of the fetus that lies over the pelvic inlet. The three types are cephalic, breech, and shoulder.

Proteinuria. The presence of protein in the urine.

Pseudocyesis. Imaginary pregnancy. Sometimes reported by women who strongly desire children. Also called false pregnancy.

Ptyalism. Profuse salivation.

Quickening. First maternal sensation of fetal movement. Occurs between the 16th and 20th week of gestation. This sign corroborates pregnancy and is used to help establish gestational age.

Rectocele. Prolapse of the rectum into the vagina. Caused by weakened muscle support.

Rh disease. A condition in which maternal antibodies produced by an Rh-positive mother cause hemolysis in an Rh-negative fetus.

Ritgen's manuever. A method of assisting the delivery. During delivery of the fetal head, forward pressure is applied to the undelivered chin of the fetus through the maternal perineum with one hand, and downward pressure is applied to the fetal occiput with the other hand.

Rooming-in. A practice that allows the newborn to stay at the mother's bedside rather than in the nursery during her postpartum hospitalization. Encourages attachment and helps the mother to master infant care.

Shoulder dystocia. A condition in which, after the birth of the fetal head, the anterior shoulder becomes impacted behind the symphysis pubis, thereby trapping the fetal body inside the pelvis.

Show. The escape of a small amount of blood-tinged mucus from the vagina, indicating the extrusion of the mucous plug that had filled the cervical os during pregnancy. Labor may ensue any time from several hours to a few days after the appearance of show.

Souffle (funic). A sharp, whistling sound that may sometimes be auscultated abdominally (synchronous with the fetal pulse). This sound is produced by the rush of blood through the fetal umbilical arteries.

Souffle (uterine). A soft, blowing sound that may be heard with the fetoscope (synchronous with maternal pulse). This sound is produced by the rush of blood through the dilated uterine vessels.

Station. The relationship between the leading edge of the presenting part and an imaginary line drawn between the ischial spines.

Subinvolution. Failure of the reproductive organs to return to their nonpregnant state. Usually secondary to infection.

Synclitism. The relationship of the fetal sagittal suture to the front and back of the maternal pelvis (when the fetal head is in the transverse position). If the suture is midway between the front and back of the pelvis, the fetal head is said to be synclitic.

Teratogen. Any substance that causes developmental malformations.

Toxemia of pregnancy. Traditional term used to indicate preeclampsia, eclampsia, or both.

Trichomonas. A flagellated, motile organism that causes vaginal pruritus, burning, and thin, bubbly, yellowish green, malodorous leukorrhea.

Trimester. The traditional method of dividing pregnancy into three equal parts — 3 calendar months or slightly more than 13 weeks each.

Ultrasound. Vibrations of the same physical nature as sound but with frequencies above the range of human hearing. Ultrasound has been adapted to monitoring fetal heart tones.

Venereal. Resulting from, or contracted during, sexual intercourse.

Wharton's jelly. Matrix of the umbilical cord, through which pass the arteries and vein.

APPENDIX D: THE PREGNANT PATIENT'S BILL OF RIGHTS

American parents are becoming increasingly aware that well-intentioned health professionals do not always have scientific data to support common American obstetrical practices and that many of these practices are carried out primarily because they are part of medical and hospital tradition. In the last 40 years many artificial practices have been introduced which have changed childbirth from a physiological event to a very complicated medical procedure in which all kinds of drugs are used and procedures carried out, sometimes unnecessarily, and many of them potentially damaging for the baby and even for the mother. A growing body of research makes it alarmingly clear that every aspect of traditional American hospital care during labor and delivery must now be questioned as to its possible effect on the future well-being of both the obstetric patient and her unborn child.

One in every 35 children born in the United States today will eventually be diagnosed as retarded; in 75 percent of these cases there is no familial or genetic predisposing factor. One in every 10 to 17 children has been found to have some form of brain dysfunction or learning disability requiring special treatment. Such statistics are not confined to the lower socioeconomic group but cut across all segments of American society.

New concerns are being raised by childbearing women because no one knows what degree of oxygen depletion, head compression, or traction by forceps the unborn or newborn infant can tolerate before that child sustains permanent brain damage or dysfunction. The recent findings regarding the cancer-related drug diethylstilbestrol have alerted the public to the fact that neither the approval of a drug by the U. S. Food and Drug Administration nor the fact that a drug is prescribed by a physician serves as a guarantee that a drug or medication is safe for the mother or her unborn child. In fact, the American Academy of Pediatrics' Committee on Drugs has recently stated that there is no drug, whether prescription or over-the-counter remedy, which has been proven safe for the unborn child.

The Pregnant Patient has the right to participate in decisions involving her well-being and that of her unborn child, unless there is a clearcut medical emergency that prevents her participation. In addition to the rights set forth in the American Hospital Association's ''Patient's Bill of Rights'' (which has also been adopted by the New York City Department of Health), the

605

Pregnant Patient, because she represents *two* patients rather than one, should be recognized as having the following additional rights:

1. *The Pregnant Patient has the right,* prior to the administration of any drug or procedure, to be informed by the health professional caring for her of any potential direct or indirect effects, risks or hazards to herself or her unborn or newborn infant which may result from the use of a drug or procedure prescribed for or administered to her during pregnancy, labor, birth or lactation.

2. *The Pregnant Patient has the right,* prior to the proposed therapy, to be informed, not only of the benefits, risks and hazards of the proposed therapy but also of known alternative therapy, such as available childbirth education classes which could help to prepare the pregnant patient physically and mentally to cope with the discomfort or stress of pregnancy and the experience of childbirth, thereby reducing or eliminating her need for drugs and obstetric intervention. She should be offered such information early in her pregnancy in order that she may make a reasoned decision.

3. *The Pregnant Patient has the right,* prior to the administration of any drug, to be informed by the health professional who is prescribing or administering the drug to her that any drug which she receives during pregnancy, labor and birth, no matter how or when the drug is taken or administered, may adversely affect her unborn baby, directly or indirectly, and that there is no drug or chemical which has been proven safe for the unborn child.

4. *The Pregnant Patient has the right,* if cesarean section is anticipated, to be informed prior to the administration of any drug, and preferably prior to her hospitalization, that minimizing her and, in turn, her baby's intake of nonessential pre-operative medicine will benefit her baby.

5. *The Pregnant Patient has the right,* prior to the administration of a drug or procedure, to be informed of the areas of uncertainty if there is NO properly controlled follow-up research which has established the safety of the drug or procedure with regard to its direct and/or indirect effects on the physiological, mental and neurological development of the child exposed, via the mother, to the drug or procedure during pregnancy, labor, birth or lactation — (this would apply to virtually all drugs and the vast majority of obstetric procedures).

6. *The Pregnant Patient has the right,* prior to the administration of any drug, to be informed of the brand name and generic name of the drug in order that she may advise the health professional of any past adverse reaction to the drug.

7. *The Pregnant Patient has the right* to determine for herself, without pressure from her attendant, whether she will accept the risks inherent in the proposed therapy or refuse a drug or procedure.

8. *The Pregnant Patient has the right* to know the name and qualifications of the individual administering a medication or procedure to her during labor or birth.

9. *The Pregnant Patient has the right* to be informed, prior to the

administration of any procedure, whether that procedure is being administered to her for her or her baby's benefit (medically indicated) or as an elective procedure (for convenience, teaching purposes or research).

10. *The Pregnant Patient has the right* to be accompanied during the stress of labor and birth by someone she cares for, and to whom she looks for emotional comfort and encouragement.

11. *The Pregnant Patient has the right* after appropriate medical consultation to choose a position for labor and for birth which is least stressful to her baby and to herself.

12. *The Obstetric Patient has the right* to have her baby cared for at her bedside if her baby is normal, and to feed her baby according to her baby's needs rather than according to the hospital regimen.

13. *The Obstetric Patient has the right* to be informed in writing of the name of the person who actually delivered her baby and the professional qualifications of that person. This information should also be on the birth certificate.

14. *The Obstetric Patient has the right* to be informed if there is any known or indicated aspect of her or her baby's care or condition which may cause her or her baby later difficulty or problems.

15. *The Obstetric Patient has the right* to have her and her baby's hospital medical records complete, accurate and legible and to have their records, including Nurses' Notes, retained by the hospital until the child reaches at least the age of majority, or, alternatively, to have the records offered to her before they are destroyed.

16. *The Obstetric Patient,* both during and after her hospital stay, has the right to have access to her complete hospital medical records, including Nurses' Notes, and to receive a copy upon payment of a reasonable fee and without incurring the expense of retaining an attorney.

It is the obstetric patient and her baby, not the health professional, who must sustain any trauma or injury resulting from the use of a drug or obstetric procedure. The observation of the rights listed above will not only permit the obstetric patient to participate in the decisions involving her and her baby's health care, but will help to protect the health professional and the hospital against litigation arising from resentment or misunderstanding on the part of the mother.

Reprinted with permission from the Committee on Patient's Rights, New York.

BIBLIOGRAPHY

Chapter 1

Maternity Center Association. A Baby is Born. Grosset & Dunlap, Inc., New York. 1977. Tenth edition.

Myles, M. F. Textbook for Midwives. Churchill Livingstone, Inc., New York. 1981. Ninth edition.

Olds, S. B., M. L. London, P. A. Ladewig, and S. V. Davidson. Obstetric Nursing. Addison-Wesley Publishing Co., Inc., Menlo Park, Calif. 1980.

Pritchard, J. A., and P. C. MacDonald. Williams Obstetrics. Appleton-Century-Crofts, East Norwalk, Conn. 1980. Sixteenth edition.

Ross Laboratories. Clinical Education Aids (Numbers 13 and 18). Columbus, Ohio. 1979.

Sandberg, E. Synopsis of Obstetrics. C. V. Mosby Co., St. Louis. 1978. Tenth edition.

Varney, H. Nurse Midwifery. Blackwell Scientific Publications, Inc., Boston. 1980.

Chapter 2

Davison, J. M. The urinary system. *In* Hytten, F. E., and G. Chamberlain, editors. Clinical Physiology in Obstetrics. Blackwell Scientific Publications, Inc., Boston. 1981. Third edition.

de Swiet, M. The respiratory system. *In* Hytten, F. E., and G. Chamberlain, editors. Clinical Physiology in Obstetrics. Blackwell Scientific Publications, Inc., Boston. 1981. Third edition.

Jensen, M. D., R. C. Bensen, and I. M. Bobak. Maternity Care: The Nurse and the Family. C. V. Mosby Co., St. Louis. 1981. Second edition.

Letsky, E. The haematological system. *In* Hytten, F. E., and G. Chamberlain, editors. Clinical Physiology in Obstetrics. Blackwell Scientific Publications, Inc., Boston. 1981. Third edition.

Moore, K. L. Before We Are Born: Basic Embryology and Birth Defects. W. B. Saunders Co., Philadelphia. 1977.

Netter, F. H. The CIBA Collection of Medical Illustrations. Vol. II. Reproductive System. CIBA Pharmaceutical Co., Summit, N. J. 1974.

Niswander, K. Obstetrics: Essentials of Clinical Practice. Little, Brown & Co., Boston. 1981. Second edition.

Pritchard, J. A., and P. C. MacDonald. Williams Obstetrics. Appleton-Century-Crofts, East Norwalk, Conn. 1980. Sixteenth edition.

Ryan, G. M., Jr., P. J. Sweeney, and A. S. Solala. Prenatal care and pregnancy outcome. *American Journal of Obstetrics and Gynecology* (August 15, 1980). 876-881.

Varney, H. Nurse Midwifery. Blackwell Scientific Publications, Inc., Boston. 1980.

Chapter 3
Clark, A., and D. D. Alfonso. Childbearing: A Nursing Perspective. F. A. Davis Co., Philadelphia. 1979. Second edition.

Clausen, J. P., M. H. Flook, and B. Ford. Maternity Nursing Today. McGraw-Hill Book Co., New York. 1977. Second edition.

Pritchard, J. A., and P. C. MacDonald. Williams Obstetrics. Appleton-Century-Crofts, East Norwalk, Conn. 1980. Sixteenth edition.

Varney, H. Nurse Midwifery. Blackwell Scientific Publications, Inc., Boston. 1980.

Chapter 4
Antle, K. Psychologic involvement in pregnancy by expectant fathers. *(JOGN Nursing) Journal of Obstetric, Gynecologic and Neonatal Nursing* (July-August 1975). 40-42.

Ascher, B. H. Maternal anxiety in pregnancy and fetal homeostasis. *(JOGN Nursing) Journal of Obstetric, Gynecologic and Neonatal Nursing* (May-June 1978). 18-21.

Benedek, T. The psychobiology of pregnancy. *In* Bardwick, J. M., editor. Readings on the Psychology of Women. Harper & Row, Publishers, Inc., New York. 1972.

The Boston Women's Health Book Collective. Our Bodies, Ourselves. Simon & Schuster, Inc., New York. 1979. Second edition.

Burst, H. V. Adolescent pregnancies and problems. *Journal of Nurse-Midwifery* (March-April 1979). 19-24.

Caplan, G. An Approach to Community Mental Health. Grune & Stratton, Inc., New York. 1966.

Ciaramitaro, B. Help for Depressed Mothers. Independent Printing Co., Ashland, Ore. 1978.

Clausen, J. P., M. H. Flook, and B. Ford. Maternity Nursing Today. McGraw-Hill Book Co., New York. 1977. Second edition.

Cohen, R. L. Maladaptation to pregnancy. *Seminars in Perinatology* (January 1979). 15-24.

Coleman, A. D., and L. L. Coleman. Pregnancy: The Psychological Experience. Seabury Press, Inc., New York. 1971.

Crandon, A. J. Maternal anxiety and obstetric complications. *Journal of Psychosomatic Research* (1979). **23**(2):109-111.

Crandon, A. J. Maternal anxiety and neonatal wellbeing. *Journal of Psycosomatic Research* (1979). **23**(2):113-115.

Curtis, F. L. S. Observations of unwed pregnant adolescents. *American Journal of Nursing* (March 1974). 100.

Falicov, C. J. Sexual adjustment during first pregnancy and postpartum. *American Journal of Obstetrics and Gynecology* (December 1, 1973). 991-1000.

Fein, R. A. The first weeks of fathering: the importance of choices for new parents. *Birth and the Family Journal* (Summer 1976). 53-58.

Jessner, L. On becoming a mother. *In* Vonbaeyer, W., and R. M. Griffith, editors. Conditio Humana. Springer-Verlag New York, Inc., New York. 1966.

Jessner, L., E. Weigert, and J. L. Foy. The development of parental attitudes during pregnancy. *In* Anthony, E. J., and T. Benedek, editors. Parenthood: Its Psychology and Psychopathology. Little, Brown & Co., Boston. 1970.

Kitzinger, S. The Experience of Childbirth. Penguin Books, Baltimore. 1972. Third edition.

Kitzinger, S. Education and Counseling for Childbirth. Bailliere Tindall, London. 1977.

Laukaran, V. H., and B. J. vanden Berg. The relationship of maternal attitude to pregnancy outcomes and obstetric complications. A cohort study of unwanted pregnancy. *American Journal of Obstetrics and Gynecology* (February 1, 1980). 374-379.

Masters, W. H., and V. E. Johnson. Human Sexual Response. Little, Brown & Co., Boston. 1966.

Melges, F. T. Postpartum psychiatric syndromes. *Psychosomatic Medicine* (January-February 1968). 95-108.

Moore, D. S. The body image in pregnancy. *Journal of Nurse-Midwifery* (Winter 1978). 17-27.

Newton, R. W., P. A. C. Webster, and P. S. Binu. Psychological stress in pregnancy and its relationship to the onset of premature labour. *British Medical Journal* (August 18, 1979). 411-413.

Pugh, T. F., B. K. Jerath, W. B. Schmidt, and R. B. Reed. Rates of mental disease related to childbearing. *New England Journal of Medicine* (May 30, 1963). 224-228.

Reedy, N. J. Nurse-midwife in complicated obstetrics: trend or treason? *Journal of Nurse-Midwifery* (January-February 1979). 11-17.

Roehner, J. Fatherhood: in pregnancy and birth. *Journal of Nurse-Midwifery* (Spring 1976). 13-18.

Rubin, R. Cognitive style in pregnancy. *American Journal of Nursing* (March 1970). 502.

Sheehy, G. Passages. E. P. Dutton Co., Inc., New York. 1976.

Standley, K., B. Soule, and S. A. Copans. Dimensions of prenatal anxiety and their influence on pregnancy outcome. *American Journal of Obstetrics and Gynecology* (September 1, 1979). 22-26.

Trethowan, W. H., and M. F. Colon. The couvade syndrome. *British Journal of Psychiatry* (January 1965). 57-66.

Wapner. J. The attitudes, feelings and behaviors of expectant fathers attending Lamaze classes. *Birth and the Family Journal* (Spring 1976). 5-14.

Westbrook, M. T. Analyzing affective responses to past events: women's reactions to a childbearing year. *Journal of Clinical Psychology* (October 1978). 967-971.

Chapter 5

Beal, V. Nutrition in the Life Span. John Wiley & Sons, Inc., New York. 1980.

Brewer, G. S. What Every Pregnant Woman Should Know: The Truth about Diet and Drugs in Pregnancy. Penguin Books, New York. 1977.

California Department of Health. Nutrition during Pregnancy and Lactation. California Department of Health, Sacramento, Calif. 1975.

Churchill, J. A., and H. W. Berendes. Intelligence of Children whose Mothers Had Acetonuria During Pregnancy. Pan American Health Organization, Washington, D. C. 1969.

Committee on Nutrition. Nutrition in Maternal Health Care. American College of Obstetricians and Gynecologists, Chicago. 1974.

Eastman, N. J., and E. Jackson. Weight relationships in pregnancy. I. The bearing of maternal weight gain and pre-pregnancy weight on birth weight in full term pregnancies. *Obstetrical and Gynecological Survey* (November 1968). 1003-1025.

Gazella, J. G. Nutrition for the Childbearing Year. Woodland Publishing Co., Inc., Wayzata, Minn. 1979.

Green, M. L., and J. Harry. Nutrition in Contemporary Nursing Practice. John Wiley & Sons, Inc., New York. 1981.

Higgins, A. C. Nutritional status and the outcome of pregnancy. *Journal of the Canadian Dietetic Association* (1976). 17-34.

Love, E. J., and R. A. H. Kinch. Factors influencing the birthweight in normal pregnancy. *American Journal of Obstetrics and Gynecology* (1976). 342-349.

Lubchenco, L. O., D. T. Searls, and J. V. Brazie. Neonatal mortality rate: relationship to birth weight and gestational age. *Journal of Pediatrics* (October 1972). 814-822.

Luke, B. Maternal Nutrition. Little, Brown & Co., Boston. 1979.

National Dairy Council. Nutrition Source Book. National Dairy Council, Chicago. 1972.

Papaevangelou, G., C. Papadatos, and D. Alexiou. The effects of maternal age, parity and social class on the incidence of small-for-dates newborns. *Acta Paediatrica Scandinavica* (September 1973). 527-530.

Rosso, P., and M. Winick. Intrauterine growth retardation. A new systematic approach based on the clinical and biochemical characteristics of this condition. *Journal of Perinatal Medicine* (1974). 2(3):147-160.

Simpson, J. W., R. W. Lawless, and A. C. Mitchell. Responsibility of the obstetrician to the fetus. II. Influence of prepregnancy weight and pregnancy weight gain on birthweight. *Obstetrics and Gynecology* (May 1975). 481-487.

Slattery, J. S., G. A. Pearson, and C. T. Torre, editors. Maternal and Child Nutrition: Assessment and Counseling. Appleton-Century-Crofts, East Norwalk, Conn. 1979.

Task Force on Nutrition. Assessment of Maternal Nutrition. American College of Obstetricians and Gynecologists and American Dietetic Association, Chicago. 1978.

U. S. Department of Health, Education and Welfare. Smoking and pregnancy. *In* Health Consequences of Smoking: A Report of the Surgeon General. U. S. Department of Health, Education and Welfare, Washington, D. C. 1971.

Varney, H. Nurse Midwifery. Blackwell Scientific Publications, Inc., Boston. 1980.

Weiss, W., and E. C. Jackson. Maternal factors affecting birth weight. *In* Perinatal Factors Affecting Human Development. Pan American Health Organization, Washington, D. C. 1969.

Worthington, B. S., J. Vermeersch, and S. R. Williams. Nutrition in Pregnancy and Lactation. C. V. Mosby Co., St. Louis. 1977.

Chapter 6

Burrow, G. N., and T. F. Ferris. Medical Complications During Pregnancy. W. B. Saunders Co., Philadelphia. 1975.

Danforth, D. N., editor. Obstetrics and Gynecology. Harper & Row, Publishers, Inc., New York. 1977. Third edition.

Jensen, M. D., and I. M. Bobak. Handbook of Maternity Care. A Guide for Nursing Practice. C. V. Mosby Co., St. Louis. 1980.

Neeson, J. D., and C. R. Stockdale. The Practitioner's Handbook of Ambulatory OB/GYN. John Wiley & Sons, Inc., New York. 1981.

Pritchard, J. A., and P. C. MacDonald. Williams Obstetrics. Appleton-Century-Crofts, East Norwalk, Conn. 1980. Sixteenth edition.

Varney, H. Nurse Midwifery. Blackwell Scientific Publications, Inc., Boston. 1980.

Chapter 7

Crane, J. P., J. P. Sauvage, and F. Arias. A high-risk management protocol. *American Journal of Obstetrics and Gynecology* (May 15, 1976). 227-235.

Diamond, F. High-risk pregnancy screening techniques — a nursing overview. *(JOGN Nursing) Journal of Obstetric, Gynecologic and Neonatal Nursing* (November-December 1978). 15-20.

Elias, S. Fetoscopy in prenatal diagnosis. *Seminars in Perinatology* (July 1980). 199-205.

Evertson, L. R., and R. H. Paul. Antepartum fetal heart rate testing: the non-stress test. *American Journal of Obstetrics and Gynecology* (December 15, 1978). 895-900.

Finster, M., and R. Petrie. Monitoring of the fetus. *Anesthesiology* (August 1976). 198-215.

Hospital of the University of Pennsylvania. Antepartum Heart Rate Testing Protocol. Department of Obstetrics and Gynecology, Department of Nursing, Hospital of the University of Pennsylvania, Philadelphia. 1979.

Huddleston, J., G. Sutliff, F. Carney, and C. Flowers. Oxytocin challenge test for antepartum fetal assessment. Report of a clinical experience. *American Journal of Obstetrics and Gynecology* (November 1, 1979). 609-614.

Jensen, M. D., and I. M. Bobak. Handbook of Maternity Care. C. V. Mosby Co., St. Louis. 1980.

Manning, F. A., L. D. Platt, and L. Sipos. Antepartum fetal evaluation: development of a fetal biophysical profile. *American Journal of Obstetrics and Gynecology* (March 15, 1980). 787-795.

Neldam, S. Fetal movements as an indicator of fetal wellbeing. *Lancet* (June 7, 1980). 1222-1224.

Olds, S. B., M. L. London, P. A. Ladewig, and S. V. Davidson. Obstetric Nursing. Addison-Wesley Publishing Co., Menlo Park, Calif. 1980.

Pearson, J. F. Fetal movements — a new approach to antenatal care. *Nursing Mirror* (April 21, 1977). 49-51.

Pearson, J. F., and J. B. Weaver. Fetal activity and fetal wellbeing: an evaluation. *British Medical Journal* (May 29, 1976). 1305-1307.

Sadovsky, E., H. Yaffe, and W. Polishuk. Fetal movement monitoring in normal and pathologic pregnancy. *International Journal of Gynaecology and Obstetrics* (1974). 75-79.

Spellacy, W. N., editor. Management of the High Risk Pregnancy. University Park Press, Baltimore. 1976.

Tucker, S. M. Fetal Monitoring and Fetal Assessment in High Risk Pregnancy. C. V. Mosby Co., St. Louis. 1978.

Chapter 8
American Nurses' Association. A Statement on the Scope of High Risk Perinatal Nursing Practice. Publication No. MCH-12. American Nurses' Association, New York. 1980.

Aubry, R. H., and J. C. Pennington. Identification and evaluation of high risk pregnancy: the perinatal concept. *Clinical Obstetrics and Gynecology* (March 1973). 13-27.

Babson, S. G., M. Pernoll, and G. Penda. Diagnosis and Management of the Fetus and Neonate at Risk. C. V. Mosby Co., St. Louis. 1980. Fourth edition.

Goodwin, J., J. Dunne, and B. Thomas. Antepartum identification of the fetus at risk. *Canadian Medical Association Journal* (October 18, 1969). 57-64.

Hobel, C., M. Hyvarinen, D. Okada, and W. Oh. Prenatal and intrapartum high-risk screening. I. Prediction of the high-risk neonate. *American Journal of Obstetrics and Gynecology* (September 1, 1973). 1-9.

Hobel, C. Prenatal Risk Assessment through POPRAS. South Bay Regional Perinatal Project, Harbor General Hospital, Torrance, Calif. 1976.

Schneider, J. The high risk pregnancy. *Hospital Practice* (October 1971). 133-143.

Spellacy, W. N., editor. Management of the High-Risk Pregnancy. University Park Press, Baltimore. 1976.

Chapter 9

Danforth, D. N. Obstetrics and Gynecology. Harper & Row, Publishers, Inc., New York. 1982. Fourth edition.

Friedman, E. A. Labor: Clinical Evaluation and Management. Appleton-Century-Crofts, East Norwalk, Conn. 1978. Second edition.

Friedman, E. A. Graphic appraisal of labor: a study of 500 primigravidae. *Bulletin of the Sloane Hospital for Women in the Columbia-Presbyterian Medical Center* (June 1955). 42-48.

Hassid, P. Textbook for Childbirth Educators. Harper & Row, Publishers, Inc., New York. 1978.

Jensen, M. D., and I. M. Bobak. Handbook of Maternity Care: A Guide for Nursing Practice. C. V. Mosby Co., St. Louis. 1980.

Oxorn, H. Oxorn-Foote Human Labor and Birth. Appleton-Century-Crofts, East Norwalk, Conn. 1980. Fourth edition.

Pritchard, J. A., and P. C. MacDonald. Williams Obstetrics. Appleton-Century-Crofts, East Norwalk, Conn. 1980. Sixteenth edition.

Varney, H. Nurse Midwifery. Blackwell Scientific Publications, Inc., Boston. 1980.

Chapter 10

Danforth, D. N. Obstetrics and Gynecology. Harper & Row, Publishers, Inc., New York. 1982. Fourth edition.

Oxorn, H. Oxorn-Foote Human Labor and Birth. Appleton-Century-Crofts, East Norwalk, Conn. 1980. Fourth edition.

Pritchard, J. A., and P. C. MacDonald. Williams Obstetrics. Appleton-Century-Crofts, East Norwalk, Conn. 1980. Sixteenth edition.

Varney, H. Nurse Midwifery. Blackwell Scientific Publications, Inc., Boston. 1980.

Chapter 11

Danforth, D. N. Obstetrics and Gynecology. Harper & Row, Publishers, Inc., New York. 1982. Fourth edition.

Oxorn, H. Oxorn-Foote Human Labor and Birth. Appleton-Century-Crofts, East Norwalk, Conn. 1980. Fourth edition.

Varney, H. Nurse Midwifery. Blackwell Scientific Publications, Inc., Boston. 1980.

Chapter 12

Brown, M. S., and S. T. Hurlock. Mothering the mother. *American Journal of Nursing* (March 1977). 439-441.

Rovinsky, J. J. Management of normal labor and delivery. Chapter 65. *In* Sciarra, J. J., editor. Gynecology and Obstetrics. Vol. II. Harper & Row, Publishers, Inc., New York. 1980.

Vorherr, H. Puerperium: maternal involutional changes — management of puerperal problems and complications. Chapter 90. *In* Sciarra, J. J., editor. Gynecology and Obstetrics. Vol. II. Harper & Row, Publishers, Inc., New York. 1980.

Chapter 13

Cooperative Birth Center Network News. Cooperative Birth Center Network, Perkiomenville, Pa. 1981.

Dobbs, K., and K. Kirkwood. Alternative birth rooms and birth options. *Obstetrics and Gynecology* (May 1981). 58.

Ernst, E. The evolving practice of midwifery. *Health Law Project Library Bulletin* (September 1979). 20-23.

Ernst, E., J. R. McTammany, T. Ebersole, M. Farr, E. Mack, and S. Perkins. The continuum concept: home, hospital and birth center. Chapter 43. *In* Stewart, D., and L. Stewart, editors. Compulsory Hospitalization: Freedom of Choice in Childbirth. National Association of Parents and Professionals for Safe Alternatives in Childbirth, Marble Hill, Mo.

Kitzinger, S. Birth at Home. Oxford University Press, New York. 1979.

Klaus, M. H., and J. H. Kennell. Parent-Infant Bonding. C. V. Mosby Co., St. Louis. 1981. Second edition.

Mann, R. San Francisco General Hospital nurse-midwifery practice: the first thousand births. *American Journal of Obstetrics and Gynecology* (July 13, 1981). 110.

Neilsen, I. Nurse-midwifery in an alternative birth center. *Birth and the Family Journal* (Spring 1977). 24.

Sumner, P. E., J. P. Wheeler, and S. G. Smith. Six years experience of prepared childbirth in a home-like delivery room. *Birth and the Family Journal* (Summer 1976). 79.

Ventre, F., E. Herman, D. Fitzgerald, and T. Long. Home Oriented Maternity Experience: A Comprehensive Guide to Home Birth. HOME, Inc., Washington, D. C. 1976.

Varney, H. Nurse Midwifery. Blackwell Scientific Publications, Inc., Boston. 1980.

Chapter 14

Aleksandrowicz, M. K., and D. R. Aleksandrowicz. The molding of personality: a newborn's innate characteristics in interaction with parents' personalities. *Child Psychiatry and Human Development* (Summer 1975). 231-241.

Anderson, C. J. Enhancing reciprocity between mother and neonate. *Nursing Research* (March-April 1981). 89-93.

Barnett, C. R., P. H. Leiderman, R. Grobstein, and M. Klaus. Neonatal separation: the maternal side of interactional deprivation. *Pediatrics* (February 1970). 197-205.

Blackburn, S. Sleep and awake states of the newborn. *In* Duxbury, M., and P. Carroll, editors. Early Parent-Infant Relationships. The National Foundation—March of Dimes, White Plains, N. Y. 1978.

Blackburn, S. State-related behaviors and individual differences. *In* Duxbury, M., and P. Carroll, editors. Early Parent-Infant Relationships. The National Foundation—March of Dimes, White Plains, N. Y. 1978.

Bowlby, J. Attachment and Loss. Attachment. Vol. I. Basic Books, Inc., Publishers, New York. 1969.

Brazelton, T. B. Does the neonate shape his environment? *Birth Defects* (1974). **10**(2):131-140.

Brazelton, T. B. Neonatal Behavioral Assessment Scale. J. B. Lippincott Co., Philadelphia. 1973.

Caplan, G. An Approach to Community Mental Health. Grune & Stratton, Inc., New York. 1961.

Clark, A., and D. D. Affonso. Infant behavior and maternal attachment: two sides to the coin. *Maternal-Child Nursing Journal* (March-April 1976). 94-99.

Curry, M. A. Contact during the first hour with the wrapped or naked newborn: effect on maternal attachment behaviors at 36 hours and three months. *Birth and the Family Journal* (Winter 1979). 227-235.

Farrar, C. A. A data collection procedure to assess behavioral individuality in the neonate. *(JOGN Nursing) Journal of Obstetric, Gynecologic and Neonatal Nursing* (May-June 1974). 15-19.

Goren, C. C., M. Sarty, and P. Y. K. Wu. Visual following and pattern discrimination of face-like stimuli by newborn infants. *Pediatrics* (October 1975). 544-549.

Gray, J. D., C. A. Cutler, J. G. Dean, and C. H. Kempe. Prediction and prevention of child abuse. *Seminars in Perinatology* (January 1979). 85-90.

Greenfield, P. M. Cross-cultural studies of mother-infant interaction: towards a structural-functional approach. *Human Development* (1972). 131-138.

Gromada, K. Maternal-infants attachment: the first step toward individualizing twins. *Maternal-Child Nursing Journal* (March-April 1981). 129-134.

Hurd, J. M. Assessing maternal attachment: first step toward the prevention of child abuse. *(JOGN Nursing) Journal of Obstetric, Gynecologic and Neonatal Nursing* (July-August 1975). 25-30.

Jenkins, R. L., and N. K. Westhus. The nurses role in parent-infant bonding — overview, assessment, intervention. *(JOGN Nursing) Journal of Obstetric, Gynecologic and Neonatal Nursing* (March-April 1981). 114-118.

Kang, R. Parent-infant attachment. *In* Duxbury, M., and P. Carroll, editors. Early Parent-Infant Relationships. The National Foundation—March of Dimes, White Plains, N. Y. 1978.

Kennedy, J. The high-risk maternal-infant acquaintance process. *Nursing Clinics of North America* (September 1973). 549-556.

Kerns, D. L., J. Cavanaugh, and B. C. Berliner. Child abuse and neglect: the hospital's expanding role in prevention, identification and management. *Connecticut Medicine* (May 1979). 293-300.

Klaus, M., R. Jerauld, N. C. Kreger, W. McAlpine, M. Steffa, and J. H. Kennell. Maternal attachment: importance of the first post-partum days. *New England Journal of Medicine* (March 2, 1972). 460-463.

Klaus, M. H., and J. H. Kennell. Maternal-Infant Bonding: The Impact of Early Separation or Loss on Family Development. C. V. Mosby Co., St. Louis. 1976.

Klaus, M. H., and J. H. Kennell. Mothers separated from their new-born infants. *Pediatric Clinics of North America* (November 1970). 1015-1037.

Klaus, M. H., J. H. Kennell, N. Plumb, and S. Zuehlke. Human maternal behavior at the first contact with her young. *Pediatrics* (August 1970). 187-192.

Korner, A. Individual differences at birth — implications for child-care practices. *Birth Defects* (1974). **10**(2):51-61.

Lamper, C. Facilitative attachment through well-baby care. *In* Hall, J. E., and B. R. Weaver, editors. Nursing of Families in Crisis. J. B. Lippincott Co., Philadelphia. 1974.

Mcrae, M. Bonding in a sea of silence. *Maternal-Child Nursing Journal* (January-February 1979). 29-34.

Neikirk, R. Crisis intervention during child-bearing cycle. *In* Hall, J. E., and B. R. Weaver, editors. Nursing of Families in Crisis. J. B. Lippincott Co., Philadelphia. 1974.

Oppe, T. E. The vulnerable baby. *Midwives Chronicle and Nursing Notes* (September 1974). 310-312.

Riesch, S. Enhancement of mother-infant social interaction. *(JOGN Nursing) Journal of Obstetric, Gynecologic and Neonatal Nursing* (July-August 1979). 242-246.

Robson, K. The role of eye-to-eye contact in maternal-infant attach-ment. *Journal of Child Psychology and Psychiatry and Allied Disciplines* (May 1967). 13-25.

Robson, K., and H. A. Moss. Patterns and determinants of maternal attachment. *Journal of Pediatrics* (December 1970). 976-985.

Rubin, R. Attainment of the maternal role. Models and referrants. Part II. *Nursing Research* (Fall 1967). 342-346.

Rubin, R. Maternal tasks in pregnancy. *Maternal-Child Nursing Journal* (Fall 1975). 143-153.

Salk, L. The role of the heartbeat in the relations between mother and infant. *Scientific American* (May 1973). 24-29.

Turkewitz, G., H. G. Birch, and K. Cooper. Responsiveness to simple and complex auditory stimuli in the human newborn. *Developmental Psychobiology* (January-March 1972). 7-19.

Wooten, B. Death of an infant. *Maternal-Child Nursing Journal* (July-August 1981). 257-260.

Yarrow, L., and M. S. Goodwin. Some conceptual issues in the study of mother-infant interaction. *American Journal of Orthopsychiatry* (April 1965). 473-481.

Young, D. Bonding — How Parents Become Attached to Their Baby. International Childbirth Education Association, Inc., Rochester, N. Y. 1978.

Chapter 15

Beneson, A. Control of Communicable Diseases in Man. American Public Health Association, Inc., Washington, D. C. 1970.

Benson, R. C. Current Obstetric and Gynecologic Diagnosis and Treatment. Lange Medical Publications, Los Altos, Calif. 1978. Second edition.

Burrow, G. N., and T. F. Ferris. Medical Complications During Pregnancy. W. B. Saunders Co., Philadelphia. 1975.

Cameron, N. Personality Development and Psychopathology. Houghton Mifflin Co., Boston. 1963.

Danforth, D. N., editor. Obstetrics and Gynecology. Harper & Row, Publishers, Inc., New York. 1982. Fourth edition.

Dickason, J., and M. Schultz. Maternal and Infant Care: A Text for Nurses. McGraw-Hill Book Co., New York. 1975.

Jensen, M., and I. Bobak. Handbook of Maternity Care: A Guide for Nursing Practice. C. V. Mosby Co., St. Louis. 1980.

Lubchenco, L. O., C. Hausman, and L. Backstrom. Factors influencing fetal growth. *In* Nutricia Symposium: Aspects of Prematurity and Dysmaturity. H. E. Stenford Kroese B. V., Leiden, The Netherlands. 1968.

Midwinter, A. Vomiting in pregnancy. *Practitioner* (January 1971). 739-745.

Monif, G. Infectious Disease in Obstetrics and Gynecology. Harper & Row, Publishers, Inc., New York. 1974.

Neeson, J. D., and C. R. Stockdale. The Practitioner's Handbook of Ambulatory Ob/Gyn. John Wiley & Sons, Inc., New York. 1981.

Nelson, B., L. Gillespie, and P. White. Pregnancy complicated by diabetes mellitus. *Obstetrics and Gynecology* (January 1953). 215-230.

Scipien, G. M., M. Barnard, M. Chard, J. Howe, and P. Phillips. Comprehensive Pediatric Nursing. McGraw-Hill Book Co., New York. 1975.

Stevenson, R. E. The Fetus and the Newly Born Infant: Influences of the Prenatal Environment. C. V. Mosby Co., St. Louis. 1977. Second edition.

Thorn, G. W., R. D. Adams, E. Braunwald, K. J. Isselbacher, and R. G. Petersdorf, editors. Harrison's Principles of Internal Medicine. McGraw-Hill Book Co., New York. 1977. Eighth edition.

Varney, H. Nurse Midwifery. Blackwell Scientific Publications, Inc., Boston. 1980.

Wallach, J. Interpretation of Diagnostic Tests: A Handbook Synopsis of Laboratory Medicine. Little, Brown & Co., Boston. 1978. Third edition.

Chapter 16

Bishop, E. H. Pelvic scoring for elective induction. *Obstetrics and Gynecology* (August 1964). 266-268.

Danforth, D. N. Obstetrics and Gynecology. Harper & Row, Publishers, Inc., New York. 1982. Fourth edition.

Oxorn, H. Oxorn-Foote Human Labor and Birth. Appleton-Century-Crofts, East Norwalk, Conn. 1980. Fourth edition.

Varney, H. Nurse Midwifery. Blackwell Scientific Publications, Inc., Boston. 1980.

Chapter 17

Aladjem, S., editor. Obstetrical Practice. C. V. Mosby Co., St. Louis. 1980.

Bolton, G. C., and F. L. Cohen. Detecting and treating ectopic pregnancy. *Contemporary Ob/Gyn* (July 1981). 101-104.

Clark, A., and D. Affonso. Childbearing: A Nursing Perspective. F. A. Davis Co., Philadelphia. 1979. Second edition.

Clausen, J. P., M. H. Flook, and B. Ford. Maternity Nursing Today. McGraw-Hill Book Co., New York. 1977. Second edition.

Hawkins, J. W., and L. P. Higgins. Maternity and Gynecological Nursing. J. B. Lippincott Co., Philadelphia. 1981.

Olds, S. B., M. L. London, P. A. Ladewig, and S. V. Davidson. Obstetric Nursing. Addison-Wesley Publishing Co., Menlo Park, Calif. 1980.

Oxorn, H. Oxorn-Foote Human Labor and Birth. Appleton-Century-Crofts, East Norwalk, Conn. 1980. Fourth edition.

Pritchard, J. A., and P. C. MacDonald. Williams Obstetrics. Appleton-Century-Crofts, East Norwalk, Conn. 1980. Sixteenth edition.

Queenan, J., R. Berkowitz, R. Creasy, and I. Merkatz. Anticipating premature labor. *Contemporary Ob/Gyn* (November 1980). 170-184.

Zuspan, F. P., and K. J. Zuspan. Strategies for controlling eclampsia. *Contemporary Ob/Gyn* (July 1981). 135-142.

Chapter 18

American Journal of Nursing. Fetal and Maternal Monitoring. Continuing Education Unit. 1978.

Columbia Presbyterian Medical Center. Guidelines for Making FHR-UC Notations. Columbia Presbyterian Medical Center, New York. 1981.

Gassner, C., and W. Ledger. The relationship of hospital acquired maternal infections to invasive intrapartum monitoring techniques. *American Journal of Obstetrics and Gynecology* (September 1976). 33-37.

Goodlin, R. History of fetal monitoring. *American Journal of Obstetrics and Gynecology* (February 1979). 323-352.

Haverkamp, J. The evaluation of continuous monitoring. *American Journal of Obstetrics and Gynecology* (June 1976). 526-540.

Hobel, C. Prenatal and intrapartum high risk screening. *American Journal of Obstetrics and Gynecology* (September 1973). 1-9.

Hon, E. Introduction to Fetal Heart Rate Monitoring. Postgraduate Division, University of Southern California, Los Angeles. 1973.

Martin, C., and B. Gingerich. Uteroplacental physiology. *(JOGN Nursing) Journal of Obstetric, Gynecologic and Neonatal Nursing* (September-October 1976). 165-258.

National Institute of Child Health and Human Development. Antenatal Diagnosis. United States Department of Health, Education and Welfare, Bethesda, Md. 1979.

Petrie, R., and K. Pollack. Intrapartum fetal monitoring. *(JOGN Nursing) Journal of Obstetric, Gynecologic and Neonatal Nursing* (September-October 1976). 520-555.

Shields, D. Maternal reaction to fetal monitoring. *American Journal of Nursing* (December 1978). 2110-2111.

Starkman, M. Psychological responses to use of the fetal monitor during labor. *Psychosomatic Medicine* (July-August 1976). 269-277.

Chapter 19

Bowlby, J. Attachment and Loss. Attachment. Vol. I. Basic Books, Inc., Publishers, New York. 1969.

Brazelton, T. B. The early mother-infant adjustment. *Pediatrics* (1963). 931-938.

Clausen, J. P., M. H. Flook, and B. Ford. Maternity Nursing Today. McGraw-Hill Book Co., Inc., New York. 1977. Second edition.

Grams, K. E. Infant nutrition. Breastfeeding: a method of imparting immunity? *(MCN) The American Journal of Maternal Child Nursing* (November-December 1978). 340.

Harris, H. E., V. I. Thomas, and G. W. Hai. Postpartum surveillance for urinary tract infection: patients at risk of developing pyelonephritis after catheterization. *Southern Medical Journal* (January 1977). 1273.

Jelliffe, D. B., and E. F. Jelliffe. Human Milk in the Modern World. Oxford University Press, Oxford. 1978.

Jensen, M. D., R. C. Benson, and I. M. Bobak. Maternity Care. The Nurse and the Family. C. V. Mosby Co., St. Louis. 1981. Second edition.

Klaus, M. H., and J. H. Kennell. Maternal Infant Bonding: The Impact of Early Separation or Loss on Family Development. C. V. Mosby Co., St. Louis. 1976.

Knowles, J. A. Excretion of drugs in milk: a review. *Journal of Pediatrics* (January 1965). 65-68.

Ludington-Hoe, S. M. Postpartum development of maternity. *American Journal of Nursing* (July 1977). 1170-1174.

Manual of Standards and Guidelines for Perinatal Nursing Care. Western and Upper Manhattan Perinatal Network, New York. 1979.

Olds, S. B., M. L. London, P. A. Ladewig, and S. V. Davidson. Obstetric Nursing. Addison-Wesley Publishing Co., Menlo Park, Calif. 1980.

Pillitteri, A. Maternal-Newborn Nursing. Care of the Growing Family. Little, Brown & Co., Boston. 1981. Second edition.

Pritchard, J. A., and P. C. MacDonald. Williams Obstetrics. Appleton-Century-Crofts, East Norwalk, Conn. 1980. Sixteenth edition.

Ziegel, E., and C. Van Blarcom. Obstetric Nursing. Macmillan Publishing Co., New York. 1972. Sixth edition.

Chapter 20

Dickey, R. P. Managing Contraceptive Pill Patients. Creative Informatics, Inc., Aspen, Colo. 1980. Second edition.

Hatcher, R. A., G. K. Stewart, F. Stewart, F. Guest, D. W. Schwartz, and S. A. Jones. Contraceptive Technology 1980-1981. Irvington Publishers, Inc., New York. 1980. Tenth edition.

Martin, L. L. Health Care of Women. J. B. Lippincott Co., Philadelphia. 1978.

Siemens, S., and R. C. Brandzel. Sexuality: Nursing Assessment and Intervention. J. B. Lippincott Co., Philadelphia. 1982.

Varney, H. Nurse Midwifery. Blackwell Scientific Publications, Inc., Boston. 1980.

Chapter 21

Alexander, M. M., and M. S. Brown. Physical examinations. Part 18. Neurological examination. *Nursing 76* (July 1976). 50-55.

Bates, B. A Guide to Physical Examinations. J. B. Lippincott Co., Philadelphia. 1979. Second edition.

Clausen, J. P., M. H. Flook, and B. Ford. Maternity Nursing Today. McGraw-Hill Book Co., New York. 1977. Second edition.

Desmond, M. M., A. J. Rudolph, and P. Phitaksphraiwan. The transitional care nursery. *Pediatric Clinics of North America* (August 1966). 651-668.

Dubowitz, L., V. Dubowitz, and C. Goldberg. Clinical assessment of gestational age in the newborn infant. *Journal of Pediatrics* (July 1970). 1-10.

Illingworth, R. S. The Development of the Infant and Young Child. Churchill Livingstone, Inc., New York. 1976. Sixth edition.

Kaye, R., F. A. Oski, and L. A. Barness, editors. Core Textbook of Pediatrics. J. B. Lippincott Co., Philadelphia. 1978.

Oehler, J. M. Family Centered Neonatal Nursing Care. J. B. Lippincott Co., Philadelphia. 1981.

Scanlon, J. W., T. Nelson, L. J. Grylack, and G. F. Smith. A System of Newborn Physical Examination. University Park Press, Baltimore. 1979.

Vaughan, V. C., and R. J. McKay, editors. Nelson's Textbook of Pediatrics. W. B. Saunders Co., Philadelphia. 1979. Tenth edition.

Waechter, E. H., and F. G. Blake. Nursing Care of Children. J. B. Lippincott Co., Philadelphia. 1976. Ninth edition.

Chapter 22

Adams, M. Early concerns of primigravida mothers regarding infant care activities. *Nursing Research* (Spring 1963). 72-77.

American Academy of Pediatrics, Committee on Nutrition. On the feeding of supplemental foods to infants. *Pediatrics* (June 1980). 1178-1181.

American Academy of Pediatrics, Committee on Nutrition. Vitamin and mineral supplement needs in normal children in the United States. *Pediatrics* (December 1980). 1015-1021.

American Academy of Pediatrics, Nutrition Committee of the Canadian Pediatric Society and Committee on Nutrition. Breastfeeding. *Pediatrics* (October 1978). 591-601.

Bender, K. J., M. W. McKenzie, and A. J. Seals. Infant formulas. *Journal of the American Pharmaceutical Association* (May 1975). 230-238.

Blake, F. G., F. H. Wright, and E. H. Waechter. Nursing Care of Children. J. B. Lippincott Co., Philadelphia. 1970. Eighth edition.

Clausen, J. P., M. H. Flook, and B. Ford. Maternity Nursing Today. McGraw-Hill Book Co., New York. 1977. Second edition.

Fitzpatrick, E., S. R. Reeder, and L. Mastroianni, Jr. Maternity Nursing. J. B. Lippincott Co., Philadelphia. 1971. Twelfth edition.

Ishida, M. C., V. Ewers, and Y. Ishida. Introducing solid foods to infants. *(JOGN Nursing) Journal of Obstetric, Gynecologic and Neonatal Nursing* (October 1973). 27-32.

Jelliffe, D. B., and E. F. P. Jelliffe. Current concepts in nutrition: "breast is best": modern meanings. *New England Journal of Medicine* (October 27, 1977). 912-915.

La Leche League International. How the Nurse Can Help the Breastfeeding Mother. La Leche League International, Franklin Park, Ill.

Mosher, M. R., and G. Meyer. PCBs and breast milk. *Nutrition Action* (November 1980). 10-13.

Newton, M., N. Newton, and R. Applebaum. Management of Successful Lactation. Child and Family, Oak Park, Ill. 1972. Reprint booklet series.

Pryor, K. Nursing Your Baby. Pocket Books, New York. 1977.

Slattery, J. S., G. A. Pearson, and C. T. Torre. Maternal and Child Nutrition: Assessment and Counseling. Appleton-Century-Crofts, East Norwalk, Conn. 1979.

Varney, H. Nurse Midwifery. Blackwell Scientific Publications, Inc., Boston. 1980.

Chapter 23

Clausen, J. P., M. H. Flook, and B. Ford. Maternity Nursing Today. McGraw-Hill Book Co., New York. 1977. Second edition.

Committee on Infectious Diseases. Report of the Committee on Infectious Diseases. American Academy of Pediatrics, Evanston, Ill. 1977. Eighteenth edition.

Committee on Standards of Child Health Care. Standards of Child Health Care. American Academy of Pediatrics, Evanston, Ill. 1977. Third edition.

Duvall, E. M. Marriage and Family Development. J. B. Lippincott Co., Philadelphia. 1977. Fifth edition.

Fomon, S. J. Infant Nutrition. W. B. Saunders Co., Philadelphia. 1974. Second edition.

Gold, A. P. Parents checklist for normal early development. *Parents' Magazine* (November 1976). 134.

Chapter ...

Curran, F. ?... So?... to ... and ?... and ?... Pollution ... ?
Index Medicus, 1971, p. ?... New York, 1972, second edition.

Gloria ... Air Pollution Disease, Report of the Committee on
Education Bureau, American Association ?... 1921, Evanston,
Ill. 1957, Chicago, edition.

Committee on Pollution, Report of the Committee on Pollution,
Health Effects, American Academy of Pediatrics, Evanston, Ill.
1957, third edition.

Davis, Robert Principles and Practice of ... J. B. Lippincott
Co., Philadelphia, 1971, fifth edition.

Harris, Joseph Air Pollution, W. B. Saunder Co., Philadelphia,
1975, second edition.

Gold, A. ?... Principles of ... for normal study, New York,
Academy Press, 1951, published 1961, 196?.

INDEX

A